B. Schwab

Oxford American Handbook of
Radiology

About the Oxford American Handbooks in Medicine

The Oxford American Handbooks are pocket clinical books, providing practical guidance in quick reference, note form. Titles cover major medical specialties or cross-specialty topics and are aimed at students, residents, internists, family physicians, and practicing physicians within specific disciplines.

Their reputation is built on including the best clinical information, complemented by hints, tips, and advice from the authors. Each one is carefully reviewed by senior subject experts, residents, and students to ensure that content reflects the reality of day-to-day medical practice.

Key series features

- Written in short chunks, each topic is concisely covered to enable readers to find information quickly. They are also perfect for test preparation and gaining a quick overview of a subject without scanning through unnecessary pages.
- Content is evidence based and complemented by the expertise and judgment of experienced authors.
- The Handbooks provide a humanistic approach to medicine – it's more than just treatment by numbers.
- A "friend in your pocket," the Handbooks offer honest, reliable guidance about the difficulties of practicing medicine and provide coverage of both the practice and art of medicine.
- For quick reference, useful "everyday" information is included on the inside covers.

Published and Forthcoming Oxford American Handbooks

Oxford American Handbook of Clinical Medicine
Oxford American Handbook of Anesthesiology
Oxford American Handbook of Cardiology
Oxford American Handbook of Clinical Dentistry
Oxford American Handbook of Clinical Diagnosis
Oxford American Handbook of Clinical Examination and Practical Skills
Oxford American Handbook of Clinical Pharmacy
Oxford American Handbook of Critical Care
Oxford American Handbook of Disaster Medicine
Oxford American Handbook of Endocrinology and Diabetes
Oxford American Handbook of Emergency Medicine
Oxford American Handbook of Gastroenterology and Hepatology
Oxford American Handbook of Geriatric Medicine
Oxford American Handbook of Hospice and Palliative Medicine
Oxford American Handbook of Infectious Diseases
Oxford American Handbook of Nephrology and Hypertension
Oxford American Handbook of Neurology
Oxford American Handbook of Obstetrics and Gynecology
Oxford American Handbook of Oncology
Oxford American Handbook of Ophthalmology
Oxford American Handbook of Otolaryngology
Oxford American Handbook of Pediatrics
Oxford American Handbook of Physical Medicine and Rehabilitation
Oxford American Handbook of Psychiatry
Oxford American Handbook of Pulmonary Medicine
Oxford American Handbook of Reproductive Medicine
Oxford American Handbook of Rheumatology
Oxford American Handbook of Sports Medicine
Oxford American Handbook of Surgery
Oxford American Handbook of Urology

Oxford American Handbook of **Radiology**

Edited by

Petra J. Lewis, MBBS
Professor of Radiology and OBGYN
The Geisel School of Medicine at Dartmouth, Hanover, NH
Vice Chair of Education
Department of Radiology
Dartmouth-Hitchcock Medical Center
Lebanon, New Hampshire, USA

Nancy J. McNulty, MD
Associate Professor of Radiology and Anatomy
The Geisel School of Medicine at Dartmouth, Hanover, NH
Associate Director of Student Education
Department of Radiology
Dartmouth-Hitchcock Medical Center
Lebanon, New Hampshire, USA

OXFORD
UNIVERSITY PRESS

OXFORD
UNIVERSITY PRESS

Oxford University Press is a department of the University of Oxford.
It furthers the University's objective of excellence in research, scholarship,
and education by publishing worldwide.

Oxford   New York
Auckland   Cape Town   Dar es Salaam   Hong Kong
Karachi   Kuala Lumpur   Madrid   Melbourne   Mexico City   Nairobi
New Delhi   Shanghai   Taipei   Toronto

With offices in
Argentina   Austria   Brazil   Chile   Czech Republic   France   Greece
Guatemala   Hungary   Italy   Japan   Poland   Portugal   Singapore
South Korea   Switzerland   Thailand   Turkey   Ukraine   Vietnam

Oxford is a registered trademark of Oxford University Press in the UK
and certain other countries.

Published in the United States of America by
Oxford University Press
198 Madison Avenue, New York, NY 10016

Copyright © 2013 by Oxford University Press.

All rights reserved. No part of this publication may be reproduced, stored in a
retrieval system, or transmitted, in any form or by any means, without the prior
permission in writing of Oxford University Press, or as expressly permitted
by law, by license, or under terms agreed with the appropriate reproduction
rights organization. Inquiries concerning reproduction outside the scope of the
above should be sent to the Rights Department, Oxford University Press, at the
address above.

You must not circulate this work in any other form
and you must impose this same condition on any acquirer.

Library of Congress Cataloging-in-Publication Data
Oxford American handbook of radiology / edited by Petra J. Lewis, Nancy J. McNulty.
   p. ; cm. — (Oxford American handbooks)
   American handbook of radiology
   Handbook of radiology
   Includes bibliographical references and index.
   ISBN 978-0-19-974413-8
I. Lewis, Petra J.   II. McNulty, Nancy J.   III. Title: American handbook of
radiology.   IV. Title: Handbook of radiology.   V. Series: Oxford American
Handbooks.
[DNLM: 1. Diagnostic Imaging—methods—Handbooks.   2. Radiology—
methods—Handbooks.   3. Technology, Radiologic—methods—Handbooks.
WN 39]
LC Classification not assigned
616.07'54—dc23
2012006853

9 8 7 6 5 4 3 2 1

Printed in China
on acid-free paper

This material is not intended to be, and should not be considered, a substitute for medical or other professional advice. Treatment for the conditions described in this material is highly dependent on the individual circumstances. And, while this material is designed to offer accurate information with respect to the subject matter covered and to be current as of the time it was written, research and knowledge about medical and health issues is constantly evolving and dose schedules for medications are being revised continually, with new side effects recognized and accounted for regularly. Readers must therefore always check the product information and clinical procedures with the most up-to-date published product information and data sheets provided by the manufacturers and the most recent codes of conduct and safety regulation. Oxford University Press and the authors make no representations or warranties to readers, express or implied, about the accuracy or completeness of this material, including without limitation that they make no representation or warranties about the accuracy or efficacy of the drug dosages mentioned in the material. The authors and the publishers do not accept, and expressly disclaim, any responsibility for any liability, loss, or risk that may be claimed or incurred as a consequence of the use and/or application of any of the contents of this material.

How to use this book

The *Oxford American Handbook of Radiology* is designed for medical students, interns, and general medical and surgical residents to be used as a guide for:
- Ordering appropriate imaging studies.
- Understanding key radiological modalities and concepts.
- Understanding how imaging fits into the clinical evaluation of patients.
- Learning basic image interpretation.
- Imaging safety issues.

It is not intended as a comprehensive textbook of radiology. The material is presented in an abbreviated format suitable for fast review and reference. It provides a framework to be built on through clinical experience. Space limitations preclude a complete review of radiological anatomy, and readers should consult other referenced texts and on-line resources for anatomy tutorials.

Many important concepts have been consolidated in the 'Essentials' chapters. These include:
- Descriptions of imaging modalities that are common to several chapters (radiography, CT, MRI).
- Contrast media (uses, allergies, prophylaxis).
- Patient risks (contrast, radiation, interventional).
- Imaging in pregnancy.
- Imaging algorithms for common clinical questions.

Grouping these topics together provides a quick resource for patient management questions.

The remainder of the handbook is arranged into a combination of organ-based and modality-based chapters:

Chest Imaging	Abdominal Imaging
Neuroimaging	Musculoskeletal Imaging
Ultrasound	Fluoroscopy
Nuclear Medicine	Interventional Radiology
Pediatric Imaging	Breast Imaging

This system was used to mimic as closely as possible the organization of most modern radiology departments, allowing students on radiology clerkships and electives easier access to key information.

We would like to express our thanks to our families who supported us with patience and tolerance of the amount of family time it took to bring this book to press. In particular, Nancy's husband Ben and sons Charlie and Cameron and Petra's husband Lionel and daughters Rhian and Katy. We would also like to thank Steven Poplack MD, Theresa Vaccaro MD and Sword Cambron MD who kindly reviewed chapters, as did medical students Joo Cho, Dana Lin, and Aja Bjerke.

Contents

Contributors *xi*
Abbreviations *xiii*

1	Radiology essentials	1
2	Chest imaging	41
3	Abdomen/pelvis imaging	115
4	Musculoskeletal imaging	183
5	Ultrasound	239
6	Pediatrics	291
7	Fluoroscopy	329
8	Neuroimaging	369
9	Nuclear medicine	419
10	Interventional radiology	449
11	Breast imaging	475

Index *507*

Contributors

Jocelyn D. Chertoff, MD, MS
Vice Chair, Department
of Radiology
Professor of Radiology and OBGYN
The Geisel School of Medicine at
Dartmouth, Hanover, NH
Department of Radiology
Dartmouth-Hitchcock Medical
Center
Lebanon, NH

Avneesh Chhabra, MD, DNB
Assistant Professor Radiology &
Orthopedic Surgery
Russell H Morgan Department of
Radiology & Radiological Sciences
Johns Hopkins University
Baltimore, MD

Julianna M. Czum, MD
Assistant Professor of Radiology
and Medicine, Section of
Cardiology
The Geisel School of Medicine at
Dartmouth, Hanover, NH
Director, Division of
Cardiothoracic Imaging
Department of Radiology
Dartmouth-Hitchcock Medical
Center
Lebanon, NH

Michael A. DiPietro, MD
John F. Holt Collegiate Professor
Department of Radiology
Director, Medical Student
Education in Radiology
University of Michigan Health
System
Ann Arbor, MI

Elizabeth W. Dann, MD
Assistant Professor of Radiology
The Geisel School of Medicine at
Dartmouth, Hanover, NH
Director of Breast MRI
Department of Radiology
Dartmouth Hitchcock Medical
Center
Lebanon, NH

Rihan Khan, MD
Assistant Professor of Radiology
Division of Neuroradiology
Department of Radiology
University of Arizona Medical
Center
Tucson, AZ

Donna Magid, MD, M.Ed
Associate Professor of Radiology,
Orthopaedic Surgery, and
Functional Anatomy and Evolution
Associate Professor of Radiology,
Orthopaedic Surgery, and
Functional Anatomy
Director, Undergraduate Medical
Student Education in Radiology
Director, Horizontal Strand in
Diagnostic Imaging
Johns Hopkins School of Medicine
Baltimore, MD

Alan Siegel, MD, MS
Professor of Radiology and
Pathology
The Geisel School of Medicine at
Dartmouth, Hanover, NH
Department of Radiology
Dartmouth Hitchcock Medical
Center
Lebanon, NH

Anne M. Silas, MD, FRCPC
Associate Professor of Radiology
The Geisel School of Medicine at Dartmouth, Hanover, NH
Radiology Residency Program Director
Department of Radiology
Dartmouth Hitchcock Medical Center
Lebanon, NH

Albert J. Song, MD
Albert J. Song, MD
Assistant Professor of Diagnostic Radiology
Stritch School of Medicine
Department of Radiology
Loyola University Medical Center
Maywood, IL

Stephanie P. Yen, MD
Assistant Professor of Radiology and OBGYN
The Geisel School of Medicine at Dartmouth, Hanover, NH
Co-Director of Ultrasound
Department of Radiology
Dartmouth Hitchcock Medical Center
Lebanon, NH

Abbreviations

2D	2 dimensional
3D	3 dimensional
AAA	Abdominal aortic aneurysm
AP	Anterior-posterior
ARDS	Acute respiratory distress syndrome
ASCVD	Atherosclerotic cerebrovascular disease
AXR	Abdominal radiograph
BAC	Bronchoalveolar carcinoma
BMR	Breast MR
CBC	Complete blood count
CECT	Contrast enhanced CT
CFA	Common femoral artery
COPD	Chronic obstructive pulmonary disease
CP	Costophrenic
CHF	Congestive heart failure
CRI	Chronic renal impairment
CSF	Cerebrospinal fluid
CT	Computed tomography
CTA	CT angiogram
CTPA	CT pulmonary angiogram
CTU	CT urography
CVC	Central venous catheter
CXR	Chest radiograph
DCIS	Ductal carcinoma in situ
DDx	Differential diagnosis
DHT	Dobhoff tube
DM	Diabetes mellitus
DVT	Deep vein thrombosis
ED	Emergency department
ETT	Endotracheal tube
EVAR	Endovascular aneurysm repair
FOV	Field of view
Fx	Fracture
GFR	Glomerular filtration rate
GI	Gastrointestinal

ABBREVIATIONS

GU	Genitourinary
HTN	Hypertension
HV	Hepatic vein
Hx	History
HU	Hounsfield unit
ICU	Intensive care unit
IMV	Inferior mesenteric vein
IV	Intravenous
IVC	Inferior vena cava
IVP	Intravenous pyelography (also called IVU- IV urography)
kVp	Kilovolt peak
LA	Left atrium
LAO	Left anterior oblique
LFTs	Liver function tests
LLL	Left lower lobe
LLQ	Left lower quadrant
LMB	Left main bronchus
LMP	Last menstrual period
LPA	Left pulmonary artery
LPO	Left posterior oblique
LUL	Left upper lobe
LUQ	Left upper quadrant
LV	Left ventricle
LVF	Left ventricular failure
mA(s)	Milliamperage(s)
MCP	Metacarpal phalangeal
MI	Myocardial infarction
MIP	Maximal intensity projection
MR	Magnetic resonance
MRA	MR angiogram
MRCP	Magnetic resonance cholangiopancreatography
MRU	Magnetic resonance urography
MSK	Musculoskeletal
MTP	Metatarsal phalangeal
MVA	Motor vehicle accident
NECT	Non-enhanced CT
NGT	Nasogastric tube
NPV	Negative predictive value
OR	Operating room
PA	Posterior-anterior

ABBREVIATIONS

PACS	Picture archiving and communication system
PE	Pulmonary emboli
PET	Positron emission tomography
PICC	Peripheral intravenous central catheter
POFT	Pulmonary outflow track
PPV	Positive predictive value
Ptx	Pneumothorax
PV	Portal vein
RA	Right atrium
RLL	Right lower lobe
RLQ	Right lower quadrant
RMB	Right main bronchus
RML	Right middle lobe
RPA	Right pulmonary artery
RPO	Right posterior oblique
RSV	Respiratory syncytial virus
RUL	Right upper lobe
RUQ	Right upper quadrant
RV	Right ventricle
SBO	Small bowel obstruction
SLE	Systemic lupus erythematosus
SMA	Superior mesenteric artery
SMV	Superior mesenteric vein
SPN	Solitary pulmonary nodule
s/p	Status post
SQ	Subcutaneous
SVC	Superior vena cava
TA	Transabdominal
TV	Transvaginal (endovaginal)
UGI	Upper gastrointestinal (fluoroscopic study)
UPJ	Uretero-pelvic junction
US	Ultrasound
UTI	Urinary tract infection
w, w/o	With, without

Chapter 1

Radiology Essentials

Rihan Khan, MD, Petra Lewis, MBBS, Nancy McNulty, MD, and Anne M. Silas, MD

The requisition *2*
Imaging modalities *2*
  Radiography *3*
  Computed tomography *6*
  Magnetic resonance imaging (MRI) *10*
  PACS systems *15*
  What makes an image look good or bad? *14*
What about contrast? *16*
  Iodinated contrast *16*
  Contrast induced nephropathy *16*
  Gadolinium agents *17*
  Intraluminal agents *18*
  Contrast allergies *17*
What are the risks of imaging? *22*
  Radiation *22*
  Interventional *25*
  MRI *25*
How do I image my pregnant patient? *27*
  Appendicitis *28*
  Pulmonary emboli *29*
  Renal calculi *29*
  Trauma *30*
How much does imaging cost? *30*
Common imaging algorithms *31*
  Chest pain *32*
  Solitary pulmonary nodule *33*
  Abdominal and pain *34*
  Jaundice *35*
  Back pain *36*
  Suspected pedal osteomyelitis in diabetic *36*
  Suspected stress or insufficiency fracture *37*
  Headache *37*
  Cerebrovascular disease *38*
  Dementia *38*
  Pediatric UTI *38*
  Suspected child abuse *39*
  Vomiting infants *39*

CHAPTER 1 Radiology Essentials

The requisition

One of the most important jobs of the ordering physician is to convey accurate, relevant information to the radiologist. This is done via a requisition; either handwritten or on a computerized ordering system. The information is vital for ensuring that the correct study is performed and the right protocol is used; to correctly interpret the study; and for billing purposes.

What should a requisition include?

Contact information:
- Ordering physicians name and contact number must be accurate.

Patient information:
- Name, date of birth, identifying medical record number.

History:
- Patient's symptoms and signs.
- Duration.
- Relevant PMH; history of cancer or immunosuppression is almost always important as are key surgeries.

> Do not write "rule out X" as the only history. Insurance companies will NOT take this as a billable indication.

Exam type:
- Type of study (i.e., CT, x-ray, nuclear medicine).
- Body part to be imaged.

What protocol do I order?

Selection of the appropriate protocol based on patient's signs and symptoms is the radiologist's area of expertise! Knowing when oral or IV contrast is indicated is also our job, although we need to know if the patient has a contraindication to contrast.

What if the patient has a contrast allergy?

Indicate this on the requisition and specify what the reaction was (e.g., hives, rash, anaphylaxis, wheezing, etc.).

Imaging modalities

This first chapter covers the basic principles of radiography, CT, and MRI. Issues specific to certain body regions are presented in the technical sections of appropriate chapters. Ultrasound and nuclear medicine are covered separately in individual chapters.

Radiography

Also known as "Plain Films," radiographs are two dimensional images that are a summation of the density of all objects through which the x-ray beam passes.

How are images acquired?
The X-ray beam

> ### Features of X-rays
> - <u>Radiant energy</u>—energy radiates from the source in all directions.
> - <u>Attenuation</u>—X-rays are absorbed (attenuated) by tissues to a varying degree based on factors including specific density, atomic number and thickness. Those that penetrate the patient and hit a detector create the image.
> - <u>Wavelength</u>—X-ray wavelength is shorter than that of visible light. The specific wavelength determines the penetrating strength of the beam.
> - The <u>strength</u> of the beam and the <u>number of photons</u> in the beam can be adjusted dependent on the properties of the target.
>   - Peak kilovoltage (kVp)—Higher kVp creates a more penetrating beam needed for dense structures like bone.
>   - Milliamperage (mAs)—Higher mAs result in more x-ray photons reaching the target and thus the detector. Needed for obese patients and thick structures such as the lumbar spine.

The detector
The x-rays that are not absorbed by the patient's tissues hit the detector and are converted into light, which exposes a photographic film (in traditional screen-film radiography) or is converted into an electrical current (digital radiograph). Virtually all radiography is now digital. For simplicity, the terms *detector* and *film* will be used synonymously.

What is scatter?
X-rays interact with matter and the energy is re-emitted as secondary photons, which scatter (deflected from their incident path) in all directions.
- Some scattered photons will hit the detector, causing image blurring.
- Scatter is a significant source of radiation to personnel.

Grids (alternating thin bands of metal) are used to absorb scattered photons.

Magnification
X-rays diverge upon leaving the generator, causing magnification.
- Standard source to detector distance is 72 inches.
- Portable films are obtained with a reduced distance of ~48 inches, resulting in greater magnification.

Views

Usually named by the angle they take through the body:
- The first word (letter) describes where the beam enters (e.g., AP – the beam enters anteriorly and exits posteriorly).

> ### Common Views
> **AP**: antero-posterior (used for spine, abdomen, extremities)
> **PA**: postero-anterior (used for chest when possible)
> **Lateral**: beam passes through right to left or left to right
> **Decubitus**: patients lie on their sides and beam passes AP or PA (used to rule out free air, evaluating pleural effusions).
> **Obliques:**
> - RPO (right posterior oblique) the right posterior body is against the detector, beam passes AP).
> - RAO (right anterior oblique) the right anterior body is against the detector, beam passes PA.
>
> **"Coned" views:** small field of view, centered only on the area of greatest concern (used in MSK to look for fractures, fluoroscopy).
> **Cross-table lateral:** the beam is horizontal (parallel to floor). Often used for MSK imaging and neonates

Factors influencing appearance

Physical properties

The density of a structure, based on its atomic number, determines how much of the incident X-ray beam is absorbed.
- Dense structures absorb more of the beam and appear white on the final image (radioopaque, radiodense).
- Lucent structures absorb less of the beam and appear black (radiolucent).

Radiolucent					⟶ Radiodense
Air	Fat	Water	Soft tissue	Bone	Metal

Thickness
Thicker structures absorb more of the beam and appear radiodense.

Shape/form
- A structure of uniform composition, if flat, will produce a uniform appearance on x-ray (see Figure 1.1).
- If it is folded, the overlapping areas will be more radiodense (see Figure 1.2).

Portable versus intradepartmental films?

> Films should always be obtained in the radiology department, unless the patient's clinical condition prohibits this.

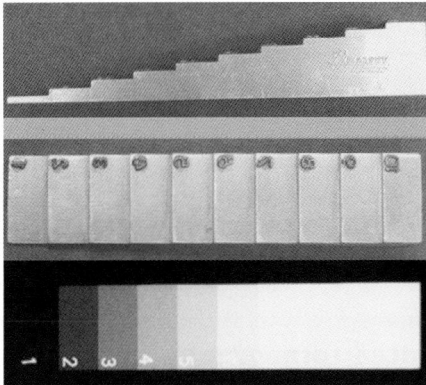

Figure 1.1 This step plate is a uniform type of metal, and is the thinnest on the left, and thickest on the right. The corresponding radiograph demonstrates that the thinner part of the plate is more radiolucent, and the thicker part more radiodense.

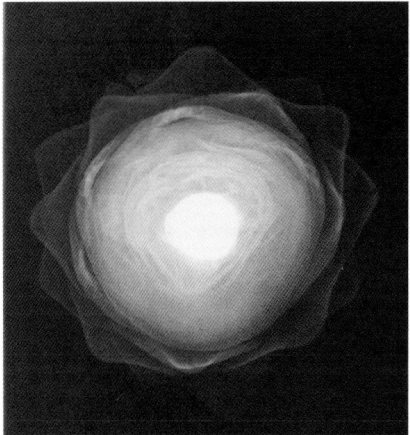

Figure 1.2 This radiograph of an artichoke was taken from above, and the density of the stem is additive, appearing white. Although each leaf is uniform in composition and thickness, where they are densely packed, they overlap and are more radiodense.

Portable radiographs are limited based on the following factors:
- <u>kVp & mA</u>: The x-ray generator in portable units cannot produce the power needed to penetrate large patients and dense areas, such as the lumbar spine. Films commonly underpenetrated (white).
- <u>Magnification</u>: Source to image distance is less with portable chest films, resulting in greater magnification.
- <u>Grids</u>: Grids are stationary on portable units and require very precise patient positioning and alignment of the beam to prevent the grid from attenuating *too much* of the incident beam. This results in poor quality image.
- <u>Positioning</u>: Positioning is variable; true upright images are hard to obtain, patients are typically sitting semi-upright, and inspiratory effort is limited.

Computed tomography

Known more commonly as "CT," computed tomography creates two dimensional (2D), grayscale images, which are "slices" through the body.

How are images acquired?
CT images are obtained using ionizing radiation. The patient lies on a table that moves slowly through a circular tube that houses the x-ray generator and a row of detectors 180 degrees opposite.
- As the table moves through the gantry, the generator and detectors spin as a unit around the patient. The generator continuously emit a thin beam of x-rays and the detectors sense those that traverse the patient.
- This produces a helix of density data on the patient.
- The detectors transmit the digital signals to a computer for interpolation and subsequent display.
  - The helix of data can be reformatted in any plane, although most commonly axial, coronal, and sagittal images are generated.

Factors influencing appearance
Physical properties
Since CT is performed with x-rays, similar factors affect the appearance of the images—tissue density being the primary factor.
- Denser structures appear whiter, or "high attenuation."
- Less dense structures appear dark, or "low attenuation."

Contrast and resolution
The excellent soft tissue contrast with CT in combination with the thin sections that can be obtained allows for discrimination of structures of similar densities that cannot be distinguished on radiography. Spatial resolution is a millimeter or less.

CT artifacts
<u>Motion</u>: Patient movement during scanning blurs the images.
<u>Streak</u>: This is a streak or line through the CT image. Causes of streak artifact: metal, edges of dense bone, sharp edge transitions (e.g., fluid/air levels in bowel).

COMPUTED TOMOGRAPHY

Hounsfield Units (HU) (aka "CT number")
This is a measure of the CT density of tissue and can be obtained by placing a "region of interest" on the digital image. These aid in characterizing tissues when interpreting CT (e.g., simple fluid-filled structures should measure < 20 HU)

Approximate Hounsfield unit values:

Air	Fat	Water	Bone
−1000	−50 to −100	0	+500 to +1500

Image display
Images are viewed on settings that limit the range of CT numbers displayed and that define how they are displayed:

Window width
The range of CT numbers displayed; this affects image contrast.
- A narrower window (less CT numbers displayed) results in greater contrast because each shade of gray will represent a wider range of densities.

Window level
The level is the HU that is depicted as the "middle" shade of gray.
- All tissues with CT numbers greater than the selected level will appear whiter/lighter and tissues with numbers lower will be blacker/darker.

Standard windows
There are "standard" window and level settings set to optimize the visualization of structures in the lungs, bones, brain, etc.

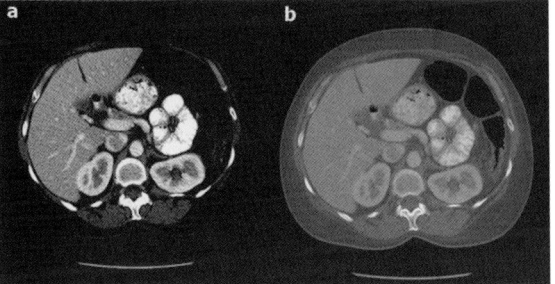

Figure 1.3 Image (a) has a window of 200, and (b) 700 (both have a level of 100). Note the greater contrast of the intraabdominal soft tissues with the narrower window; however, the intrabdominal and subcutaneous fat are black and cannot be evaluated.

Contrast enhancement
- An iodine based dye is injected intravenously. The dye is high attenuation and makes blood vessels and organs, which concentrate the dye, appear higher in attenuation on CT.
- Injection volume and rate vary with the CT protocol being utilized.
- Enhancement is defined as an increase in HU *by at least 10 HU* from unenhanced to enhanced images.

(Also see "What about contrast?" p. 16)

Technology

Multidetector CT (MDCT)
Current CT scanners have rows of multiple parallel detectors (8–64), allowing for a greater length of the patient to be scanned with each rotation of the gantry than was possible with single detector scanners.
- Enables faster scanning.
- Enables acquisition of images rapidly enough to keep up with flowing blood, allowing for diagnostic exams of the arteries (CT angiography (CTA), see below).
- Each detector is 0.5–0.625 mm in width, enabling thin section high spatial resolution images to be obtained.

CT reformatting techniques:
The helix of data can be reformatted in many ways:
- Multiplanar reformats (MPR): 2D images with any slice thickness desired. Most commonly axial, sagittal, and coronal.
- Curved planar reformats: A sub-type of MPR that aligns the imaging plane to follow an anatomic structure, such as the pancreatic duct or a tortuous aorta. This produces excellent images of the structure in question, but distorts all surrounding structures (see Figure 1.4).
- Maximum intensity projection (MIP): A 2D image that displays only the highest attenuation structure in the slice. Used most commonly for CT angiography. Slice thickness can be tailored to the clinical question:
  - Thin sections—useful to evaluate branch vessel ostia in CTA.
  - Thick sections—useful to see entire course of small vessels, like in CTA of the brain to evaluate for aneurysms or stenoses.
- Minimum intensity projection (MinIP): A 2D image that displays only the lowest attenuation structures in the slice. Used for airway evaluation and CT colonography.
- 3-Dimensional: 3D images are created by a variety of methods. These images display only the surface of a structure, and are shaded to give the appearance of depth. They can be rotated in any plane, and show the 3D relationships of structures. This is commonly done to evaluate complex fractures and for CT angiography.

COMPUTED TOMOGRAPHY

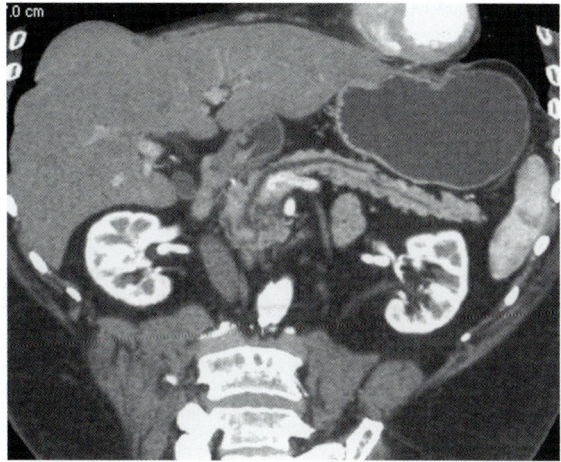

Figure 1.4 Curved MPR along the pancreatic duct. The second portion of the duodenum, pancreatic head, body, and tail are all seen in one plane, however, note the distortion of the surrounding structures.

What is "volume averaging"?
Standard CT images display the mean attenuation of structures that are superimposed on the slice. For example:
- If a 10 mm slice contains all liver, the attenuation of structures is uniform, and is accurately displayed.
- If the 10 mm slice through the liver contains a 5 mm cyst, the low density of the cyst (~ 0 HU) will be "averaged" with the density of the liver (~100 HU), and the resulting displayed attenuation in the cyst will be ~50 HU. Thus, the cyst will falsely appear higher density than it should.

Protocols

General
A protocol is the way the CT images are obtained. Each protocol stipulates the following:
- IV contrast: injection rate and volume.
- Oral contrast: type and duration of ingestion.
- Scan delay: how to time scan acquisition.
- Number of acquisitions.

Multiphase scanning
MDCT is so fast that it allows multiple scans of the same body part to be obtained during the IV contrast bolus. This increases the ability of CT to

accurately characterize lesions, but it comes at the price of higher radiation doses. Primary indication is identification of masses in solid organs.

CT Angiography (CTA)
CT is acquired while the contrast is located within the arteries, before it has had time to pass through to the capillary phase and into the veins. Reformats are an integral part of this study:
<u>Curved MIP reformats</u>: Along the long axis of the vessel. These are also called "centerline" reformats, which straightens tortuous vessels and presents them in a straight line, enabling accurate measurements of regions of stenosis or aneurysmal dilatation.
<u>3D images</u>: Useful to demonstrate tortuosity. Beware, densely calcified atherosclerotic plaques can obscure stenoses, and 3D images cannot be interpreted in isolation.

Magnetic resonance imaging

Images are generated based on the inherent magnetic properties of protons in the body, and their interaction with an external magnetic field. Unlike CT and radiography, ionizing radiation is not used; MRI capitalizes on the molecular composition of tissues to generate an image.

How are images acquired?
Brief outline of how MRI works
The patient lies on a table within the bore of a 1.5 or 3 Tesla (T) magnet. For reference:
- 1.5 T = 10,000 G (Gauss).
- Refrigerator magnet has a strength of 10 G.
- Odd numbered protons (e.g., hydrogen) in the body have their own magnetic field and align themselves parallel to the external magnetic field. This is longitudinal magnetization.
- A radiofrequency pulse (RF) is applied, disrupting the proton alignment and causing them to transiently assume a high energy state.
- Over time, the protons relax back to their baseline and emit radiofrequency waves (the "echo"), which the MRI machine records.
- This signal is used to determine spatial localization and signal intensity, and to create the image.

T1 and T2 Relaxation
After the RF pulse is applied, the protons begin to re-align themselves with the external magnetic field. This is called "relaxation." Different tissues relax back to baseline at different rates. There are two types of relaxation:
- <u>T1</u>: The realignment of protons parallel to the external magnetic field, thus re-gaining the longitudinal magnetization.
- <u>T2</u>: Loss of the transverse magnetization that is caused by the RF pulse.

Different tissue types have different inherent T1 and T2 relaxation properties, which allows them to be differentiated on MRI.

What generates the MRI signal?
Only molecules with an odd number of protons have their own magnetic field; it is these molecules that interact with the external magnetic field and generate the MRI signal.
- Hydrogen atoms in water are the most abundant protons in the body, and produce most of the signal in clinical MRI.

Technology
MRI coils
A coil is basically an antenna that senses the emitted MRI signal. The coil is positioned as close as possible to the item being examined, and come in a variety of shapes and sizes depending on the area to be imaged (e.g., head coil, breast coil).

Image acquisition
Images can be acquired directly in the axial, coronal, or sagittal plane.

3D acquisition & reformatting
Data can be acquired as a volume rather than as discrete slices. This data can then be reformatted into any plane.
- This is most commonly performed in MR angiography & MRCP.
- 3D images can also be generated, which display the surface of structures. This, too, is most commonly done for MR angiograms.

MR spectroscopy
Technique to identify relative amounts of specific chemicals (e.g., choline, N-acetylaspartate) in tissue. Used for problem solving in specific circumstances (e.g., to differentiate tumor from inflammation). It is used clinically in neuroimaging, but other uses are currently investigational.

Functional MRI
Uses MRI to localize the region of cerebral cortex that controls a specific function. Based on signal changes caused by the increase in oxygen levels that occurs in areas of activated cortex. Not used routinely clinically, but there are emerging indications.

3T imaging
3T images can be acquired more quickly, and have improved soft tissue contrast in most areas in comparison to 1.5 T. Pitfalls of 3T imaging include higher cost, louder scans, increased artifacts (susceptibility/metal, chemical shift, field inhomogeneity) and potential for heating-related complications.

Factors influencing appearance
Tissue composition
- Tissues that emit a lot of signal are termed "high signal intensity" and look white/bright on the images.
- Tissues that do not emit much sign are termed "low signal intensity" and look dark.
- Tissues with a high concentration of odd numbered protons, such as water, emit much of the MRI signal.
- Tissues devoid of water, such as cortical bone, emit little signal and are low signal intensity.

Pulse sequences
MRI sequences ("pulse sequences") are created by machine settings that control multiple factors, including:
- TR–the length of time between administered radiofrequency pulses.
- TE–the time delay for the machine to "listen" for the echo.

By calibrating TR and TE settings, imaging sequences of varying T1 and T2 weighting are created.
- T1 weighted images: short TR, short TE.
- T2 weighted images: long TR, long TE.

In an MRI exam, multiple pulse sequences are acquired. Each of these has a unique name, appearance, and sensitivity. Some of these are machine vendor-dependent.

> **Most commonly used pulse sequences:**
> **T1 weighted**: water dark, fat bright, good for anatomy
> **T2 weighted**: water bright, fat bright, good for edema/pathology
> **Proton density (PD)**: weakly T2 weighted, water is gray, good for tendons, ligaments, and cartilage
> **FLAIR**: Free water dark, edema/pathology bright, good for brain
> **Diffusion**: restricted water diffusion is bright, good for CVA, indications in the abdomen & elsewhere are being developed.
> **STIR**: inherent fat suppression, T2 weighted image. Good for spine, bones

Fat saturation
Images can be acquired such that the signal from fat is suppressed and is dark on the images. Uses of fat saturation ("fat sat"):
- <u>T2 fat sat:</u> Edema/pathology has high signal intensity; more conspicuous when fat is dark. Useful in MSK, neck, and abdominal applications.
- <u>T1 fat sat:</u> Can differentiate blood products (often T1 bright) from fat (e.g., fatty ovarian mass versus hemorrhagic cyst).
- <u>T1 fat sat postcontrast:</u> Increases the conspicuity of pathologic enhancement.

Some pulse sequences, such as STIR images, have inherent fat saturation.

Contrast enhancement
Images are obtained prior to and following administration of IV contrast. The pre-contrast image can be subtracted from the post-contrast, to increase visualization of subtle areas of enhancement (see "Contrast" p. 18).

Protocols
General
Standard ways of performing an MRI scan have been developed for specific indications; these are called protocols.
- In general, most MRI scans include several different pulse sequences, which provide different but complimentary information.

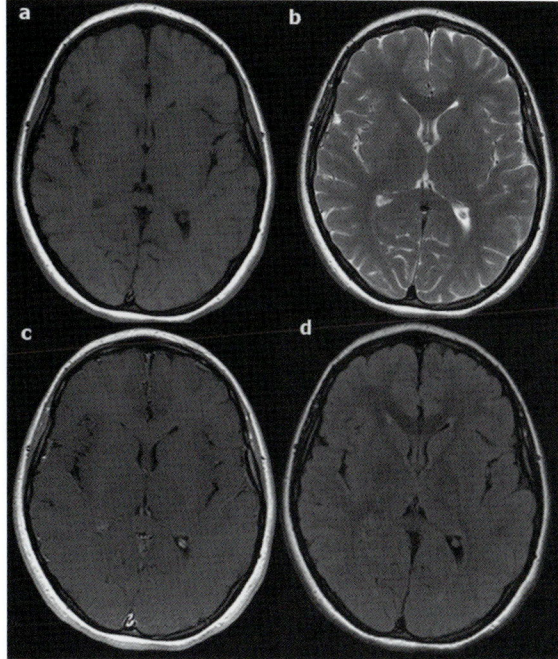

Figure 1.5 Common pulse sequences used in brain MRI. T1 weighted (a), T2 weighted (b), T1 post contrast (c), and FLAIR (d) images. Note that fluid (CSF) is dark on T1 and FLAIR, and bright only on T2. Note that the signal intensity of gray versus white matter is the opposite on T1 versus T2.

MR angiography (MRA)
MRA is an excellent non-invasive way to evaluate the vasculature, and can be used to assess arteries and veins. One of the strengths of MRA is that it can be performed with or without IV contrast.

MRA without contrast
Relies on the properties of flowing blood and flow velocity to image the vasculature. Several imaging techniques have been developed:

<u>Black-blood</u> (flowing blood appears black):
- Can assess intraluminal and mural abnormalities (flaps, clot).
- Long acquisition time.

<u>Phase-contrast</u> (flowing blood appears white):
- Yields anatomic and velocity data, used to evaluate stenoses.

<u>Time of flight (TOF) (2D or 3D):</u>
- Signal intensity is proportionate to flow velocity; flowing blood is high signal intensity.
- Longest acquisition time; limits the field of view of coverage possible.
- Used to evaluate vascular stenoses.

MRA with contrast
Using gadolinium allows for faster and clearer vascular imaging with fewer artifacts than non-contrast methods.
- Contrast enhanced vessels are bright on T1 weighted images.
- Fat saturation is typically performed to increase vascular conspicuity.

<u>3D acquisition:</u>
- Allows data acquisition in single breath hold.
- Data can be reformatted in any plane, including curved.
- 3D images can be generated.

<u>2D acquisition:</u>
- Axial, coronal, or oblique images are acquired directly.
- Thin sections are acquired to assess small branch vessels.
- These do not produce similar high quality MIP reformats, and 3D images cannot be generated from these data sets.

MRI safety
The safety of patients in MRI magnets is paramount, and there are several potential risks to them. See p. 25 for further details.

What makes images look good or bad?

Signal-to-noise ratio
The ratio of desirable signal to the background noise from all sources influences the quality of the image. High signal to noise ratios result in clearer, less "grainy" images.

Portable radiographs: Often produce films that are underpenetrated, with low signal to noise ratio (see p. 4, "Radiography").

Radiography, CT: The "signal" on the final image is dependent on the strength of the beam strength used.
- Higher mAs produces more transmitted photons to create a better image, but at the cost of higher radiation dose to the patient.
- Higher kVp creates a more penetrating beam; this can be desirable, such as in an obese patient, but it may not be helpful otherwise.

MRI: Factors that influence the final MR image include the field strength (higher strength generally results in better resolution) and the sampling frequency.

Motion
Radiography: Motion is particularly a problem in mammography, where fine calcifications must be identified.

CT: Only the slices that were obtained while the patient was moving look blurred; the rest of the images will not be affected.

MRI: Due to the way images are acquired, the entire sequence will have blurring. Since MRIs are long exams, they are particularly prone to be affected by patient motion; the table can become uncomfortable after a time.

Obesity

Obese patients attenuate more of the x-ray beam, and as a result, radiographs can appear underpenetrated (too white, too little information reaching the detector). In CT, the images may look "grainy." Increasing the dose can overcome this to some degree, but again, at a cost of increased radiation exposure.

What is "PACS"?

PACS = "Picture Archiving and Communication System". PACS is the computer network used for digital image storage, image review, and manipulation. It has replaced the traditional screen-film and film library format used in the pre-digital era. PACS systems vary between vendors.

> **Benefits of PACS:**
> - *Image storage*: all of a patient's studies are immediately available for review and comparison.
> - *Image review*: can be performed remotely for conferences and consultations, available in procedure areas such as the operating rooms.
> - *Image manipulation*: window/level, contrast and brightness can be adjusted to highlight the area of interest. Images can be magnified, annotated, and measurements can be made and stored. Some PACS also enable multiplanar and 3D reformatting.

PACS workstations have high quality, high resolution monitors conforming to national (DICOM) standards and a range of software tools to allow image manipulation.
- Monitor resolution depends on the images that are being viewed.
- Resolution required: mammograms>radiographs>CT/MR/US

> **What is DICOM?**
> "Digital Imaging and Communications in Medicine"; a standard for handling, storing, printing, and transmitting information in medical imaging. It enables the integration of scanners, workstations, printers, servers, and network hardware from multiple manufacturers into a PACS system.

In many institutions, images can also be viewed on a Web browser/stand-alone software on standard PCs, allowing for more widespread accessibility.
- These displays do not typically conform to the DICOM standard.
- Resolution is typically lower and should not be used for diagnosis, especially of radiographs and mammograms.

What about contrast?
- Modalities that use x-rays (radiography, CT, fluoroscopy) use contrast agents that contain high atomic number atoms (e.g., iodine, barium) to absorb x-rays and increase the density of organs and tissues.
- MRI contrast agents change the magnetic properties of tissues.
- Ultrasound uses compounds that increase the echoes in tissues (e.g., microbubbles).

Intravenous iodinated contrast agents
- Used in CT, angiography and in some fluoroscopy studies (e.g., IVPs). They are predominantly eliminated via the kidneys.

Risk: contrast induced nephropathy (CIN)
Defined as the deterioration of renal function in the absence of other etiologies; temporally associated with the administration of IV iodinated contrast media.
- Risk of CIN rises proportional to the degree of pre-existing renal impairment as well as to the number of pre-existing risk factors
- GFR > 45, risk CIN < 1%.
- GFR < 45, risk CIN 10%.
- Risk is greatest in patients with both renal impairment and diabetes.

Screening for CRI before intravenous contrast administration
- Screening of out-patients aims to identify patients with clinical history/risk factors that have the highest association with elevated serum creatinine, including: chronic renal impairment (CRI), proteinuria, prior renal surgery, hypertension, gout and diabetes mellitus (DM).
- Patients with any risk factor should have a serum creatinine checked before administering IV contrast.

Prevention of contrast induced nephropathy
Perform an alternative exam:
- Does this exam need to be done?
- Could US, MRI, or other study answer the clinical question?
- Would a non-contrast study give sufficient information?

Administer nephroprotective agents:
Although studies are limited, several nephroprotective strategies have been suggested to be beneficial:
- Hydration with volume expansion (oral water or IV NS). This is the best established and simplest method.
- Bicarbonate infusion.
  - Sodium bicarb 150 mEq in 850 cc D5W at 3 ml/kg/h × 1 h, then 1 ml/kg/h × 6 h.

WHAT ABOUT CONTRAST? 17

- N-acetyl cysteine administration.
  - 600 mg PO q12h BID the day prior to and day of study.
- Use of low osmolar IV contrast e.g., Visipaque™.
  - Controversial; likely benefit in patients with CRI or DM.

Risk: contrast allergy
Please see p. 20.

Relative contraindications to administering IV iodinated contrast
- Renal impairment: no specific creatinine threshold exists, however at Cr of >1.5, risk/benefits must be assessed especially if diabetic.
- Known prior severe (anaphylactoid) iodinated contrast allergy.
- Myeloma: high risk of nephropathy if Bence-Jones proteinuria.
- Current metformin therapy: increased risk of lactic acidosis
  - Stop for 2 days after contrast and check renal function before re-starting.
- Pheochromocytoma: theoretical risk of hypertensive crisis but case studies show non-ionic contrast is safe.

Gadolinium-based contrast agents (GBCA)
These agents are used almost exclusively in MRI. Gadolinium is a paramagnetic agent and shortens the longitudinal relaxation time (T1), leading to increased signal on T1 images of structures that contain it.

Extracellular agents
- Gadolinium chelated to an organic compound circulates and then freely distributes in the *extracellular* fluid compartment.
- Elimination is primarily renal.

Hepatobiliary specific MRI agents
- These are gadolinium-based agents that are taken up by hepatocytes and partially excreted through the biliary tree (50%).
- Lesions containing hepatocytes and bile become T1 bright.
- In addition to the typical post-contrast images obtained, a delayed "hepatocyte" phase image is also acquired, from 20 minutes to several hours post-contrast.
- Clinical applications include:
  - MR cholangiography (e.g., r/o leak, evaluate obstruction, anatomy).
  - Characterization of liver lesions—only hepatocyte-containing lesions will retain contrast on hepatocyte phase images; all other lesions will appear hypointense.

Risks
Allergic reactions
Very uncommon.

Nephrogenic systemic fibrosis (NSF)
A disabling fibrosing condition that has been associated with GBCA. Skin and internal organs including heart and muscle become fibrotic, thickened and contracted.
- Renal insufficiency prohibits clearance of free gadolinium.
- Risk increases with degree of renal impairment and the cumulative dose of gadolinium:
  - GFR >60 ml/min (normal renal function): no risk.
  - GFR >30 ml/min, but < 60 ml/min: the "gray zone." The risks/benefit of GBCA must be assessed.
  - GFR<30 ml/min: significant renal impairment, at risk for NSF. Incidence of NSF estimated 3% previously in these patients but now <1% with newer agents + lower doses.

NSF prevention strategies:
- Assess for most appropriate imaging exam required and whether GBCA is actually required.
- Screen for acute or chronic renal failure with measurement of GFR in patients who will receive GBCA.
- Same day dialysis following MRI is advised for patients with renal failure who must receive GBCA.

Intraluminal agents
Used to optimize imaging of the GI tract in fluoroscopy, CT and MRI. These agents can be administered PO or per rectum.

Indications
Fluoroscopy (further details see p. 331 fluoro chapter):
- To coat the lumen for double contrast studies.
- To fill the lumen and render it radiopaque and, therefore, visible.
- Used for mucosal evaluation, luminal caliber, and GI tract anatomy.

CT
- Distinguish hollow viscus from fluid collection and/or abscess.
- Distinguish bowel loops from mass lesion, lymph nodes.
  - Positive—barium or iodine-based, high attenuation.
  - Negative—water or other agents, low density.

MRI
- Can be used to increase signal or eliminate signal from the bowel.
  - Positive—increases signal, used to evaluate bowel lumen, pathology.
  - Negative—eliminates signal, used to reduce artifacts and signal from bowel, such as in MRCP.

Types
Positive agents

> Oral full strength barium causes extensive streak artifacts on CT; don't perform a fluoroscopic GI study prior to a CT!

Barium sulfate:
- The primary contrast agent for evaluation of the upper and lower GI tract in fluoroscopy. Used less frequently for CT and MRI.
- Barium comes in different forms: thick, thin, and dilute. See "Fluoro" p. 331 for more details on barium compounds.

Water soluble agents:
Used in suspected leaks—reabsorbed if extravasates, used in single- contrast enemas.
- <u>High osmolarity</u> contrast media (HOCM, or ionic), e.g., Renograffin™ or Gastrograffin™, which contains a soap.
- <u>Low osmolarity</u> contrast media (LOCM, or non-ionic) non-ionic water soluble, e.g., Omnipaque™.

> Some of these oral agents taste awful! Often, particularly for CT, the agent is mixed with a flavoring to improve taste. However, these are typically powder drink mixes that contain sugar. This cannot be given to diabetic patients and instead, they can be given very dilute barium.

Negative agents
Air:
- Distends the lumen in double contrast studies and CT colonography.
- Used for enemas in children with suspected intussusception (see pediatrics chapter p. 307).

Gas:
- Effervesent granules are swallowed, which create gas to distend the UGI tract for esophagrams and UGI studies.

Methylcellulose:
- Used in enteroclysis, a fluoroscopic study of the small bowel. It retains fluid in the bowel lumen, preventing reabsorbtion.

Water:
- Distends the bowel only slightly as some is reabsorbed.
- Increases conspicuity of bowel wall enhancement.
- Cheap, well tolerated, and widely available.

VoLumen®:
- A suspension containing very dilute barium sulfate, natural gums, sorbitol and simethicone. Achieves bowel distension and prevents resorption. Bowel distension is better than with water.
- Looks radiolucent and accentuates visualization of mural enhancement.
- Used in CT and MRI enterography.

What about oral agents for MRI?
Oral contrast agents in MRI are confusing because the same agent may be a positive agent on T2 images and a negative agent on T1 images

(e.g., water). Water and 2% barium solutions are the most commonly used. Features of desirable MR oral contrast agents:
- Reduce signal on T1 to increase visualization of mural enhancement.
- Are bright on T2 to evaluate luminal caliber.
- Cause slight bowel distension and are not reabsorbed.

Risks and contraindications of intraluminal contrast agents
Barium sulfate
- Spill of barium into the peritoneal cavity results in chemical peritonitis, which may require surgical washout; use with caution in suspected leaks; water soluble is preferred.
- In the mediastinum can cause fibrosis.
- Should not be used intrathecally.

Water-soluble agents
- Contraindicated when aspiration is suspected because this can result in chemical pneumonitis and cause acute pulmonary edema.
  - Use barium—small aspirated amounts are harmless (but persist on CXR almost indefinitely), larger aspirations can cause pneumonia.
- Allergic reactions very rare to intraluminal contrast administration, even if there is a history of prior contrast allergies to IV use.
- Non-ionic agents should <u>never</u> be used intrathecally as they cause severe neurological problems. Non-ionic agents are safe.

Other uses of contrast
Contrast may be administered into any cavity: natural (e.g., bladder) or pathologic (e.g., fistula), with imaging performed with radiography, fluoroscopy (including C-arm in the OR), CT, or MRI.
- Water soluble iodinated contrast (ionic or non-ionic) is used for:
  - Cystograms, urethrograms, hysterosalpingograms, arthrograms, sinograms, ERCP, cholangiography, sialography, ductography (breast).
- Barium is used for GI tube checks.
- Gadolinium used for MR arthrograms.

Contrast allergies

Allergies to contrast media are not true allergies because no antibodies have been identified. These reactions are termed "anaphylactoid." Physicians administering these contrast media must be knowledgeable in and prepared to treat these contrast reactions.

Risk factors for iodinated contrast allergy
- History of prior allergic reaction to contrast.
- History of severe atopy or asthma.

> History of shellfish allergy alone is NOT a risk factor for IV contrast allergy; patients are allergic to a protein in the fish, not the iodine.

Allergic reactions

Minor 0.2–0.7% incidence	Moderate	Severe 0.01–0.02% incidence
Urticaria, pruritis	Vaso-vagal reaction	Pulmonary edema
Nausea, vomiting	Bronchospasm	Cardiac/respiratory arrest
Diaphoresis	Facial/laryngeal edema	Seizures
		Death

Prevention of contrast reactions

Generally only minor contrast reactions have benefited from pretreatment strategies. Life threatening contrast reactions have not been shown to benefit from premedication.

> **Pretreatment protocols for IV iodinated contrast**
> 1. Prednisone 50 mg PO 13 hr, 7 hr and 1 hr prior, plus diphenhydramin 50 mg IM/IV/PO 1 hr prior to contrast administration.
> *or*
> 2. Methylprednisolone 32 mg PO 12 hr and 2 hr prior, plus diphenhydramine 50 mg IM/IV/PO 1 hr prior to contrast administration.

Treatment of allergic contrast reactions

Urticaria
Diphenhydramine 25–50 mg oral or IM/IV.
Cimetidine 300 mg IV slowly.

Hypotension
IV fluids, elevate legs, oxygen.
Atropine 0.6 mg IV; repeat if necessary to 3 mg total if bradycardia

Bronchospasm or laryngeal edema
Oxygen, IV saline.
Epinephrine 1:1000 0.1–0.2 ml SQ or
Epinephrine 1:10,000 1 ml IV slowly.
Albuterol 2–3 puffs.

Seizures
Diazepam 5 g IV slowly.

Anaphylaxis
Oxygen, IV saline.
Epinephrine 1:10,000 1 ml IV, slowly.
Diphenhydramine 25–50 mg IV.
Cimetidine 300 mg in 20 ml slow IV.
Solumedrol 1 gm IV.
If on β-blockers, add glucagon 1–5 mg IV.

Contrast extravasation/infiltration
When an IV or vein "blows," injected contrast may infiltrate into the tissues. The severity of the ensuing inflammatory reaction is dependent on the type of contrast and the volume extravasated. Skin ulceration and necrosis can occur.

Treatment
- Elevation of the extremity and application of ice or cold compresses.
- Observation for ~ 2 hours.
  - Assess distal extremity perfusion, pulses, sensation.
- Consider injection of hyaluronidase (for large volume extravasation).
  - Breaks down hyaluronic acid, a component of connective tissue, and allows for dissipation of the exravasate over a larger region, facilitating rapid absorption. *Effectiveness is controversial.*
- Surgical consultation to be considered if
  - Ionic contrast—volume >30 ml.
  - Nonionic contrast—volume >100 ml.

What are the risks of imaging?

Risks associated with contrast administration
See p. 20.

Radiation
Ionizing radiation has been shown to cause tissue damage and increased risk of cancer in those people exposed to very high doses of radiation, such as atomic bomb survivors. At present, there are very few conclusive studies that have shown definite measurable increased risks of cancer from medical imaging that uses ionizing radiation (CT, x-ray, nuclear medicine). However:
- Most scientists agree that even small doses of ionizing radiation increase the risk of cancer by a finite degree.
- CT scans are responsible for a large and increasing amount of the medical radiation exposure in the United States.
- CT scans have been estimated to be the future cause of 1.5–2% of all cancers in the United States at current usage rates.

Thus, it is very important to follow the ALARA (As Low As Reasonably Achievable) principle for radiation exposure.

Radiation doses from X-rays (CT, fluoroscopy, radiography, angiography)
Modes of measurement
Radiation dose to humans is usually measured in one of two ways:
- <u>Absorbed Dose</u>: Describes how much radiation has been absorbed but does not consider where in the body, or what type of tissue has been affected.
  - Measured in rads or grays (Gy = SI units).
  - 100 rad = 1 Gray.

WHAT ARE THE RISKS OF IMAGING?

- <u>Effective Dose</u>: Takes into account the radiation risk over the entire body, and allows comparison of risk to reference standards such as background radiation or other radiological tests.
  - Measured in rems or Sieverts (Sv = SI units).
  - 100 rem = 1 Sievert.

Background radiation

For perspective, the <u>average</u> citizen of the United States is exposed to roughly 3 mSv of background radiation per year. This includes cosmic radiation and naturally occurring radiation (i.e., radon).

A PA chest x-ray of (0.1 mSv) is roughly the equivalent to 10 days of background radiation.

Comparative effective doses of various radiological studies

Table 1.1 compares the effective doses of various studies to that of natural background radiation.

Procedure	Approximate effective radiation dose	Comparable to natural background radiation (time)
Abdominal region		
CT Abdomen and Pelvis	10 mSv	3 years
CT Colonography	10 mSv	3 years
Intravenous Pyelogram (IVP)	3 mSv	1 year
Barium enema	8 mSv	3 years
UGI study	6 mSv	2 years
Bone		
Radiograph spine	1.5 mSv	6 months
Radiograph extremity	0.001 mSv	Less than 1 day
Central Nervous system		
CT Head	2 mSv	8 months
CT angiogram intra and extracranial vessels	5 mSv	20 months
Myelography	4 mSv	16 months
Chest		
CT Chest	7 mSv	2 years
CT Chest Low Dose	1.5 mSv	6 months
PA CXR	0.1 mSv	10 days
Children's imaging		
Voiding Cystourethrogram	5–10 yr. old: 1.6 mSv	6 months
	Infant: 0.8 mSv	3 months

(Continued)

Table 1.1 (Cont'd)

Face and neck		
CT Sinuses	0.6 mSv	2 months
Heart		
Cardiac CT for Calcium Scoring	2 mSv	8 months
Women's Imaging		
Bone Densitometry (DEXA)	0.001 mSv	Less than 1 day
Mammography	0.7 mSv	3 months

*Estimated doses as of January 2011

Pediatric patients*

- Children are more sensitive to ionizing radiation than adults. The younger the child, the greater the risk. 6–11% of CT scans are performed in children.
- The risk is roughly logarithmic, with children <1 year having an estimated risk of 0.14% additional lifetime cancer risk from a single abdominal CT (compared to 0.02% for a 35 year old).
- Experts have estimated that a single CT in a young child may have a risk of 1:500–1:1000 of causing a <u>fatal</u> cancer over a lifetime.
- Baseline risk of dying of cancer is 1:4–1:5.

*The "Image Gently" campaign, put forth by the Alliance for Radiation Safety in Pediatric Imaging, is centered on reducing radiation exposure to children (http://www.pedrad.org/associations/5364/ig/)

How to reduce radiation dose
Does the study really need to be done?

- Was it performed recently at your facility or elsewhere? Avoid duplication.
- Always consider "how will this change my management of this patient?"

Can an alternative study be substituted?

- Can MRI or ultrasound answer the question instead and avoid ionizing radiation exposure?

Reducing dose from CT scans

- Scan only the necessary body parts (i.e., don't order CT of the abdomen and pelvis if you only really need the pelvis).
- Avoid multiphase studies unless definitively indicated.
- Use pediatric protocols that appropriately decrease the dose.
- Use appropriate shielding (i.e., breast and eye shields) which can decrease dose.
  - Developing breasts (e.g., teenage girls) are very sensitive to radiation, and bismuth shields can reduce the breast dose significantly, though it does affect image quality.

WHAT ARE THE RISKS OF IMAGING?

Interventional procedures and fluoroscopy
Procedures performed with CT or fluoroscopic guidance can result in large radiation doses. Radiation burns have occurred with lengthy procedures. Fluoroscopy is used in the cardiac catheterization lab, orthopedic OR, etc., and often used by clinicians with little or no training in radiation safety.

Reducing radiation dose during procedures
- Frequently reposition the x-ray tube during the procedure to decrease dose to any given area of tissue (e.g., change tube angulation so skin entry site is varied).
- Use the least amount of fluoroscopy needed—TAKE YOUR FOOT OFF THE PEDAL!
- Digital pulsed fluoroscopy reduces dose.
- Reduce the air gap by keeping the image intensifier close to the patient.
- Use magnification sparingly: it increases the dose considerably.
- Use appropriate patient shielding.

MRI
MRI risks are mostly due to ferromagnetic objects within the magnetic field:
- In the patient (e.g., implanted devices, surgical clips).
- On the patient or attendants (e.g., keys in one's pocket, electrodes).
- Brought into the room (e.g., IV stands, oxygen tanks).

These objects may do any or all of the following:
- Move: aneurysm clips have come off the vessel, orbit perforations from intraorbital metal (very very rare).
- Heat: 3° burns have occurred from metallic leads or skin patches.
- Malfunction: defibrillators deploying, pacemaker no longer pacing.
- Impair image quality: metal causes an artifact that can significantly impair image interpretation.

> The MRI scanner is ALWAYS on, not just when a scan is being acquired. Therefore, everyone must always be cognisant of what metallic items they have on or in them before entering the MRI room.

What can't come into the scanner?
Inside the patient
- Pacemakers and automated implantable cardioverter-defibrillators (AICDs). Under rare circumstances scans are done with cardiac monitoring and cardiologist supervision.
- Metal in patient's eyes.

<u>Determining if implanted metallic structures are safe:</u>
The safety of any implanted device must be assessed prior to performing an MRI on the patient. Depending on the composition of a device or substance, they may be safe, unsafe, or conditional for MRI.
- *Conditional* means that a device may be safely scanned only if certain conditions can be met.

> **Need to know if your patient's device is safe?**
> Check "The List" at www.mrisafety.com to see if it has tested "safe," "conditional," or "unsafe" in a 1.5T and/or 3.0T clinical scanner, or check with the manufacturer.

The patient
<u>Claustrophobia</u>: The patient may not want to get into the scanner! The bore of the machine is relatively narrow. Consider oral sedation or if necessary, anesthesiology assistance for sedation.

<u>Pregnancy:</u> If exam is necessary, the patient must consent to have the exam done. See more in "How do I image my pregnant patient?" p. 27.

<u>Obesity</u>: Most MRI scanners have a weight limit of ≈300lb, and a narrow bore, which patients might not fit in. "Open" MRIs have a higher weight/size limit but a lower field strength, and, therefore, lesser quality images.

Outside the patient
Any metallic object on the patient's body or in their clothes cannot come into the scanner. This includes piercings, hearing aids, dentures.

<u>Orthopedic hardware</u> is safe, but the artifact produced may significantly impair images if hardware is within the field of view. For example, a hip arthroplasty will not affect a brain MRI, but will a pelvic MRI.

How to reduce risk
Patient screening
- Each patient must undergo MRI screening (usually filling out a written form) to make sure that they are safe to go in the magnetic field.

Device screening
- Implanted devices must be checked to see if they are safe for MRI.
  - Many times the patient will carry a card stating the exact device and product number that they have implanted.
  - If the patient does not know, confirm the exact implanted device with the hospital where it was implanted.
  - Once the exact device is known, check for MRI compatibility.

Check the surroundings
- Patient's have died or been hurt by metallic objects flying into the middle of the scanner and striking the patient (i.e., oxygen tanks).
- Be familiar with the MRI suite and where you cannot go and remove all metal objects and equipment from your person.

> If you are part of a code team and called to the MRI scanner:
> <u>DO NOT RUSH INTO THE MRI ROOM!!</u>
> Wait until they pull the patient out. **The scanner is always on.**

How do I image my pregnant patient?

Ultrasound is the study of choice if a gynecological problem is suspected. When a non-gynecological etiology is suspected, CT, MRI, and ultrasound can be considered, and each has advantages and disadvantages.

Relative risks of different exams
General considerations
- Main fetal risk is that from ionizing radiation, with the potential increased risk of birth defects and childhood cancer.
  - Childhood cancer risk is theoretical and there is no assumed safe threshold level.
- Maternal abdominal/pelvic studies incur maximum fetal radiation exposure.
- Teratogenic threshold: Believed to be somewhere between 50–100 mGy.
  - After 10-week gestational age, the brain is the critical organ. There is no dose threshold for potential neurological impairment.
- Majority of routine diagnostic studies produce < 20 mGy to the uterus.
  - Single-phase CT scan of the abdomen and pelvis: < 35 mGy.
  - Interventional fluoroscopically guided procedures may incur >100 mGy.

If any doubt about pregnancy status, do a urine pregnancy test prior to imaging.

Radiography
- Some radiographic studies have such low exposures that pregnancy status need not be considered prior to imaging. Maternal abdomen is lead-shielded whenever possible e.g., for:
  - Chest x-ray in 1st, 2nd trimester.
  - Skull/face/neck radiographs.
  - Extremity radiographs (except the hips).
  - Mammograms.
- Single KUBs (kidneys, ureters, bladder) also very low exposure, but higher radiation studies such as lumbar spine series should be avoided.

Fluoroscopy
- Avoid fluoroscopy of the abdomen unless critical for maternal health.
- Limited studies, e.g., one image ("shot"), IVPs can sometimes be performed.

CT
- Recommend obtaining informed consent prior to necessary imaging.
- Lead-shield abdomen in chest CT studies.
- Only perform abdomen/pelvis studies when no alternative (e.g., trauma).
- Iodinated contrast *can* be given in pregnancy.

MRI
- No adverse outcomes have been shown to the fetus from MRI with low field strength MRI (1.5 Tesla). Higher field magnets have not been well studied yet.
- Avoid in first trimester if possible because theoretical risks of heating embryos (no human studies).
- Used in 2nd/3rd trimester routinely to evaluate fetal anomalies.
- Gadolinium administration in a pregnant female is *not* recommended unless there is overwhelming benefit to the mother that outweighs the risk to the fetus (animal data showing teratogenicity).
- Risk of Nephrogenic Systemic Fibrosis (NSF) from free gadolinium in the amniotic fluid is unknown. (Refer to "Contrast" p. 18.)
- Recommend obtaining informed consent prior to necessary imaging

US
- No risk known to fetus.

Nuclear studies
- Avoid where possible, especially in first trimester.
- Tc-99m agents produce relatively low fetal doses in later pregnancy, reduced further by hydration and regular bladder emptying.
- I-131, Ga-67, Tl-201 and other long half-life agents are contraindicated.
- Breast-feeding may need to be delayed or stopped in the postpartum period for many radioisotopes. These are the only radiological studies that affect breast-feeding.

Risk to the mother
- Always remember that with a pregnant woman, you are dealing with two patients!
- Always weigh the risks and benefits of each study, considering both the mother and fetus. A dead or seriously sick mother does not help the fetus.

Common clinical scenarios—ways to reduce risk
The following are imaging options for common conditions in the pregnant female. The ACR Appropriateness Criteria (www.acr.org/ac) have more information about imaging in specific scenarios in pregnancy.

Appendicitis
Ultrasound
- Worth attempting as first study.
- Transabdominal ultrasound has variable sensitivity and specificity, but appendicitis can be diagnosed in a number of cases.
- Sensitivity reduced in later pregnancy.
- The appendix may not be seen in normal patients (50–87% even when not pregnant), and appendicitis is not excluded.

MRI
- Increasingly used as exam of choice.
- Appendicitis identified with high sensitivity (100%) and specificity (94%) and normal appendix commonly identified (83–90%).
- Limitation is lack of immediate availability at most centers.

CT

- Ionizing radiation: MRI, or US preferred.
- In pregnancy, high sensitivity (95–100%) and specificity (87–98%) for detection of appendicitis.
- Normal appendix can be seen on CT almost always, so appendicitis can be effectively ruled out.
- Oral and IV contrast usually given.

Pulmonary emboli
CXR

- Always do first to exclude other cause of symptoms, e.g., pneumonia.
- Dose to fetus very small
- Lead-shield abdomen.

CT

- Very high sensitivity and specificity ("gold standard")
- Dose to fetus ≈ half that of a VQ (ventilation/perfusion) scan.
- Dose to breasts significantly higher than VQ.
- Can diagnose other causes of symptoms.

VQ scan

- Normal study <1% chance of PE, may be good option if no underlying respiratory disease and normal CXR.
- If normal perfusion scan, ventilation scan not necessary.
- Lower sensitivity and specificity than CT.
- Not available at all centers.

Renal calculi
Ultrasound

- Initial study of choice.
- Renal and/or ureteral stones (if at ureterovesical junction) may be seen.
- Ureters and renal pelvices may be physiologically enlarged due to gravid uterus and may mimic ureteral obstruction. Usually R>L.
- Look for ureteric jets in bladder to show ureteric patency.
- A normal renal sonogram is useful in excluding renal colic

IVP

- "One-shot" IVP (single image after contrast injection) sometimes performed.

MRI

- Physiologic ureteral dilatation can be distinguished from ureteral obstruction, as perinephric fluid and renal enlargement only occur with pathology.

CT

- Patients often treated presumptively for stones if there is high clinical suspicion, and CT reserved for complex cases/non-resolution.
- Non-contrast CT has high sensitivity for detection of renal calculi (sensitivity 96%, specificity 93–98%) and nephroureteral obstruction.

Trauma
CT and Radiographs
- Primary imaging modalities to assess for traumatic injury.
- Both involve ionizing radiation, CT significantly more.
- In mild trauma, physical exam with or without radiographs may be enough to clear the patient.
- In more severe trauma, CT is indicated to exclude maternal injury.

> If there is significant mechanism of chest/abdominal injury, CT should be performed. A dead mother does not save the fetus.

MRI
- Used secondarily after CT, primarily in neuroimaging to look for: spinal ligamentous injury, spinal cord contusion, compression, transection, cerebral shear injury, infarct and spinal fractures that are occult on CT.

Ultrasound
- Some trauma surgeons will do a FAST (Focused Assessment with Sonography in Trauma) scan to look for free fluid in the abdomen.
- If patient is low risk with no free fluid, then you may avoid CT.
- Note, gravid uterus impairs evaluation for small amounts of intraperitoneal fluid.

How much does imaging cost?

Imaging is extremely expensive, and it is important to have some idea of the costs of imaging studies when you are ordering them. If patients do not have insurance, they may be liable for the whole cost of the study. Patients are often responsible for high deductibles and co-pays.

Appropriate indications for imaging
Most insurance companies will only pay for studies with an appropriate medical indication (defined by them, but usually follow Medicare guidelines).
- There is a cost to society as well as to an individual for inappropriate imaging.
- Precertification for an exam may be needed (which is usually obtained by the requesting physician's office) for some exams, e.g., CT, MRI, PET.
- Exams denied by insurance will be charged to the patient.

Costs, charges, and reimbursement
What an imaging exam *costs* to perform (includes costs of the technology, contrast, technical and radiologist staff, building costs, lighting, heating, etc.) and what is *charged* for a study are very different.

Charges
- Charges vary highly between institutions, in different areas of the country, and may be dependent on the patient's insurance coverage.
- Charges are usually split into technical fees (from the hospital) and interpretative (professional) fees (from the radiologist).
  - Patients often get two bills, which may be confusing for them.
  - Technical fees vary most and are generally higher except for some procedures.

Typical charges
Table 1.2 gives an indication of the average global (technical plus professional) charges in the United States of some common imaging exams, and the range (10%–90% nationally) relative to the average charge for a PA and lateral CXR in 2012. (C = contrast.)

Table 1.2

Exam	Average charge 2012 $	Range charges relative to CXR
CXR (2 view)	313	0.7–1.6x
AXR (KUB)(1 view)	279	0.8–1.4x
Chest CT -C	1777	5.3–10.5x
Abdo-pelvic CT +C	3369	7.1–16.7x
Brain MRI +C	3,094	9.1–16.5x
RUQ ultrasound	723	2.3–4.2x
Bone scan	1,515	4.3–8.7x
PET/CT scan	4,763	12.4–24x
MRI abdomen +C	2,839	8.3–15.8x

Reimbursement
- How much insurance companies will reimburse for a particular study also varies between companies and geographical area.
- The reimbursement by Medicare and Medicaid is significantly less than most insurance companies ($\approx$30 cents on $1 charged).
- Most institutions have contractual agreements with individual insurance companies and reimbursement is modified accordingly.

Common imaging algorithms

These imaging algorithms are modified from the July 2010 version of the American College of Radiology Appropriateness Criteria® (ACR AC; see p. 40).*
- Only the primary imaging recommendations (i.e., procedures rated as *usually* appropriate) and alternatives (i.e., procedure rated as *may be appropriate*) are included in this truncated list.

CHAPTER 1 Radiology Essentials

- Other patient factors (e.g., allergies, obesity, claustrophobia, age, and co-morbidities) as well as study availability may influence study choice.
  - The ACR AC presents these factors in the narrative portion of the topic or in the comments section of the rating table.

The ACR AC specific topic should be consulted for the complete presentation at www.acr.org/ac

RRL = Relative Radiation Level of estimated effective radiation doses to patients produced by different exams.
- Expressed as scale of 0 to ☢☢☢☢☢
- See www.acr.org/ac for more details.
- Reprinted with permission from the American College of Radiology.

*The ACR AC are evidence-based guidelines reviewed by panels of clinical and radiology experts. The most current and complete version of the ACR AC is available at www.acr.org/ac in both a searchable pdf and a mobile format. The ACR AC include references and the relative radiation levels (RRL) for different examinations.

Chest
Chest pain

Suspected aortic dissection

Imaging test 1:
- CXR: to exclude other causes of chest pain. Not diagnostic *RRL*☢

Imaging test 2:
- CT angiogram chest (p. 104). *RRL*☢☢☢☢

Alternatives:
- MR angiogram if patient has contraindication to IV contrast (p. 112). *RRL* 0
  - Not if hemodynamically unstable.
- Transesophageal echo (TEE) if hemodynamically stable. *RRL* 0
  - If skilled operator available.

Suspected pulmonary embolus

Imaging test 1:
- CXR: to exclude other causes of chest pain. RRL☢

A negative D-dimer in patients with a low clinical pretest probability of PE effectively excludes PE.

Imaging test 2:
- CT pulmonary angiogram (p. 106). *RRL*☢☢☢
  - +/− CT venography if high suspicion for DVT (deep venous thrombosis) and no/inconclusive ultrasound of lower extremities.

Alternatives:
- US lower extremity with Doppler (p. 286). *RRL* 0
  - If clinical suspicion of DVT.
- VQ scan if CTPA contraindicated (p. 445). *RRL*☢☢☢

COMMON IMAGING ALGORITHMS

- Pulmonary angiography (right heart catheterization). RRL☢☢☢☢
  - High clinical suspicion and CT pulmonary angiogram inconclusive
- MR pulmonary angiography. RRL 0
  - Not routine currently, but technical developments may allow it to be an alternative to CTPA.

ACUTE cardiac-type chest pain – low pretest probability coronary artery disease.

Imaging test 1:
- CXR to assess for other causes and failure. Not for diagnosis. RRL☢

Imaging test 2:
- SPECT rest-stress/vasodilator myocardial perfusion scan (p. 437) RRL☢☢☢☢

Alternatives:
- Coronary CT angiogram (p. 108). RRL☢☢☢☢
- Stress cardiac MRI (p. 110). RRL 0
  - If local expertise in technique available.
- Noncardiac CT/CT angiogram if noncardiac cause suspected. RRL☢☢☢/☢☢☢☢
- Transthoracic echocardiogram (rest). RRL 0

CHRONIC cardiac chest pain – low to intermediate pretest probability coronary artery disease

Imaging test 1:
CXR to assess for other causes and failure. Not for diagnosis. RRL☢

Imaging test 2 (these are weighted equally):
- SPECT rest-stress/vasodilator myocardial perfusion scan. RRL☢☢☢☢
- Or coronary CT angiogram. RRL☢☢☢☢
- Or stress transthoracic echocardiography. RRL 0

Alternatives:
- Stress cardiac MRI. RRL 0
  - If local expertise in technique available.

Solitary pulmonary nodule (SPN) diagnosed on CXR
ALWAYS OBTAIN PRIOR CXRs AS INITIAL STEP

SPN > 1 cm
Imaging test 1:
- CT non-contrast (p. 85) RRL☢☢☢

Imaging test 2:
- PET FDG scan (p. 425) RRL☢☢☢☢

Alternatives:
- CT/fluoro guided needle biopsy RRL variable.
- Usually if PET+ or CT suspicious.

SPN < 1 cm
See management according to Fleischner Society Criteria, p. 86.

Abdomen and pelvis
Abdominal/pelvic pain

Flank pain, suspected renal calculi

Imaging test 1:
- CT non-contrast abdomen and pelvis (p. 173). RRL☢☢☢☢

Alternatives:
- IVP. RRL☢☢☢
- US (+/− abdominal radiograph). *RRL☢☢ if radiograph is performed.*
  - First choice in pregnancy.
  - Consider for repeat imaging in patient with history of stones.

RUQ pain with fever and ↑WBC, +Murphy's sign

Imaging test 1:
RUQ ultrasound (p. 254) *RRL 0*

Imaging test 2:
- Hepatobiliary scan (p. 440). *RRL☢☢*
  - For inconclusive ultrasound.

Alternatives:
- CT with contrast abdomen. *RRL☢☢☢*
  - Use if diagnosis other than acute cholecystitis is likely.

RUQ pain no fever, normal WBC

Imaging test 1:
- RUQ ultrasound. *RRL 0*

Imaging test 2: (dependant on clinical suspicion).
- Hepatobiliary scan (p. 440). *RRL++.*
  - With sincalide to evaluate gallbladder ejection fraction.
- CT with contrast abdomen. *RRL+++.*
  - To assess for nonbiliary causes.
- MRI abdomen. *RRL 0*
  - If common duct stone or pancreatic abnormality suspected.

RLQ pain suspected appendicitis (fever, ↑WBC, focal RLQ tenderness) in adults

(For pregnant woman see "How do I image my pregnant patient" p. 28).

Imaging test 1:
- CT with contrast abdomen (p. 161). RRL☢☢☢

Alternatives:
- CT non – contrast abdomen. *RRL☢☢☢*
- RLQ ultrasound with graded compression. *RRL 0*

RLQ pain suspected appendicitis (fever, ↑WBC, focal RLQ tenderness) in child <14 years.

Imaging test 1:
- RLQ ultrasound with graded compression. RRL 0

Imaging test 2:
- CT with contrast abdomen. RRL☢☢☢

Alternatives:
- Abdominal radiograph. RRL☢☢
  - To exclude other causes.

Left lower quadrant pain, suspected diverticulitis in older or male patients

Imaging test 1:
- CT with contrast of abdomen and pelvis (p. 161). RRL☢☢☢☢

Alternatives:
- CT non-contrast of abdomen and pelvis. RRL☢☢☢☢

Left lower quadrant pain or pelvic pain in woman of childbearing age

Imaging test 1:
- Transvaginal US pelvis. *RRL 0*
  - +/– transabdominal pelvic US as needed. *RRL 0*

Imaging test 2:
- MRI pelvis +/– abdomen. RRL 0
  - Use if US nondiagnostic.

Alternative:
- CT with contrast pelvis +/– abdomen *RRL*☢☢☢☢
  - USE ONLY IF PREGNANCY TEST NEGATIVE.
  - Consider as first test if non-gynecological etiology suspected.

Management of jaundice

Jaundice with acute pain and at least one symptom of:
- Fever.
- History of gallstones.
- Biliary surgery.

Imaging test 1:
- Abdominal US. *RRL 0*

Alternatives:
- CT with contrast of abdomen. *RRL*☢☢☢☢
- MRI of abdomen with MRCP. *RRL 0*

Jaundice with non-obstructive clinical profile

Imaging test 1:
- Abdominal US. *RRL 0*

Alternatives:
- MRI of abdomen with MRCP (p. 153). *RRL 0*
- CT with contrast of abdomen. *RRL*☢☢☢☢

> **Painless jaundice with weight loss, fatigue, or anorexia (any symptoms >3 months).**
> Imaging test 1:
> CT with contrast of abdomen. RRL☢☢☢☢
>
> Alternatives:
> - Abdominal US. RRL 0
> - MRI of abdomen with MRCP. RRL 0
> - ERCP. RRL☢☢☢
>   - Use as follow up to imaging

MSK
Back pain

> **Acute back pain +/− radiculopathy, but NONE of the following red flags:**
> - Recent significant trauma, or milder trauma, age >50.
> - Unexplained weight loss or fever.
> - Immunosuppression/Hx cancer or IV drug use.
> - Prolonged use of corticosteroids, osteoporosis.
> - Age >70.
> - Focal neurologic deficit with progressive or disabling symptoms.
> - Duration longer than 6 weeks.
> Imaging test 1:
> No imaging recommended.
>
> **Low back pain with one of red flags above or prior to surgery**
> Imaging test 1.
> - MRI lumbar spine. *RRL 0*
>   - With contrast if suspicion/risk of infection or tumor.
>
> Alternatives:
> - CT, non-contrast lumbar spine. RRL☢☢☢
> - Radiographs lumbar spine. RRL☢☢☢
> - CT myelography lumbar spine. RRL☢☢☢☢
>   - Use if surgery is considered.
>   - Use if MRI is contraindicated or nondiagnostic.

Suspected osteomyelitis in foot of diabetic patient

> Imaging test 1:
> - Radiographs foot. RRL☢
>
> Imaging test 2:
> - MRI with contrast of foot. RRL 0

Alternatives:
- Combined Tc-99m MDP bone scan and In-111 labeled WBC scan. (p. 447). RRL☢☢☢☢
  - Use if MRI is contraindicated.

Suspected stress or insufficiency fractures

Imaging test 1:
- Radiographs of area concern. *RRL variable.*

Imaging test 2:
- Repeat radiographs in 7+ days. *RRL variable.*

Imaging test 3:
MRI non-contrast of area of concern. *RRL 0*

Alternatives
- Tc-99m MDP bone scan. *RRL*☢☢☢☢
  - Usually used if MRI contraindicated.

Nervous system
Imaging of headache

Chronic headache, no new features
Imaging unlikely to be helpful.

Chronic headache with new clinical features
Imaging test 1:
- MRI with contrast of brain. *RRL 0*

Alternatives:
- MRI non-contrast of brain. *RRL 0*

Acute severe headache
Imaging test 1:
- CT, non-contrast head *RRL* ☢☢☢

Imaging test 2:
- CT angiogram head. *RRL*☢☢☢
- Or MR angiogram brain. *RRL 0*

Alternatives:
- Cerebral angiography. *RRL*☢☢☢
- MRI non-contrast of brain. *RRL 0*

Cerebrovascular disease

Asymptomatic patient at high risk or with bruit
Equally weighted:
Imaging test 1:
- US carotid arteries. *RRL0*.
- Or MR angiogram of neck (p. 13). *RRL 0*

Alternatives:
CT angiogram of neck. *RRL☻☻☻*

History of transient ischemia attack
Equally weighted:
Imaging test 1
- MRI of head plus MR angiogram of head and neck. *RRL 0*
- Or CT of head plus CT of angiogram neck. *RRL☻☻☻*

New fixed or worsening focal neurological defect
Equally weighted:
Imaging test 1
- CT, non-contrast head (p. 389). *RRL☻☻☻*
- Or MRI head plus MR angiogram head and neck (p. 390). *RRL 0*

Alternatives:
CT with contrast head with CT angiogram of head and neck. *RRL☻☻☻*

Imaging of dementia

Suspected Alzheimer disease
Imaging test 1:
- MRI non-contrast brain. *RRL 0*

Alternatives:
- MRI with contrast brain. *RRL 0:*
- FDG PET brain scan. *RRL☻☻☻☻*
  - Used for questionable case

Pediatrics
One or more UTIs

Imaging test 1:
- US of kidneys and bladder. *RRL 0*
  - Usually only test required if 8+ yrs.

Imaging test 2:
- VCUG (p. 360). *RRL☻☻*
  - Boys 0–7 yrs.
- Radionuclide cystogram (p. 431). *RRL ☻*
  - Girls 0–7 yrs.
  - Follow up of reflux.

Alternatives:
- VCUG. *RRL*☢☢
  - Girls 0–7 yrs especially if anatomical abnormality suspected.
- +/–DMSA scan (renal cortical scintigraphy) (p. 431). *RRL*☢☢☢
  - 0–2-year-olds (even if low fever).
  - 2–7-year-olds if fever >38.5°C

Child with suspected child abuse

Child with no focal neurological signs or symptoms
Imaging test 1:
- Radiographic skeletal survey. *RRL*☢☢☢
  - If child >24 months, may just do area of concern.
- CT with contrast of abdomen and pelvis +/– chest. *RRL*☢☢☢☢
  - Use if intra-abdominal/thoracic injury suspected.

Imaging test 2:
- CT, noncontrast head. *RRL*☢☢☢
- Especially if high risk, <6 months old, or history of head trauma.

Alternative:
- MRI of head. RRL .0
  - Use if head CT is abnormal.

Child with neurological signs or symptoms
Imaging tests 1:
- Radiographic skeletal survey. *RRL*☢☢☢
  - If child >24 months, may just do area of concern.
- CT, non-contrast of head. *RRL*☢☢☢
- CT with contrast of abdomen and pelvis +/– chest. *RRL*☢☢☢☢
  - Use if intra-abdominal/thoracic injury suspected.

Imaging test 2:
- MRI head. *RRL* 0
  - Do not delay CT if symptomatic, but MRI may be needed even if CT is negative.

Vomiting infants <3 months

Bilious vomiting ≤ 1 week old
Imaging test 1:
- Abdominal radiograph. *RRL*☢☢☢

Imaging test 2:
- UGI study (p. 311). *RRL*☢☢☢
Alternatives:
- Contrast enema. *RRL*☢☢☢☢

Bilious vomiting 1 week – 3 months old
Imaging test 1:
- UGI study. *RRL*☢☢☢

Imaging test 2:
- Abdominal radiograph. *RRL*☢☢☢

Intermittent non-bilious vomiting since birth
Imaging test:
- UGI study. *RRL*☢☢☢

New onset projectile non-bilious vomiting
Imaging test 1:
- Ultrasound abdomen (pylorus) (p. 311). *RRL 0*

Alternatives:
- UGI study. *RRL*☢☢☢
  - Usually used only if US indeterminate (or repeat US in 1 week).

References

ACR Appropriateness Criteria®. www.acr.org/ac

ACR Manual on Contrast Media · Version 7, 2010. http://www.acr.org/SecondaryMainMenuCategories/quality_safety/contrast_manual/FullManual.aspx

Barrett BJ, et al. Preventing Nephropathy Induced by Contrast Medium. NEJM 2006; 354(4):379–386.

Brenner DJ et al. Computed Tomography: An increasing source of radiation exposure. NEJM 2007;357:2277–2284.

Fetal radiation wizard from Duke University. (http://www.safety.duke.edu/Radsafety/fdose/fd_wizard/wiz_intro.htm)

Ledneva E, et al. Renal Safety of Gadolinium-Based Contrast Media in Patients with Chronic Renal Insufficiency. Radiology 2009;250(3):618–628.

Chapter 2

Chest Imaging

Petra Lewis, MBBS and Juliana M. Czum, MD

Radiography 42
How are images acquired? 42
Normal anatomy 47
How do I read a CXR? 52
Patterns of disease 55
   Airspace opacification 55
   Interstitial patterns 58
   Volume loss 61
   Patterns of lobar collapse 61
   Lung masses/nodules 64
   Mediastinal masses 68
   Air that shouldn't be there 68
   Pleural and pericardial fluid 72
Chest CT 77
How are images acquired? 77
Normal anatomy 79
How do I read a chest CT? 80
Patterns of disease 81
   Air that shouldn't be there 81
   Lung abnormalities 82
   Mediastinal abnormalities 87
   Vascular abnormalities 88
   Pleural abormalities 89
   Pericardial abnormalities 90
Common conditions 91
   Pulmonary edema 91
   Infection 94
   COPD and emphysema 99
   Bronchiectasis 101
   Sarcoidosis 101
   Lung cancer 102
   Aortic dissection 104
   Blunt traumatic aortic injury 105
   Pulmonary emboli 106
Cardiac imaging 107
Applications for cardiac CT 108
Coronary calcium scoring 108
Coronary CTA 108
Cardiac MRI 110
Vascular MRA 112
Don't miss diagnoses 113

Radiographs

How are images acquired?
Views

Posterior-Anterior (PA) chest radiographs
These are the ideal view. The x-ray beam passes from the source (72 inches away) through the back to the front of the patient and then to the image receptor/film. Image is obtained with patient upright.
- Minimizes radiation dose to the breasts and thyroid.
- Reduces the magnification of the heart and mediastinum.

Technical considerations:
- The study must be obtained in the radiology department.
- Patients must be able to stand with their front against the image receptor/film cassette.
- Arms are brought forward when possible to rotate scapula away from the lungs.

Anterior-Posterior (AP) chest radiographs
May be acquired within the radiology department or as portable studies. The x-ray beam passes from the source (72 inches, or 48 inches away for portable studies) through the front of the patient to the image receptor/film behind them.
- AP projections magnify the heart and mediastinum as they are further from the image receptor device (see Figure 2.1).

Technical considerations:
- All portable studies are AP.
- All studies when the patient cannot stand unaided are AP.
- Studies may be acquired erect, supine, or semi-upright. The patient position makes a significant impact on how abnormalities such as pleural effusions and pneumothorax appear.
  - AP studies should always be annotated with the patient's estimated position (e.g., 30° upright). Some AP studies have an "inclinometer" marking to show position.

Lateral chest radiographs
Obtained with the patient's left side against the image receptor.
- The right side of the patient will be magnified as it is further from the image receptor.
- Lateral films may be obtained with patient standing or sitting.
- Portable lateral films are often of poor quality.

Lateral decubitus chest radiographs
These are AP views, which are obtained with patients lying on their side. Terminology defined by the "down" side, that is, "L lateral decubitus" is when the patient is lying left side down.

Indications:
- To assess for the presence or mobility of pleural effusions (put the abnormal side <u>down</u>) (see Figure 2.2).
- To assess for the presence of a pneumothorax (put the abnormal side <u>up</u>).
- To assess for foreign body evaluation (bilateral decubitus). See p. 307.

RADIOGRAPHS 43

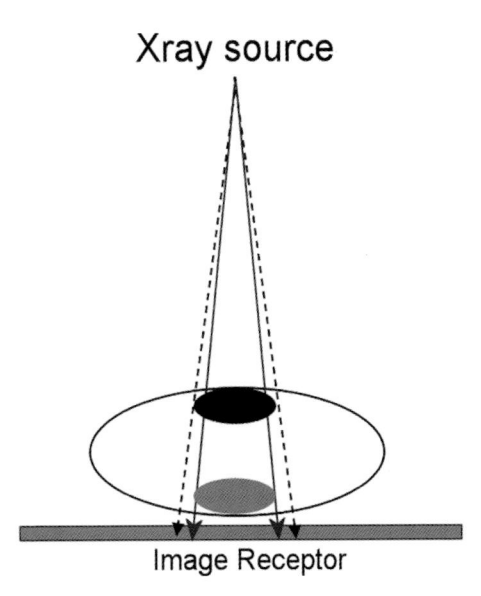

Figure 2.1 shows how objects further from the image receptor are magnified. Note how the heart in this image will appear larger on the AP study as it is further from the image receptor.

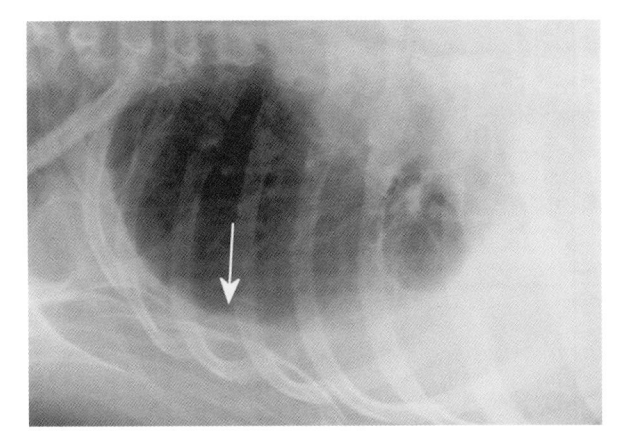

Figure 2.2 R lateral decubitus study shows a layering effusion.

Lordotic chest radiographs
Obtained with the patient leaning backwards, so the x-ray beam is directed up to the lung apices.
- The first ribs and clavicles will project superior to the lungs.
- Obtained if there is a question of apical lesion versus superimposition of structures.

Inspiration versus expiration
Inspiratory studies
Chest radiographs are ideally obtained on maximal inspiration.
- Minimizes vascular "crowding."
- Diaphragms should be at level of approx. 10th posterior rib.
- Provides the clearest visualization of subtle pulmonary opacities.

Low lung volumes produce: (see Figure 2.3).
- Artifactual cardiac and mediastinal widening.
- Increased vascular prominence.
- Basilar subsegmental atelectasis.

Causes of low lung volumes:
- Position: sitting, supine and semi-supine studies.
- Abdominal distension e.g., pregnancy, ascites.
- Ventilated patients.
- Pleuritic chest pain or shortness of breath.
- Restrictive lung disease.
- Diffuse lung consolidation.
- Morbid obesity.

See p. 99 for discussion of increased lung volumes.

Expiratory studies
Chest radiographs may be obtained on maximal expiration to:
- Evaluate for a pneumothorax (see p. 68).
- Evaluate for an aspirated foreign body (see p. 307).

> Radiographs obtained within the radiology department will always be of higher quality than those obtained portably (as long as the patient is able to be safely transported).

Patient position
The best evaluation of chest abnormalities can be made when they are acquired with the patient upright (preferably standing), but this is not always possible.

Effect of supine and semi-supine films
- Lung volumes are smaller.
- Heart and mediastinum appear wider.
- The normal gravity dependent vascular distribution pattern is changed so upper lobe vessels are more distended.
- Pleural effusions layer posteriorly.
- Pneumothoraces may be seen at the bases ("deep sulcus sign," see p. 70) rather than at the apices.

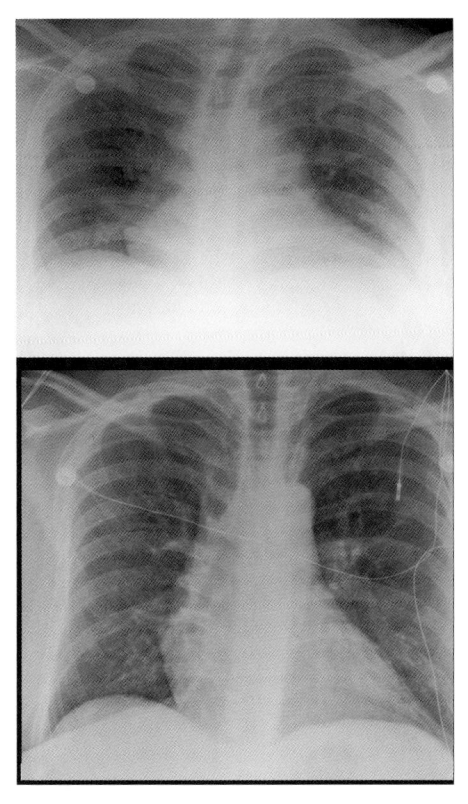

Figure 2.3 Same patient, two AP CXRs that show the effect of low lung volumes (top), compared to normal lung volumes (bottom).

Patient rotation
Rotated studies
- Make the mediastinum appear wider and different in contour.
- Produce a diffuse increase in density over one hemithorax from the superimposed chest wall muscles and breast tissue.

How to assess for rotation
- In adults, the degree of rotation can be assessed by looking at the symmetry of the position of the thoracic spinous process between the anterior ends of the clavicles
- On the lateral study, if you can see ribs curving posterior to the spine the study is rotated.
- In children, look for the symmetry of the anterior ends of the ribs.

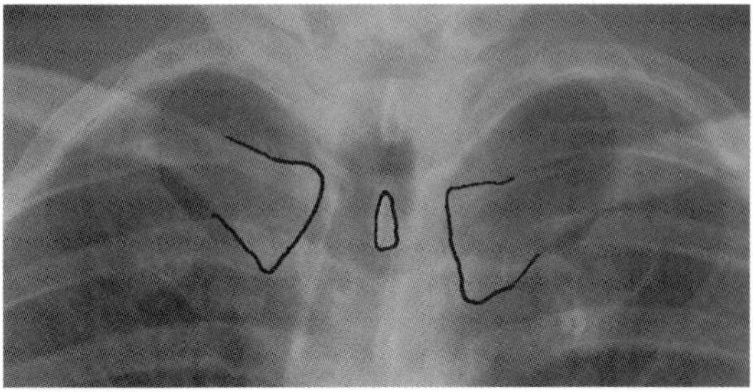

Figure 2.4 An upper thoracic spinous process should be midway between the anterior ends of the clavicles in a non-rotated CXR.

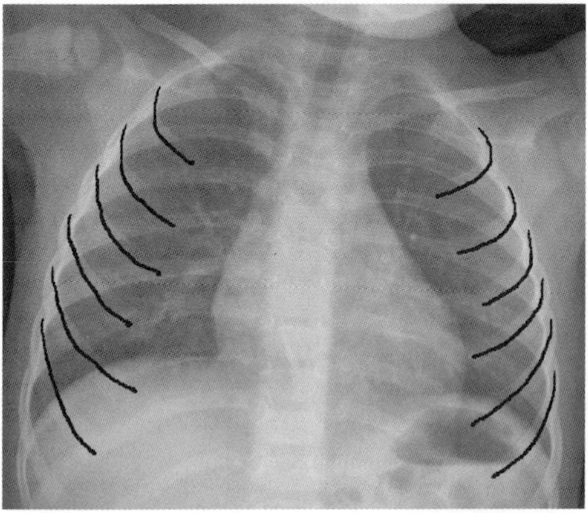

Figure 2.5 In pediatric patients the anterior ends of the ribs should look symmetrical in a non-rotated CXR.

Study penetration
- This is how black the CXR appears and is related to how much and what energy radiation was used (mAs and kVp, respectively) as well as the size and density of the thorax.
- On a properly exposed frontal CXR you should be able to see the spine through the heart, but it should not look like a spine study (see Figure 2.6).
- <u>Over-penetrated studies:</u> are too black (too lucent), and you may not see detail in the lung parenchyma.
- <u>Under-penetrated studies:</u> are too white (too opaque), and you may not see detail in the mediastinum or identify tube positions.
- Digital images allow adjustment of contrast and brightness which will overcome this to some degree.

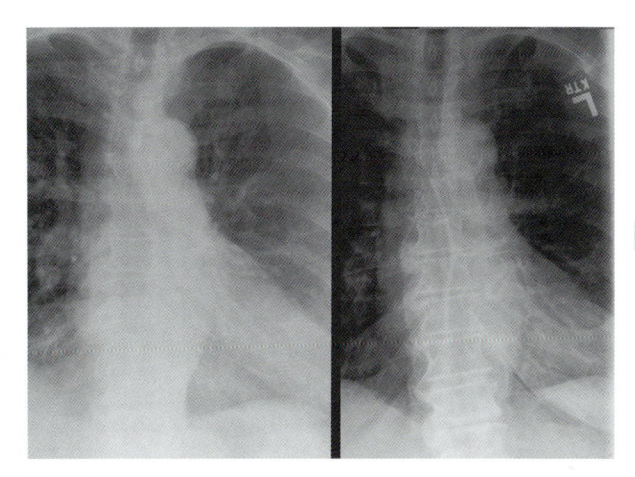

Figure 2.6 Figure showing correct degree of penetration for a CXR (left) compared to a spine study in the same patient (right).

Normal anatomy

To learn what normal looks like on a CXR, you need to look at as many normal CXRs in different age/sex/size patients as possible. There is no single "normal"!

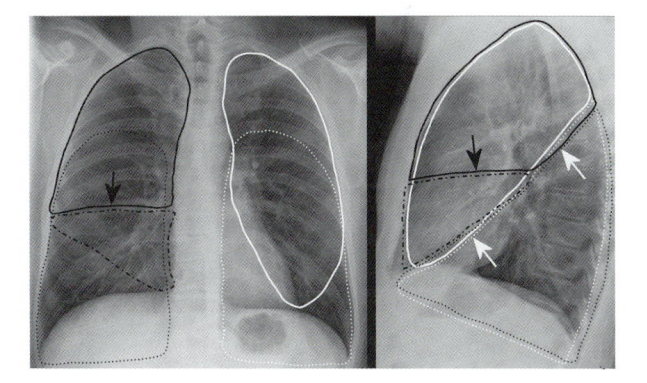

Figure 2.7 Normal lobar anatomy. The approximate projections of the lobes of the lung are shown on the frontal and lateral radiographs. Black arrow = horizontal fissure; white arrow = oblique fissure; black solid line = RUL; black dashed line = RML; black dotted line = RLL; white solid line = LUL; white dotted line = LLL.

CHAPTER 2 Chest Imaging

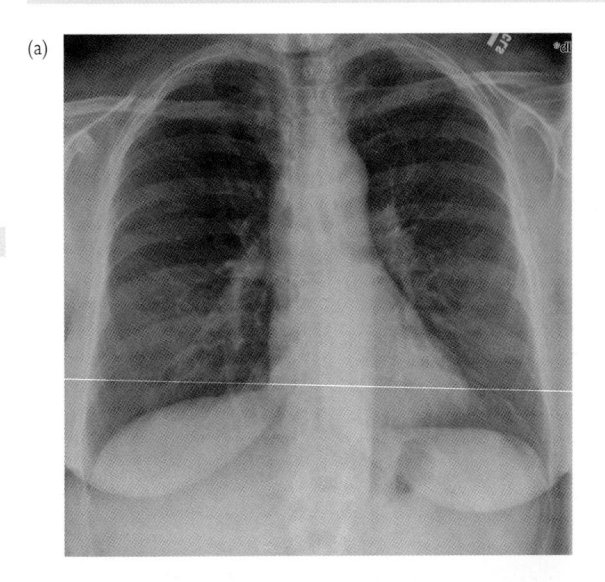

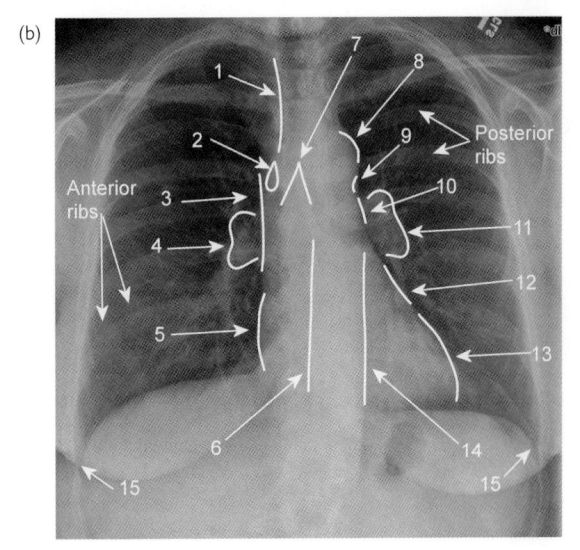

Figure 2.8 a and b Normal mediastinal anatomy on the frontal radiograph.

Key to Figure 2.8 (see p. xiii for Abbreviations):

1. R paratracheal line	<5 mm wide. Increased in adenopathy, e.g. lung cancer, lymphoma, sarcoidosis.
2. Azygous vein. Runs over the RMB into the SVC. Adjacent normal azygous node	<10 mm wide. Increased in R heart failure, fluid overload, adenopathy.
3. SVC	Expected course of central venous catheters.
4. R hilum (RPA branches)	Should be lower than L hilum. Enlarged with adenopathy, primary lung cancers. Elevated with RUL collapse.
5. R atrium	Enlarged in tricuspid valve disorders, R heart failure.
6. Azygoesophageal line	Formed by interface R lung against the esophagus and azygous vein. Deviated in esophageal disorders e.g., hiatal hernia
7. Carina	<90°. Widened with LA enlargement, adenopathy.
8. Aortic arch	Enlarged in aortic aneurysm, aortic rupture.
9. Aorto-pulmonary (AP) window	Should be concave, convex with adenopathy, other masses.
10. Main pulmonary artery	Enlarged in pulmonary hypertension, pulmonic stenosis, L to R shunts.
11. L hilum (LPA branches)	LPA. Should be higher than R hilum. Enlarged with adenopathy, primary lung cancers.
12. L atrial appendage	Becomes convex with LA enlargement e.g., mitral valve disorders.
13. L ventricle	Enlarged with LV failure. Border lost with LUL consolidation/atelectasis, mitral regurg, aortic regurg.
14. Para-aortic line	Obliterated with aortic rupture, L lower lobe consolidation or atelectasis, L pleural effusions.
15. Lateral costophrenic angle	Lost with effusions, scarring.

CHAPTER 2 Chest Imaging

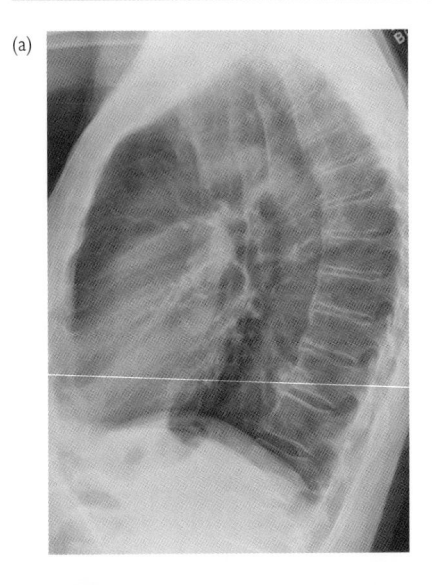

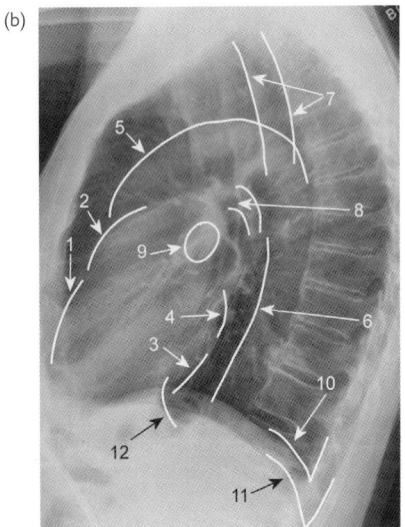

(a)

(b)

Figure 2.9 a and b Normal anatomy on the lateral chest radiograph.

Key to Figure 2.9 (see p. xiii for Abbreviations):

1. R ventricle	Should occupy less than 1/3 of the retrosternal space.
2. R ventricular outflow track	
3. L ventricle	Enlarges posteriorly and inferiorly in LVF. Border lost with LLL consolidation/atelectasis/fluid.
4. L atrium	Enlarges posteriorly in mitral valve disorders.
5. Ascending aorta and aortic arch	Enlarged in ascending aortic aneurysms.
6. Descending aorta	More tortuous and visible with age, may not see in young pts as against spine. Enlarged in aortic aneurysms. Obliterated in LLL consolidation, atelectasis, effusions.
7. Scapulae	Seen edge-on as 2 vertical lines.
8. L pulmonary artery	Higher, and more posterior than the RPA. Runs parallel and under aortic arch. Enlarged in pul.HTN and pulmonic stenosis, L to R shunts.
9. R pulmonary artery	Seen as an oval anterior and inferior to LPA, enlarged in pul.HTN, L to R shunts but not in pulmonic stenosis.
10. Posterior L costophrenic angle	
11. Posterior R costophrenic angle	The R side of the thorax is magnified and more posterior than the L as further from the x-ray source.
12. IVC	Curvilinear line approximately 3 cm anterior to posterior LV

CHAPTER 2 Chest Imaging

How to tell which diaphragm is which on the lateral study?
- Is one diaphragm much higher than other on the frontal study?
- Is there a gas bubble under one hemidiaphragm?
- The R hemidiaphragm can usually be seen up to the anterior chest wall; the heart abuts and obscures the L hemidiaphragm anteriorly.
- The R ribs are more posterior and magnified. Follow them down to the diaphragm (see 10 and 11 on Figure 2.9).
- Sometimes the horizontal and oblique fissures can be seen and followed down to the R hemidiaphragm (see spine sign p. 57).

How do I read a CXR?

Initial quality check

Is it the correct study?	Check patient name, study date.
Are there comparison studies?	Open the last study and an older one.
How were the images taken?	AP or PA, patient position (upright, semi-upright, supine, decubitus, etc.).
What is the study quality?	Degree of inspiration and patient rotation (p. 45). Penetration (p. 46). Any patient movement? Any areas of thorax not included (e.g., costophrenic angle)?

Search patterns
There are many different search patterns that you can utilize to effectively read a chest radiograph, but the best one is the one that works for you. It is important to always:
- Be systematic, to ensure that abnormalities are not missed.
- Compare to priors—both the last study and at least one older (preferably 1–2 years) if possible to assess for slowly developing abnormalities.

Essential elements that must be included in your search:

Lines and tubes
These are good to check first before you forget! Carefully check all lines, wires, and tube positions:
- What is this line (tube, wire)? Where does it enter the patient?
- Where does it end? Is it in the expected location or malpositioned?
- Look for associated complications (pneumothorax, hemothorax).
- See p. 114 for link to interactive lines and tubes module.

> **Lines and tubes**
> If you cannot prove a line/wire is ON the patient (e.g., clearly non-anatomical path), assume it is IN the patient. **The same applies to all other foreign bodies.** Visually check your patient!

Lungs
- Search each lung from top to bottom, and compare upper, mid, and lower lung zones between the L and R lungs.
- Look for symmetry in lung size, opacity, and vascular markings.
- Are there any <u>diffuse</u> or <u>focal</u> opacities?
- Are there abnormal areas of lucency (ptx, bulla)?
- Are vascular markings normal, increased, or decreased?

Table 2.1 Optimal position of tips of tubes and wires

Oral/naso-gastric tubes*	Tip and side-hole in body of stomach.
Dobhoff/feeding tubes* with weighted tips (appear dense)	Optimally, 3rd portion of duodenum; body or antrum stomach is okay. Often malpositioned in esophagus or trachea (p. 113, Figure 2.67).
Endotracheal tubes (ETT)	4–7 cm above carina. (Approx. bottom clavicles to mid aortic arch). Often malpositioned in main bronchus, occasionally in trachea (p. 114, Figure 2.68).
Tracheostomy tube	At level of clavicles (higher than ETT).
Central venous catheters & PICC	In SVC or at cavo-atrial junction.
Pacemaker wire	Variable, usually single lead RV apex or RVOT, two lead also has one in RA (appendage), three lead usually also one in a coronary vein via coronary sinus.
Automatic implantable cardioverter defibrillator (AICD)	Proximal electrode in SVC/brachiocephalic vein, tips as for pacemakers.
Intra-aortic balloon pump	Just distal to aortic arch.
Chest tubes	Tip at apex for ptx, base for pleural effusion drainage. Side-holes within pleural cavity.

*Gastric/feeding tubes are best visualized on an upper abdominal radiograph that includes the lower chest in case of malpositioning.

Airway
Tracheal deviation (e.g., mediastinal mass)?

Pleura
- Thickening/masses along expected course of pleura?
- Fluid: are the CP angles sharp?

Hila
- Position (L should always be higher than R, if not, look for signs of RUL volume loss or less common RLL hyperexpansion e.g., bulla).
- Size and shape – compare with old.

Mediastinum and diaphragm
- Look for widening/deviation of the mediastinal lines (see p. 48 and p. 50, Figures 2.8 and 2.9).
- Evaluate diaphragm clarity and position.

Heart
- Assess heart borders for specific chamber enlargement (see Figure 2.10).
- Evaluation of heart size using the cardiothoracic ratio (CTR):
  - Measure widest part of heart (exclude pericardial fat pad), and *widest internal diameter of thorax*.
  - Should be <0.5 for an adult (0.6 on AP).

- On AP study, heart is definitely enlarged if touching lateral chest wall.
- A reduced cardiomediastinal silhouette is seen in emphysema, leading to underestimation of the cardiac size.

A CTR <0.5 only applies to well positioned PA radiographs in full inspiration and is an inaccurate measure of cardiomegaly with many false positives.

What can produce artifactual "cardiomegaly"?
Apparent increase in the cardiothoracic ratio but with a normal size heart.
- AP projection, esp. portable study, with supine patient.
- Rotated projection.
- Low lung volumes.
- Pectus excavatum.
- Large pericardial fat pads.
- Pericardial effusion.

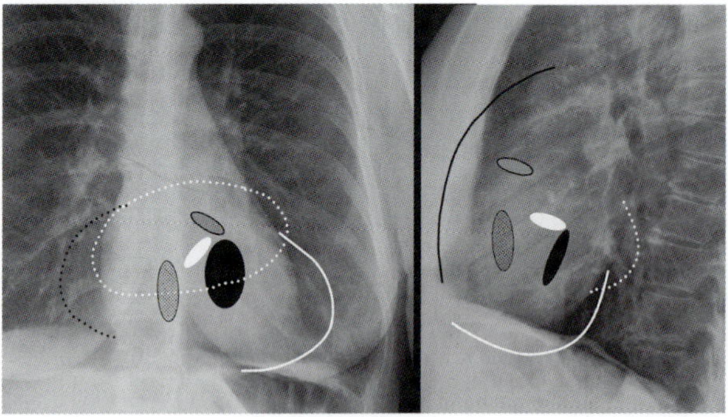

Figure 2.10 Cardiac valve positions and cardiac chamber enlargement. Lines show how individual cardiac chambers enlarge. RA: black dotted; LA: white dotted; RV: black solid; LV: white solid. Black ellipse = mitral valve; white ellipse = aortic valve; gray ellipse = pulmonary valve; dotted ellipse = tricuspid valve.

Bones
- Scan ribs, spine, shoulders, and clavicles for:
  - fractures, dislocations, arthritis.
  - lytic and sclerotic lesions.

Suspected rib fractures:
If you clinically suspect a rib fracture in a patient following trauma, most times imaging is unnecessary.
- If you are concerned about either a PTX or a hemothorax from a rib fracture, perform a PA and lateral CXR.
- Rib studies add little other than radiation dose, and are frequently false negative.

Soft tissues
- Gastric bubble (position, masses).
- Air under the diaphragms (perforation, surgery, bowel).
- Breasts (present/absent).

Lateral radiograph
These structures are best (or only) seen on the lateral study:
- Spine (fractures, arthritis).
- Posterior costophrenic sulci (effusions, kyphosis, spine sign (see p. 57))
- Retrosternal space (masses, mediastinal air).
- LA and LV enlargement.
- Retrocardiac masses and consolidation.
- Pulmonary artery enlargement (pulmonary hypertension).

Patterns of disease

Often a specific diagnosis cannot be made from a chest radiograph. However, by being able to identify the pattern of abnormality, one can significantly narrow the differential. Including the history, physical examination, and older-study comparison will further direct you to a specific diagnosis in many cases.

Airspace opacification
When air in alveoli is replaced by fluid or cells (pus, blood, edema, tumor cells), the abnormality is seen as a poorly marginated opacity of variable density ("airspace or alveolar opacity") (see Figures 2.46 and 2.47). Sharp margins are only seen at pleural margins and fissures.

Differential diagnosis
- Pneumonia.
- Pulmonary edema or ARDS.
- Pulmonary hemorrhage, infarct, trauma.
- Bronchoalveolar carcinoma, lymphoma.

May involve a small area, lobe, entire lung, or both lungs. The distribution (e.g., lobar, bilateral, peripheral, perihilar) can narrow the differential diagnosis.

Subtypes
- <u>Ground glass opacity</u>: Partial replacement of the air gives a hazy, less dense appearance where vascular structures can still be seen. Some atypical pneumonias also give this appearance.
- <u>Consolidation</u>: Complete filling of the alveoli. Vascular structures are obscured (see Figure 2.46).

Ground glass "fake outs"
As well as partial filling of the alveoli, other conditions can cause a "ground glass opacity."
- Posterior layering effusion on a supine study (see Figure 2.30).
- L upper lobe atelectasis (see Figure 2.18).
- Chest wall abnormalities, e.g., cellulitis, mastectomy patients (the side with the remaining breast appears relatively diffusely opaque).

Air bronchograms

In the normal lung, only the most proximal bronchi are seen. When the lung is consolidated, more-peripheral air-filled bronchi are seen as black branching lines in contrast to the opacified airspaces (see Figure 2.11).
- If fluid or cells extend into bronchi, air bronchograms will be lost.
- More commonly seen with air space processes, but can be seen occasionally in atelectasis.
- Not pathognomic for pneumonia.

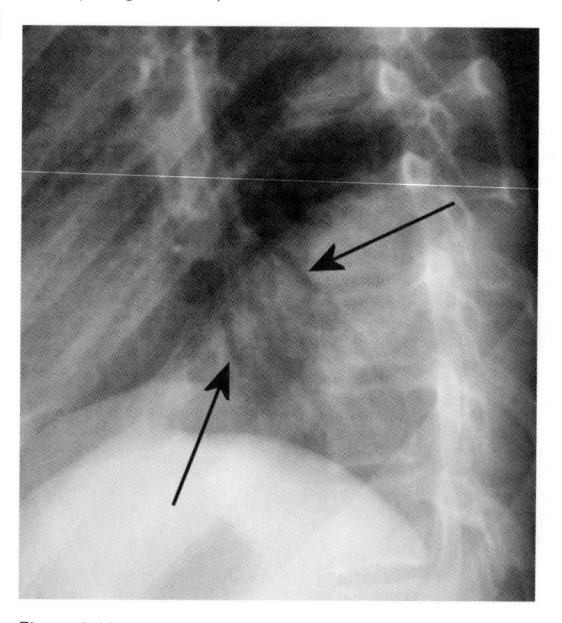

Figure 2.11 Air bronchograms in a patient with RLL pneumonia. Note also the silhouette sign of the loss of the R hemidiaphragm.

Silhouette sign

Normal soft tissue structures in the chest are visualized due to being "silhouetted" against the air in the lungs or other tissues of significantly different density. When a pathological process (fluid, consolidation or mass) replaces the air in the lungs, this normal silhouette is lost = the silhouette sign.

<u>Normal silhouettes:</u>
- Diaphragms.
- Cardiac borders.
- Aortic arch and descending aorta (L lateral border).
- R paratracheal stripe.

How to use the silhouette sign to localize an abnormality
Loss of:
- L heart border = lingular pathology.
- R heart border = RML pathology (and in pectus excavatum).
- Posterior heart border = LLL pathology.
- Anterior heart border = RML pathology.
- R/L hemidiaphragm = RLL/LLL pathology and diaphragmatic rupture.
- R paratracheal stripe = RUL pathology.

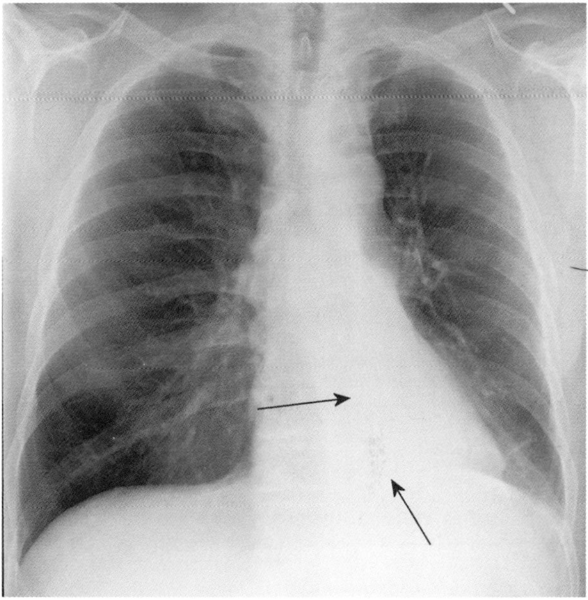

Figure 2.12 Silhouette sign. Partial loss of the L hemidiaphram and L para-aortic line caused by LLL atelectasis.

Spine sign
The spine sign is only seen on the lateral film, as an opacity in the posterior costophrenic angle of the lung. Most commonly due to a small lower lobe pneumonia, but can also be a mass.
- The spine generally appears more lucent (black) from cranial to caudal until the first hemidiaphragm is reached.
- If there is lower lobe opacity, the spine will appear more opaque (white), the diaphragmatic silhouette that is lost identifies the side of the pneumonia (see p. 52).

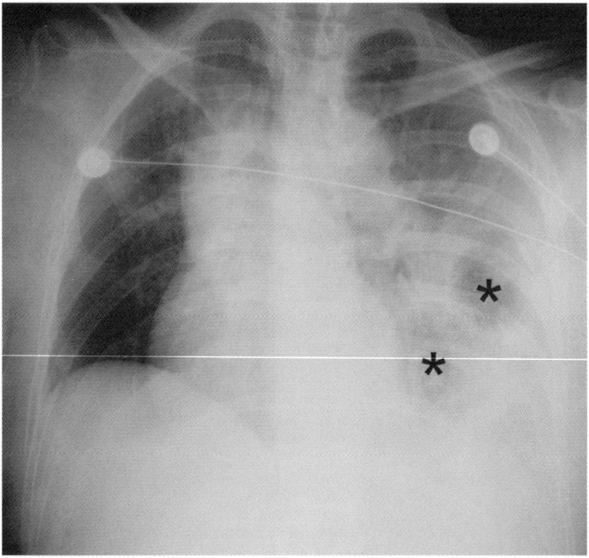

Figure 2.13 Diaphragmatic rupture. Loss of visualization of the left hemidiaphragm due to diaphragmatic rupture and upward herniation of bowel loops (see *). Note mass effect. White lines and circles = EKG electrodes.

Interstitial patterns

An interstitial pattern is sometimes known as a *reticular* or *reticulo-nodular* (if there are micronodules as well as lines) pattern. There are "too many" linear markings in the lungs, which may radiate out from the hilum or which are peripheral and perpendicular to the pleural surface. The pattern is caused by thickening of the interstitium of the lung, whereas the alveoli remain aerated.

<u>Differential diagnosis</u> (not limited to):
- Interstitial lung disease: e.g., usual interstitial pneumonia [UIP], sarcoidosis, amiodarone toxicity, end-stage pulmonary fibrosis, cystic fibrosis.
- Atypical pneumonias: e.g., mycoplasma pneumonia.
- Early pulmonary edema (see Figure 2.45).
- Lymphangitis carcinomatosis: A combination of micrometastases involving the lymphatics and lymphatic obstruction producing interstitial (Kerly B) lines.

Sometimes a combination of interstitial and airspace patterns co-exist. Causes of this include pulmonary edema, interstitial pneumonitis & atypical pneumonias.

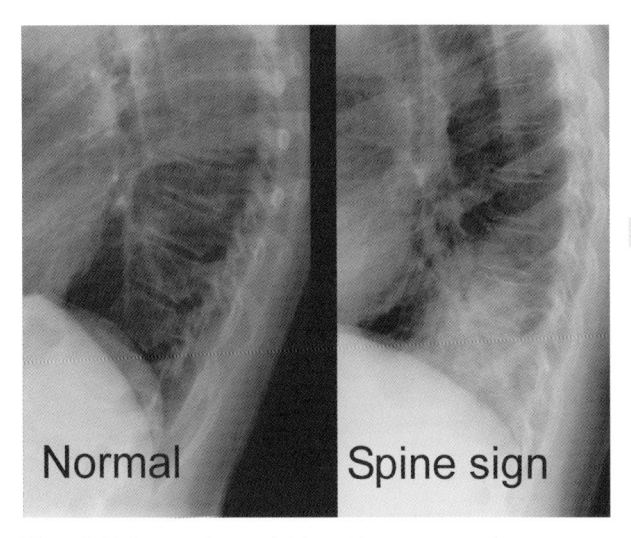

Figure 2.14 Spine sign showing a left-lower-lobe pneumonia producing opacification over the lower spine.

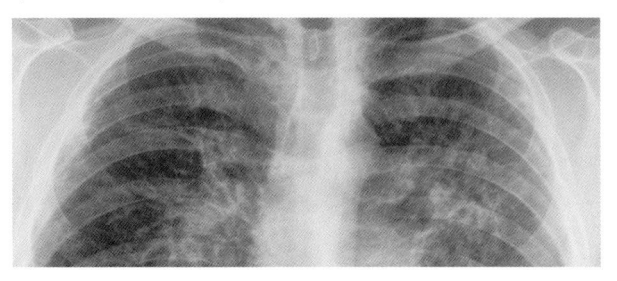

Figure 2.15 Cropped CXR from patient with advanced sarcoidosis showing increased interstitial markings.

Bronchovascular markings

The "bronchovascular markings" in the lungs are due to a combination of the pulmonary arterial and venous branches, and the thin walls of the bronchi (adjacent to the hila). Some conditions can make one or more of these structures more prominent.

<u>Pulmonary arteries:</u> Pulmonary hypertension (markings are increased centrally but attenuated peripherally); L to R shunts.

<u>Pulmonary veins:</u> Pulmonary venous hypertension from elevated L atrial pressures.

Bronchi: Peribronchial inflammation (e.g., viral infections) or thickening (chronic bronchitis, bronchiectasis, sarcoidosis, cystic fibrosis).

Kerley lines

Kerley lines are due to thickening (usually with fluid) of the interlobular septa. 3 types are seen:
- Kerley A lines: 2–5 cm long oblique lines directed toward the hilum.
- Kerley B lines: Most common of the three types. 1–3 cm long horizontal lines perpendicular to the pleural surface, typically in the bases.
- Kerley C lines: variable length with random distribution and angles.

Etiologies:
- Interstitial pulmonary edema is by far the most common.
- Mycoplasma pneumonia.
- Lymphangitis carcinomatosis. Diffuse malignant involvement of the lymphatic system of the lungs, most commonly lung, breast, pancreatic cancer. In lymphangitis carcinomatosis, Kerley B lines are often unilateral or asymmetric.

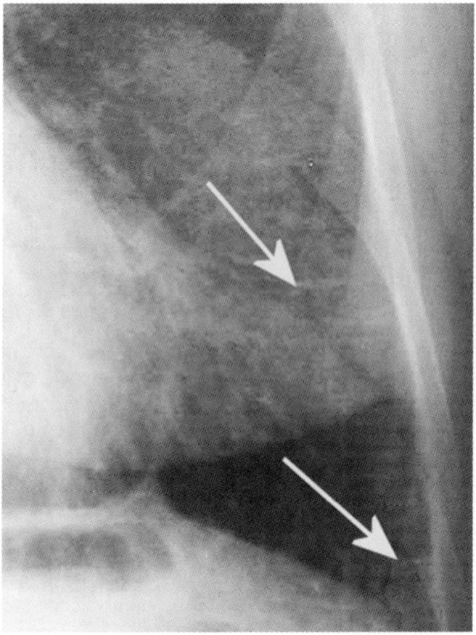

Figure 2.16 Kerly B lines in a patient with pulmonary edema.

Volume loss
Volume loss can be due to obstruction of an airway (e.g., mass or mucus plug), compression of lung (e.g., due to pleural effusion) or reabsorbtion of air (linear atelectasis).
Consolidation and atelectasis often appear similar and can be difficult to differentiate. *When an opacity is seen in the lung, check for the presence of volume loss, which usually indicates atelectasis.*
The radiographic signs of volume loss vary, and depend on:
- The lobe involved.
- The amount of lung involved.
- The compliance of the remaining lung, chest-wall structures, and mediastinum.

Signs of volume loss
- Diaphragmatic elevation.
- Tracheal deviation and hilar elevation (more common than depression).
- Cardiac deviation.
- Movement of fissures (e.g., elevation of the horizontal fissure).
- Ribs closer together.

> Rapid changes (appearance/disappearance) of an opacity are likely due to atelectasis secondary to mucus plugging/underventilation.

Patterns of lobar atelectasis/collapse
There are relatively specific findings of lobar atelectasis, but they will vary depending on the cause and how complete the collapse is.

Right upper lobe
Common in adults, children, and babies. May be benign (e.g., intubated patients, RSV) or due to proximal RUL bronchus tumor.
- R paratracheal wedge-shaped opacity with widening of R paratracheal line.
- Elevation of R hilum +/− elevation or tenting of R hemidiaphragm.
- Deviation of trachea to R.
- +/− R hilar mass.
- Lateral: opacity anterior and posterior to trachea.

Right middle lobe
Usually has a benign cause, though may be due to an obstructive lesion including bronchial adenomas, carcinoid.
- R heart border appears triangular due to the adjacent opacity.
- May see wedge shaped opacity extending laterally, base at heart.
- RML is small and, therefore, few signs of volume loss occur.
- On lateral: wedge shaped opacity overlying heart extending from hilum.

Right lower lobe
Can be due to mucus plug or neoplasm.
- Triangular opacity adjacent to R heart border from hilum to diaphragm.

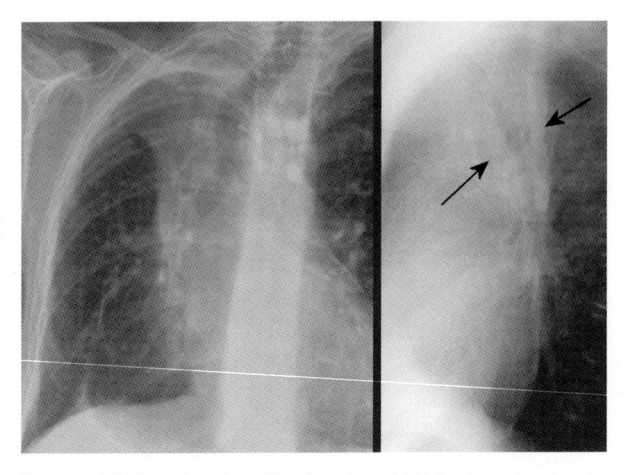

Figure 2.17 RUL atelectasis on AP (left) and lateral (right) radiographs. Note the opacity anterior and posterior to the trachea on the lateral film.

- Loss of R hemi-diaphragm with preservation of R heart border.
- May have elevation of R hemi-diaphragm and deviation of heart to R.
- On lateral: triangular opacity posteriorly and loss of R hemi-diaphragm.

Left upper lobe
Rarely has benign cause, usually due to neoplasm, so CT indicated unless in acute ICU setting. Look for associated hilar mass.
- Diffuse "ground glass" opacity over upper or middle of L hemithorax.
- Loss of L heart border on frontal.
- If L lower lobe becomes hyperinflated, L apex may be aerated.
- Diaphragm elevated and tracheal deviation to L.
- On lateral: curvilinear retrosternal opacity usually extending through entire retrosternal area.

Left lower lobe
Usually benign, and seen very commonly in post-operative and ICU patients due to mucus plugging.
- Retrocardiac wedge shaped opacity.
- Loss and elevation of L hemi-diaphragm silhouette.
- Elevation may be difficult to assess in supine patient due to lack of stomach bubble, thus limiting distinction from LLL pneumonia.
- On lateral: triangular opacity over spine ("spine sign") and loss of L hemi-diaphragm silhouette.

Entire lung atelectasis
Can be due to mucus plugging or neoplasm, or rarely foreign body aspiration (usually chronic). Appears similar to pneumonectomy (look for post-surgical changes such as resected rib or clips).
- Total or near total opacification of a hemithorax.

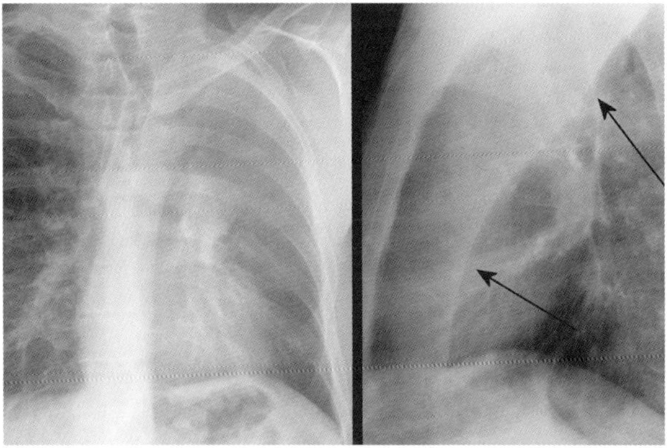

Figure 2.18 LUL atelectasis. PA (left) and lateral (right) radiographs. Note the loss of the L heart border on the PA and the retrosternal opacity on the lateral. Black arrows indicate the displaced oblique fissure.

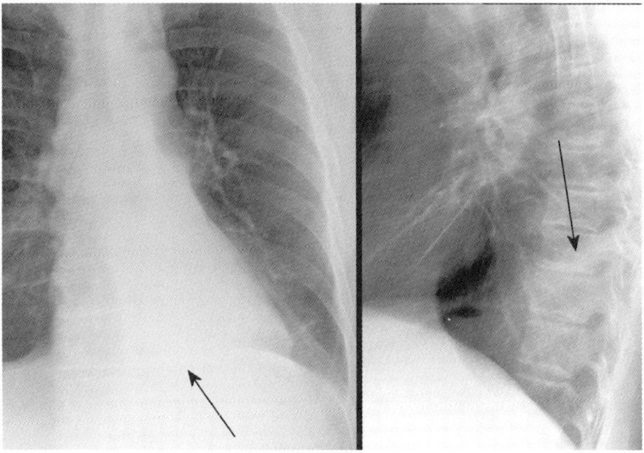

Figure 2.19 LLL atelectasis. PA (left) and lateral (right) radiographs. Note loss of the L diaphragm silhouette on PA (arrow) and spine sign on lateral (arrow).

- Loss of diaphragm silhouette.
- Tracheal and mediastinal deviation toward opacified side.
- Diaphragmatic elevation and stomach bubble may be elevated if L lung atelectasis.
- Contralateral lung hyperinflated and extends across midline.
- On lateral: complete lack of visualization of one hemidiaphragm.

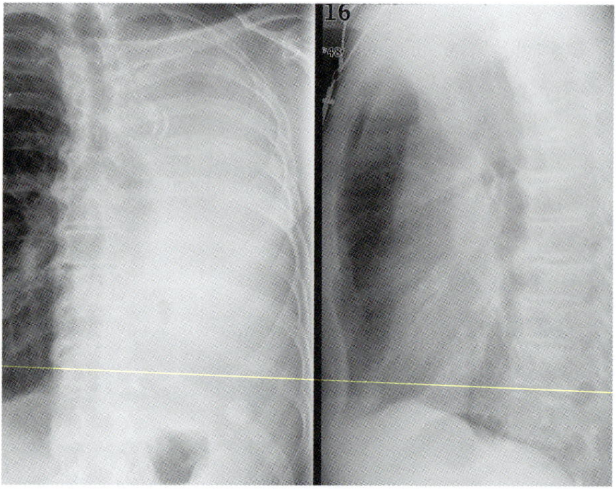

Figure 2.20 Complete L lung atelectasis (due to a bronchial carcinoma). PA (left) and lateral (right) radiographs. Note how only the R hemidiaphragm is seen on the lateral.

> ### Differential diagnosis of complete opacification of a hemithorax ("white out")
> Obviously the history and examination may help!
> - *Complete lung collapse* (mediastinal shift *toward* opacity, decreased size of hemithorax).
> - *Pneumonectomy* (as above, plus surgical clips, +/− rib resection).
> - *Large pleural effusion* (mediastinal shift *away* from opacity. Drain effusion before CT if needed to assess for underlying mass).
> - *Extensive pneumonia* (no shift, air bronchograms, may be small areas aerated lung).
> - Aplasia/agenesis of lung (Rare! Usually diagnosed in infancy, shift toward opacity, no aerated lung seen, no major ipsilateral bronchus).

Linear or subsegmental atelectasis
If only small areas of the lung collapse, they appear as thick horizontal or oblique lines (directed toward hilum), with little or no signs of volume loss. These may rapidly appear and disappear.
- Very common postoperatively or associated with viral infections.

Masses and nodules in the lung
Nodules as small as 3–4 mm are easily seen on CT, but usually have to be >8 mm to see reliably on a CXR unless calcified. See CT section p. 85 for more details.

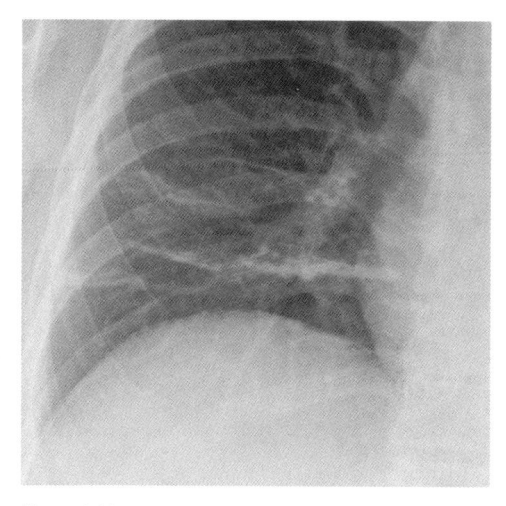

Figure 2.21 Cropped image showing areas of linear atelectasis in the R lower lung in a postoperative patient.

Worrisome features
- New or enlarging.
- Irregular or spiculated borders.
- Not calcified (small dense nodules are usually granulomas).
- High risk patients (e.g., smokers, older patients, known malignancy).
- Large size (>5 cm 95% are malignant).

Differential diagnosis
- Primary lung cancer.
- Metastases.
- Benign mass: hamartoma, granuloma, intrapulmonary lymphnode – usually <1 cm.
- Focal infection (rapid changes).
- Focal atelectasis (usually more linear).
- Superimposed normal anatomy: e.g., vessels crossing ribs.
- Nipple shadows (repeat study with nipple markers).
- Rib or other chest wall lesions projecting over the lungs.

Primary lung cancer versus metastases
<u>Characteristics of metastases</u>
- Small, round, and multiple.
- Size of nodules often varies.
- Bases > apices; peripheral>central.

Breast, colorectal, renal, head and neck cancer most common.

Management

Radiologist may recommend:
- Repeat CXR for low suspicion lesions felt to be likely superimposition, infection, or atelectasis.
- Fluoroscopy or oblique views; can be helpful for confirming superimposition.
- Repeat with nipple markers if felt to be nipple(s).
- If moderate to high concern for lung neoplasm or metastases in high risk patient: non-contrast CT (in larger masses addition of contrast may be helpful).

Mediastinal masses

Mediastinal masses usually have obtuse angled borders (merge with) the mediastinum rather than the acute borders of lung masses (see Figure 2.22).

Mediastinal masses have a wide differential, depending on where they originate. Determining origin is difficult, and CT is often required.
- Where is the center of the mass?
- Which mediastinal contour is lost?

Anterior mediastinal masses

Anterior to the heart and great vessels, below the level of the clavicles.

<u>Radiographic findings:</u>
- Often only seen on the lateral radiograph as a bulge in the retrosternal space (see Figure 2.23).
- Should not obscure aortic arch.

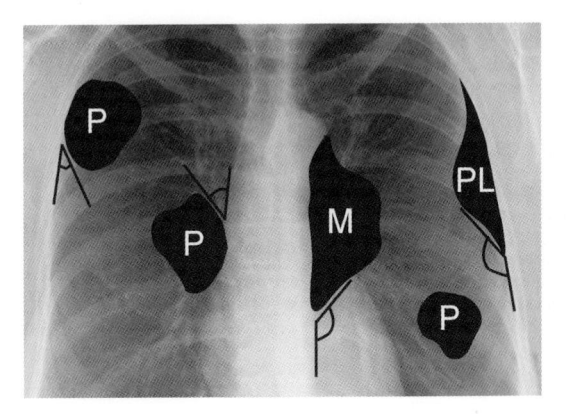

Figure 2.22 Where does the mass originate? Pulmonary masses (P) have acute angled borders with the mediastinum and pleura, while mediastinal masses (M) and pleural masses (P) have obtuse angled borders.

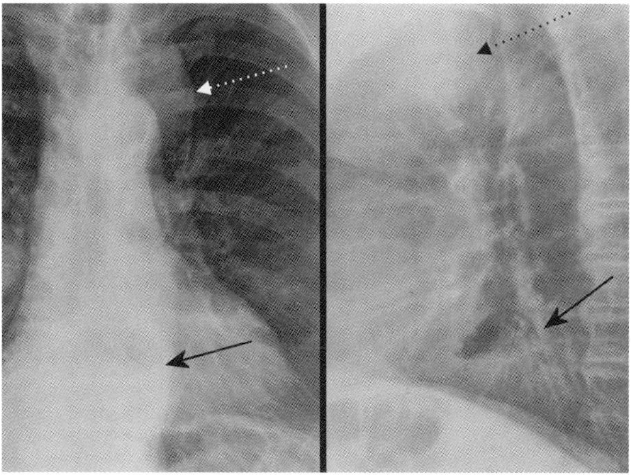

Figure 2.23 PA (L) and lateral (R) CXR in patient with anterior mediastinal mass due to lymphoma (dotted arrows) and posterior retrocardiac mass due to hiatal hernia. Note air-fluid level (solid arrows). Note how the anterior mass does not go above the clavicles and the aortic arch is still clearly seen.

Differential diagnosis:
- "The 4 Ts": teratoma, thyroid, thymoma, and "terrible lymphoma" (and lymphadenopathy).
- Goiters and lymphoma most common.
- Goiters may displace trachea laterally on frontal study.

Middle mediastinum
Includes heart, great vessels, trachea.
- <u>Aortic origin</u>: Ascending aorta or arch aneurysms or dissection.
  - These will alter the contour of the aorta. May have rim calcification. May cause widening of superior mediastinum (though is non-specific and requires CT for evaluation).
- <u>Pulmonary artery origin</u>: Pulmonary hypertension or stenosis.
  - Enlarged central pulmonary arteries.
  - In pulmonary stenosis, only L is enlarged.
- <u>Cardiac origin</u>: Pericardial cysts, L ventricular aneurysms.
  - Abnormal cardiac contour, will merge with the mass.
  - Aneurysms may have rim calcification.
- <u>Adenopathy</u>: Metastatic cancer, sarcoidosis, infectious.
  - Hilar—large lobular hila (see Figure 2.57).
  - R paratracheal—widening of the R paratracheal stripe.
  - Subcarinal—widening of carinal angle.
  - AP window—nodes produce a convexity there.
- <u>Tracheal or bronchial origin</u>: Bronchogenic cysts (large, sharply marginated, close to hilum). Bronchogenic carcinomas, especially small cell.

Posterior mediastinum
Includes esophagus, descending aorta, spine & paraspinal tissues. Can be seen above clavicles on frontal study.
- <u>Esophageal</u>:
  - Hiatal hernia (see Figure 2.23) – Seen as a rounded mass containing an air-fluid level in the retrocardiac region. Loss of normal azygo-esophageal stripe (see Figure 2.8).
  - Esophageal neoplasms—rarely seen, but gastric pull-ups following esophageal resection can produce a tubular mediastinal density.
- <u>Aorta</u>: Descending aortic aneurysms—fusiform or saccular dilatation of the descending aorta. Bulge or lobularity of para-aortic stripe.
- <u>Neurogenic masses and cysts</u>: Paragangliomas, neurogenic cysts.
  - Usually well-defined posterior masses that merge with spine. MRI most helpful to evaluate.

Air that shouldn't be there
Abnormal air on a CXR can be in the pleural cavity (pneumothorax); in the mediastinum (pneumomediastinum); in the pericardium (pneumopericardium); within a bulla, pneumatocele (see Figure 2.54), cavitating mass, or cavitating pneumonia in the lung; in the peritoneal cavity (pneumoperitoneum—see chapter 3) or within the soft tissues (subcutaneous emphysema). Air will appear as a lucency (black), its distribution and shape depending on where it is.

Pneumothorax
<u>Pneumothorax on upright images:</u>
Small pneumothoraces can be difficult to see, especially in the apex where they can be confused with ribs (see Figure 2.24).
- Look for a very thin white line with absent lung markings peripheral to it. It is usually parallel to the chest wall.
- Sometimes you will need to do an expiratory or a decubitus film to confirm a pneumothorax.
- Skin folds can "fake" a PTX especially in neonates and the elderly. They cannot be followed over the apex and are a wider "white band" rather than a thin pleural line (see Figure 2.25).

> #### Hints for seeing small pneumothoraces
> - Adjust the contrast and brightness (usually lighter and more contrast helps).
> - Zoom the image over the apex.
> - Invert the display to black on white.
> - Put on a CLAHE filter or other high-contrast filter.
> - Follow the contours of the upper ribs and see if any lines do not match ribs.
> - Do an expiratory or decubitus study (abnormal side up).

RADIOGRAPHS 69

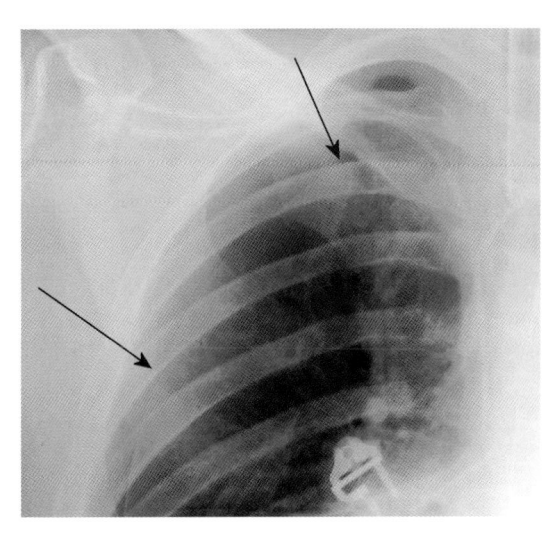

Figure 2.24 Cropped view of the R lung apex in a patient with a pneumothorax. Note fine white line (arrows) with absent lung markings peripheral to line.

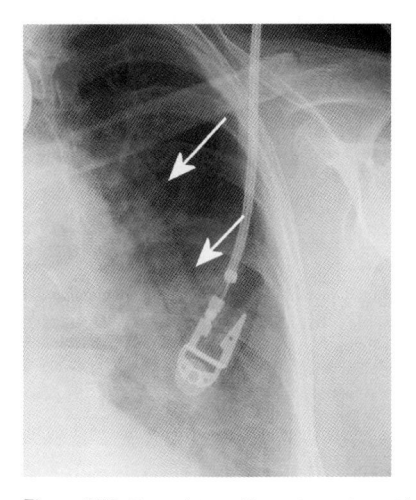

Figure 2.25 Cropped view of L apex in a patient with multiple skin folds. Note the thicker white lines that fade off inferiorly (arrows), with preservation of lung markings peripherally.

Pneumothorax on supine images:

In a supine patient, air in the pleural space accumulates anteriorly and at the base (the most non-dependent portion of the pleural space in a supine patient). It appears as a deep, hyper-lucent costophrenic sulcus (the "deep sulcus sign").

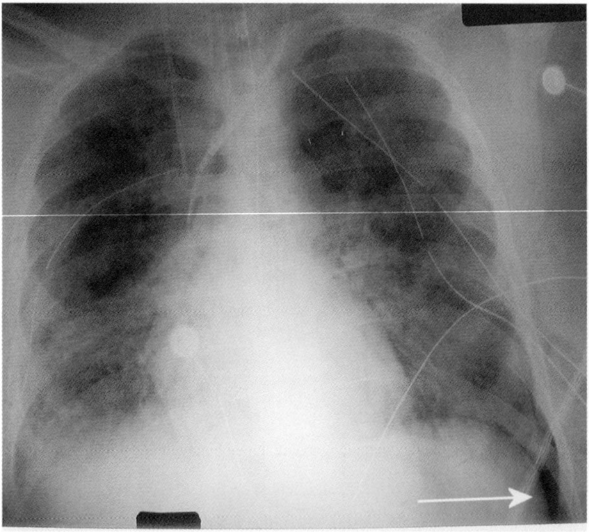

Figure 2.26 Deep sulcus sign on the L in a supine ICU patient with a pneumothorax.

Tension pneumothorax:

Tension pneumothorax is a life-threatening medical emergency. The air must be decompressed urgently to prevent rapid cardiorespiratory arrest (via needle aspiration or chest tube placement) (see Figure 2.27).

Radiographic findings:
- Signs of the pneumothorax (hyperlucency, pleural edge).
- Mediastinal shift away from the pneumothorax.
  - Compare to old films—shift can be subtle.
- Diaphragmatic depression, or even inversion.
- Lung collapse—PTX is usually large (lung collapse may not be marked if the lungs are "stiff," e.g., pulmonary fibrosis or edema).

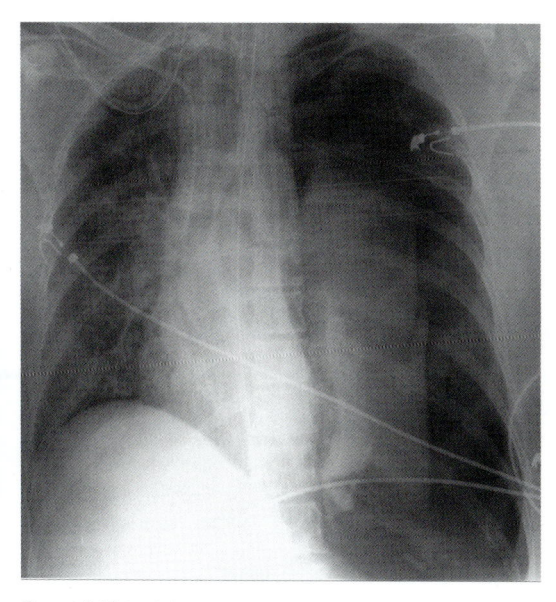

Figure 2.27 L sided tension pneumothorax. Note mediastinal shift to right and left diaphragmatic depression.

> **Key points about pneumothorax:**
> You won't see them unless you look carefully!
> - In a supine patient look for the deep sulcus sign.
> - Always look for associated signs of tension.

Pneumomediastinum

Radiographic findings:
- Lucent streaks within the mediastinal soft tissues that may extend into subcutaneous tissues (see Figure 2.28).
- Usually vertically oriented, extending into the neck or following the edges of mediastinal structures such as the aorta, trachea, major bronchi or pericardium.
- Sometimes best seen on the lateral film outlining the aorta.
- Continuous hemidiaphragm—air adjacent to the central diaphragm means both hemidiaphragms are seen as one continuous line.

Etiologies:
- Post surgical (CABG, mediastinoscopy).
- Extension from pneumothorax.
- Barotrauma from ventilator.
- Idiopathic.
- Ruptured esophagus, or rarely, major airway.

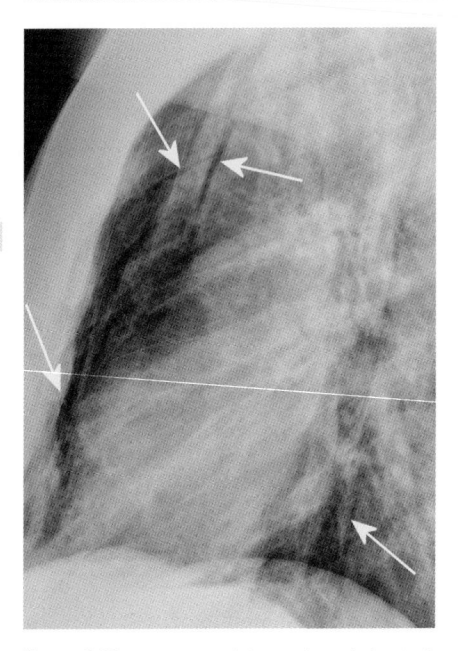

Figure 2.28 Cropped lateral chest radiograph showing lucent streaks of air within the mediastinum in a patient with pneumomediastinum.

Pneumopericardium
Air can surround the pericardial sac in a pneumomediastinum, or be located within it in a pneumopericardium. Can produce fatal tamponade.

Etiologies:
- Extension of a pneumomediastinum.
- Penetrating trauma or surgery.
- Rarely due to fistula with a gas-filled viscus or anaerobic infection.

Pleural and pericardial fluid
Fluid within the pleural or pericardial cavity may be simple (water density), proteinaceous (e.g., due to tumor), blood (e.g., traumatic), or pus (empyema). Effusions may be mobile or loculated.

Pleural effusions—upright radiographs
- Need approximately 150–200 cc to see on frontal upright, 50 cc on lateral, 10 cc on CT.
- Appear as density in the lateral or posterior costophrenic sulcus.

RADIOGRAPHS

- Small effusions have a meniscus (horizontal line with curved edges) in the costophrenic angles. Best seen on the lateral study.
- Larger effusions will obliterate the normal silhouettes of mediastinal structures and the diaphragm ("the silhouette sign," see p. 56).
- Very large effusions can have mass effect with mediastinal shift away from effusion.

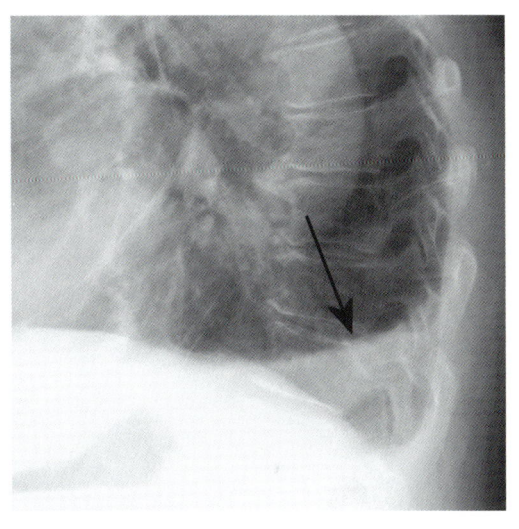

Figure 2.29 Small L sided pleural effusion, not seen on PA study.

> **Effusions can sometimes be difficult to distinguish from consolidation or atelectasis.**
> - Look for air bronchograms (pneumonia).
> - Look for signs volume loss (atelectasis).
> - Do a decubitus study (abnormal side DOWN).
> - Do an ultrasound e.g., if immobile, ICU patient, child.
> - CT scan if still in doubt.

Pleural effusions—supine radiographs

When the patient is supine or semi-upright, the fluid appears as "ground glass opacity" as it layers posteriorly with aerated lung anteriorly, becoming denser at the bases (see Figure 2.30).

- Sometimes the fluid can track up the lateral chest wall.
- Appearance will depend on:
  - Position of the patient (the more upright the denser the effusion inferiorly and the more diaphragm is obscured).
  - Amount of fluid.

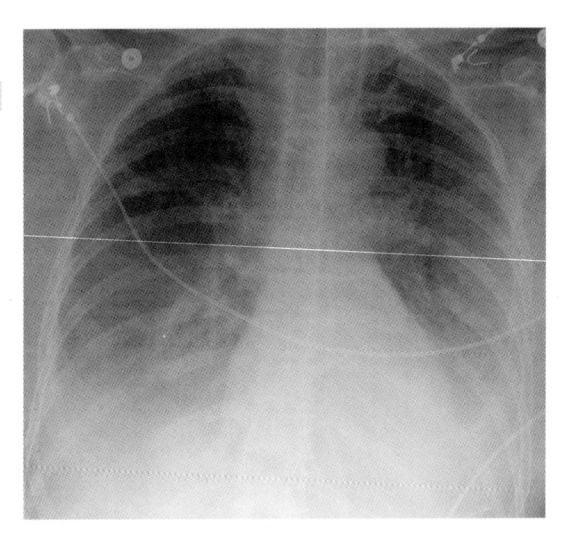

Figure 2.30 Large bilateral effusions in a nearly supine patient. Notice how the vascular markings are superimposed over the hazy densities, which increases from apices to the bases.

Types of effusions

Hydropneumothorax:
This occurs when there is air and fluid in the pleural cavity. Recognized by a straight horizontal line (the air fluid level) (see Figure 2.31).
- Commonly seen post-op (e.g., lobectomy, pneumonectomy) and when chest tubes are present.

Loculated effusions:
Effusions may become loculated (separated by septations, not free flowing), especially if infected, bloody, proteinaceous, chronic, or in patients with pleural scarring.
- Decubitus views are useful to assess (see Figure 2.2).

Subpulmonic effusions:
Occasionally fluid can accumulate UNDER the lung, pushing the lung up rather than surrounding the lung.
- This gives the appearance of a raised hemidiaphragm. The costophrenic angle may remain sharp.

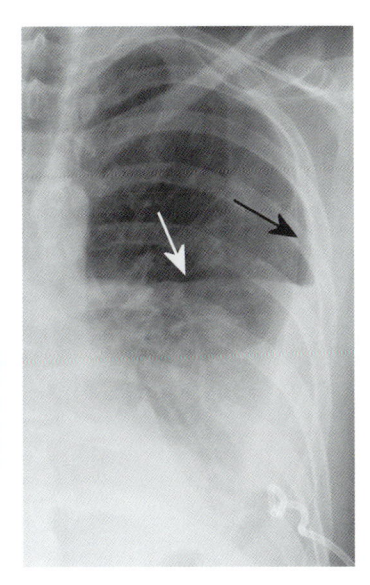

Figure 2.31 Cropped image of a hydropneumothorax. Notice the horizontal air fluid level (white arrow) and the small pneumothorax (black arrow).

- The lung/fluid interface is shaped differently than a normal diaphragm, with the 'dome' displaced laterally (sometimes called 'Rock of Gibraltar sign').
- Decubitus views, US or CT can confirm diagnosis.

Pseudotumor:
Fluid can accumulate focally in a fissure, such that it gives the appearance of a mass.
- On the lateral study it is typically elliptical and aligned parallel to a fissure.

Empyema
Infected effusions generally cannot be diagnosed on CXR, although they may be loculated and may contain pockets of air. See CT p. 89.

Pericardial effusions
Fluid accumulating in the pericardial sac (with or without tamponade) produces diffuse cardiomegaly, sometimes described as a "waterbottle" (wide and flat looking) shaped heart. Look for sudden changes in the size of the cardiac silhouette.
- The CXR is rarely diagnostic.

Calcifications

Densities that are as "white" as bone are calcifications. These may be in the lung, mediastinum, pleura, or extrathoracic. They are far more likely to be benign than malignant, though the latter do occur.

Common types of calcifications

Lung:
- Granulomas (solitary or multiple), usually 3–5 mm, round.
- Silicosis (small, multiple, upper lobes and eggshell hilar node calcs).
- Bronchial and tracheal cartilage calcification.
- Prior varicella pneumonia (multiple, punctuate).
- Rarely metastases, e.g., osteosarcoma, thyroid.

Mediastinum:
- Calcified lymph nodes (especially in prior granulomatous disease, TB, treated lymphoma, silicosis).
- Aortic atherosclerosis and aneurysms (rim around aorta).
- Pericardial calcifications.
- Myocardial calcifications.
- Calcified aortic or mitral valves (stenosis) or annulus (common).
- Coronary (also stents!). Best seen on CT.

Pleural:
- Asbestos exposure (calcified pleural plaques and diaphragmatic calcifications are pathognomonic, see Figure 2.32).

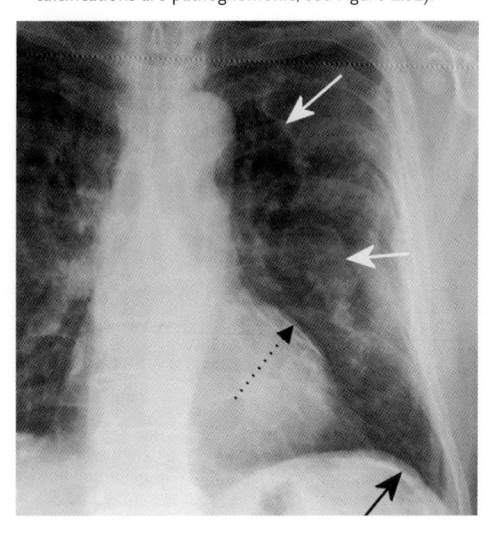

Figure 2.32 Patient with history of asbestos exposure with calcified pleural plaques seen on the diaphragms (solid black arrow), pericardium (dotted black arrow) and "en face" (white arrows) projecting over the lungs.

- Prior empyema including tuberculous, or hemothorax.
- Prior surgery, including pneumonectomy.

Extrapulmonary:
Non-thoracic calcifications in carotid arteries, shoulder joints, gallbladder, spleen, and so on are commonly seen on CXRs.

> **Remember**: anything in the thoracic wall or soft tissues may be projected over the lungs, and appear as a pulmonary mass. Think "skin to skin." Extrapulmonary calcifications such as healing rib fractures or costochondral calcifications may look like lung masses.

Chest CT

Chest CT scans are ordered for a wide variety of reasons including respiratory symptoms, cancer staging, and evaluation of abnormalities on CXRs.

How are images acquired?
See chapter 1, Radiology Essentials. The chest CT may be part of a chest/abdomen/pelvis study or acquired alone.

Common Protocols
Intravenous contrast-enhanced chest CT (CECT)
IV contrast is indicated when the vascular structures need to be well seen, such as when evaluating for hilar lymphadenopathy, or in CT angiography. Most studies are obtained on inspiration. Oral contrast is rarely needed unless the esophagus is being evaluated.
- <u>"Standard" CECT:</u> Uses a smaller, slower bolus so that contrast is in both the pulmonary and aortic circulation. Used for cancer staging, pneumonia evaluation, and other miscellaneous indications. Slice thickness usually 3–5 mm.
- <u>Pulmonary angiogram (CTPA):</u> High injection rate and early imaging to catch the bolus of contrast in the pulmonary circulation to look for PEs. Thin slices obtained (typically 1.25 mm).
- <u>Aortic angiogram (CTA):</u> Similar technique to CTPA, but scan acquired slightly later, when bolus of contrast has reached the aorta. Used for trauma, aortic dissection, aortic aneurysm studies, etc.
- <u>Cardiac angiogram</u> protocols (see p. 107).

Non-enhanced chest CT (NECT)
Performed when the lung parenchyma is of primary concern rather than mediastinal or hilar structures.
- <u>Low dose NECT:</u> Indicated for lung cancer screening, nodule follow-up, evaluation of questionable CXR abnormalities, and pediatric studies where possible. May be limited to area of concern (e.g., nodule).
  - Uses a lower dose of radiation; adequate to evaluate the lungs, but inadequate for evaluation of mediastinal structures.

- <u>High resolution NECT</u>: Provides thin, high resolution images of the lung parenchyma in patients with suspected or known interstitial lung disease.
  Images are obtained in inspiration, and may also be obtained in:
  - Expiration—to look for air trapping.
  - Prone—to differentiate dependent atelectasis from lower lobe pathology.

Algorithms and image viewing

Chest CT scans will be reconstructed by at least 2 algorithms (software reconstruction methods) and viewed on at least 2 window settings (see p. 7 chapter 1, Radiology Essentials).

Algorithms

<u>Lung</u> —This uses a high contrast ("noisy") algorithm, which accentuates lines and edges, and gives the best contrast and resolution for lung parenchyma and airways. View lungs on this algorithm.
<u>Soft tissue</u>—standard, images look smoother. Used for non-lung structures.

Windows

<u>Lung</u>—only good for lungs; all other structures appear white.
<u>Mediastinal</u>—to look at the mediastinal structures, chest wall, and upper abdomen.

Accessory series

Depending on the clinical question, there may be other images to view:
- 3D reconstructions of vascular anatomy (e.g., patients with aortic aneurysms, coarctation, or arch anomalies).
- MIP reconstructions for CTA of the aorta.
- Pulmonary artery reconstructions for PE studies (usually coronal)

CHEST CT

Normal anatomy

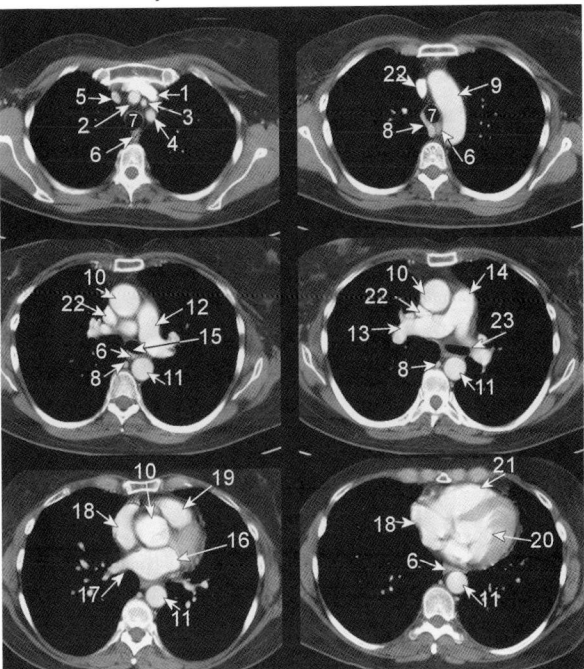

Figure 2.33 Selected normal mediastinal anatomy on chest CT.

Key to Figure 2.33

1	L brachiocephalic vein	12	L pulmonary artery
2	Brachiocephalic artery	13	R pulmonary artery
3	L common carotid artery	14	Main pulmonary artery
4	L subclavian artery	15	Carina
5	R brachiocephalic vein	16	L atrium
6	Esophagus	17	Pulmonary vein
7	Trachea	18	R atrium
8	Azygous vein	19	R ventricle outflow tract
9	Aortic arch	20	L ventricle
10	Ascending aorta	21	R ventricle
11	Descending aorta	22	Superior vena cava
		23	L main bronchus

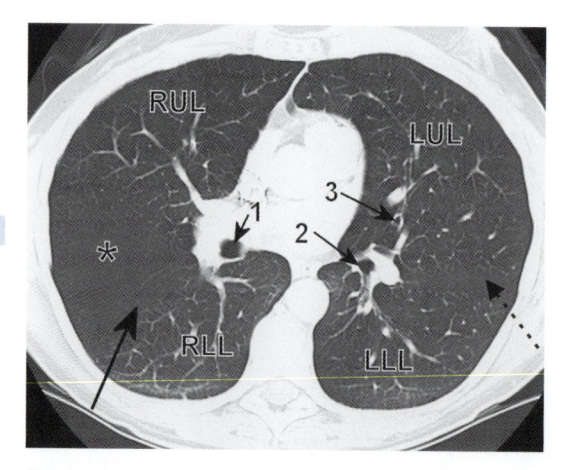

Figure 2.34 Normal lung anatomy on CT. R oblique fissure (solid arrow), L oblique fissure (dotted arrow), Horizontal fissure (*) seen as relatively lucent area on axial images. 1 = R bronchus intermedius (intermediate) 2 = LLL bronchus 3 = LUL bronchus.

How do I read a Chest CT

Chest CTs should be looked at on both lung and mediastinal windows and other reconstructions depending on clinical question (see protocols earlier).

Search strategies

Two basic strategies (use combination of both):
Slice by slice: searching each slice for abnormalities.
- Most useful on lung windows. Start at top and work down.

Structure by structure: scroll up and down following each structure over multiple slices then returning to top to follow the next structure.
- Best for mediastinum/chest wall.

What are you looking for?

Lungs:
- *Lung window:* nodules, masses, air space, and ground glass opacities, interstitial and emphysematous changes, pneumothorax, pneumomediastinum.
- *Mediastinal window:* pleural effusions, calcifications.

Airways:
- *Lung window:* Tracheal and major bronchial narrowing and intra-luminal masses, mucus and aspirated debris, bronchiectasis.

Lymph nodes:
- Enlargement, abnormal enhancement, calcifications (see patterns of disease later).

Aortic arch vessels:
- Dilatations, stenoses, occlusions, anomalous vessels.

Aorta:
- Diameter, mural and intra-luminal abnormalities including plaque, thrombus, and flaps; peri-aortic fluid or hemorrhage.

Pulmonary arteries:
- Diameter. Intra-luminal filling defects (emboli).

Heart:
- Size of individual chambers, calcifications including coronary, focal dilatations (aneurysms), masses, pericardial effusions.

Thyroid:
- Goiter, nodules.

Esophagus:
- Dilatation, masses, hiatal hernia.

Chest wall:
- Bones: fractures, sclerotic/lytic lesions.
- Soft tissues: air, masses and hematomas.

Pitfalls and problems
- Using the wrong windows
  - If looking for vascular intra-luminal abnormalities (e.g., PE, aortic dissection), window the study so the IV contrast is not too "bright" or abnormalities will be obscured.
  - Small pulmonary nodules and subtle opacities may not be seen on the mediastinal/soft tissue reconstruction *algorithm*, even if viewed on the lung *window* display.
- Forgetting to check the chest wall for abnormalities of the bones and soft tissues.
- Cardiac, respiratory, and aortic motion can produce "pseudo-lesions" that may simulate pathology such as ascending aortic dissection or PEs.

Patterns of disease

Air that shouldn't be there
CT is exquisitely sensitive for air, which is best visualized on the lung windows.
- Air will be the only material that is "black" on lung windows outside of the major airways (or air within a large bulla).
- Very small pneumothoraces will be seen as crescent shaped lucencies anteriorly.
- Pneumomediastinum will show air tracking around mediastinal structures.
- Air in the soft tissues usually follows fascial planes and along muscle fibers (see Figure 2.35).

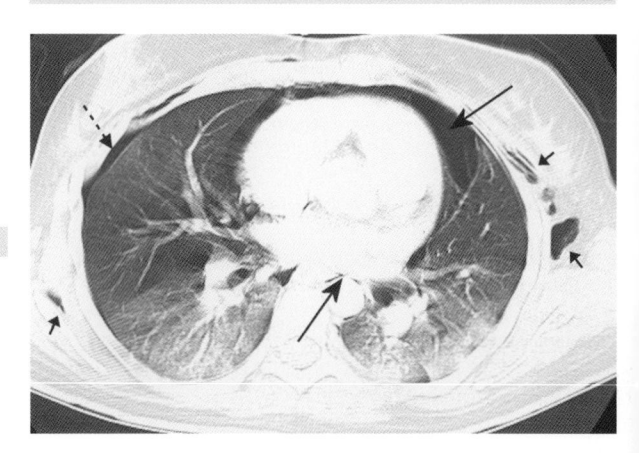

Figure 2.35 Patient with a small R pneumothorax (dashed arrow), pneumomediastinum (solid arrows) and subcutaneous air (short arrows).

Lung abnormalities
CT has increased sensitivity and specificity compared to CXRs.

Alveolar or airspace opacities
Produced when the alveoli are filled with fluid (e.g., pulmonary edema, ARDS), blood (e.g., pulmonary infarct, contusion, or hemorrhage), pus (pneumonia), or abnormal cells (e.g., bronchoaveolar carcinoma).

<u>CT findings:</u>
- Increased attenuation of the lung; may be focal, multifocal, or lobar.
- Usually ill-defined, but not spiculated, borders.
- Air bronchograms may occur with any cause, but are variable.
- The normal vascular markings are obscured.
- Not usually round or masslike (note: rare exception of "round" pneumonia, most common in children see p. 307).
- Often sharply marginated at border with pleura (e.g., fissures) but does not tether pleura (see Figure 2.36).
- Similar to CXRs, partial alveolar filling can give a "ground glass" appearance, when vascular markings are still seen (see Figure 2.37).

The distribution of the opacities as well as the clinical history are clues to the diagnosis.

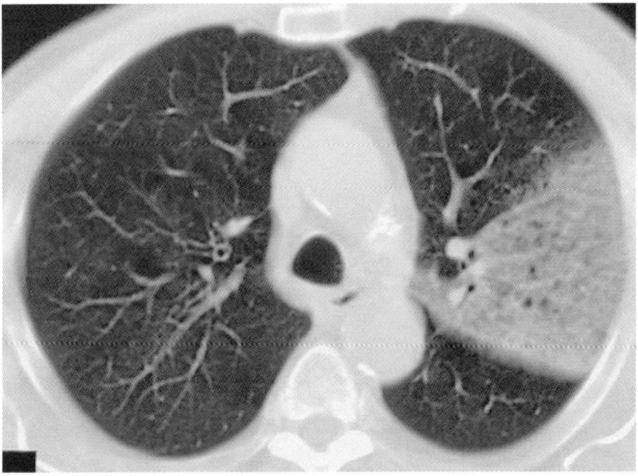

Figure 2.36 Bronchoalveolar carcinoma in the L upper lobe on CT producing an airspace opacity appearing similar to pneumonia.

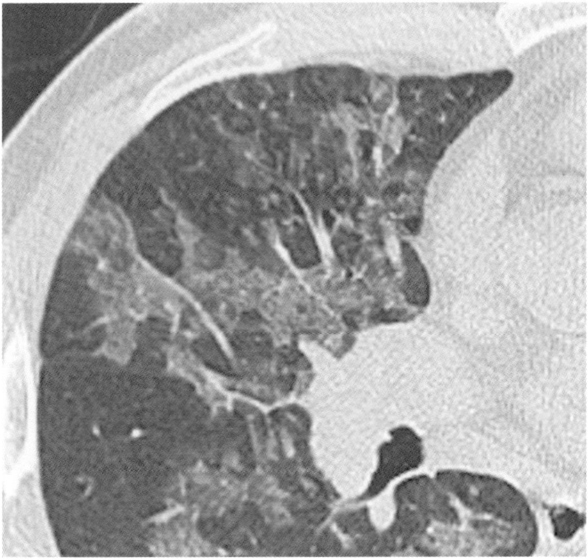

Figure 2.37 Ground glass opacities on a CT due to extrinsic allergic alveolitis.

Interstitial abnormalities

Pulmonary abnormalities that affect the interstitium of the lung rather than filling the alveoli.

<u>CT findings</u> (see Figure 2.38):
- Linear bands of tissue and thickening of the interlobular septa—you should not usually see these (solid arrows).
- Bronchiectasis (dashed arrow).
- "Honeycombing" in advanced disease due to a combination of fibrosis and subpleural blebs (curved arrows).

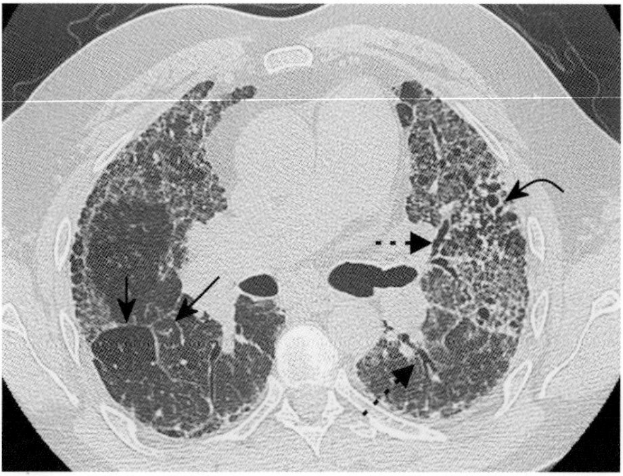

Figure 2.38 High resolution CT scan in a patient with pulmonary fibrosis due to advanced usual interstitial pneumonitis. See text for explanation.

Atelectasis

Atelectasis, or collapsed lung, appears on CT as areas of increased lung opacity, usually wedge shaped with the apex toward the hilum and the base extending out toward the pleura.
- Frequency: Subsegmental/segmental >lobar>whole lung.
- Usually fairly dense opacity depending on degree of atelectasis.
- Lack of peripheral air bronchograms, but central air bronchograms are commonly seen.
- +/− rapid changes on sequential imaging.
- Signs of volume loss (depending on volume of lung involved):
  - Mediastinal deviation toward side of atelectasis.
  - Ipsilateral diaphragmatic elevation.
  - Hilar elevation/depression on coronal images.
  - Deviation of major and minor fissures toward atelectasis.

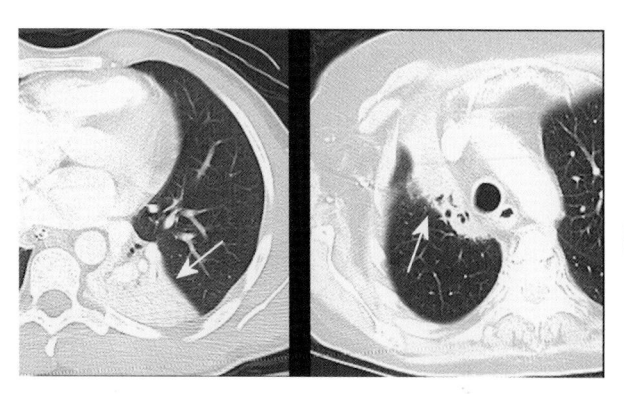

Figure 2.39 Two patients, one with LLL atelectasis (L) and one with RUL atelectasis (R).

Pulmonary nodules and masses

<u>Definitions:</u>
- By convention, a mass < 3 cm is called a "nodule."
- A single lesion < 3 cm is a "solitary pulmonary nodule" or SPN.

Nodules as small as 2–3 mm can be seen on a high quality CT scan and these small nodules are very common:
- Nodules >4 mm are found on about 50% of chest CTs in smokers >50 years of age.
- Common benign nodules: granulomas, hamartomas, and intrapulmonary lymph nodes.
- Common malignant nodules: bronchogenic carcinoma, metastasis.

<u>Important characteristics of lung nodules/masses:</u>
These factors influence the level of concern for malignancy, and they affect the management of a mass/nodule within the lung:
- Size (larger more likely malignant).
- Density.
- Border characteristics:
  - Chance malignancy: spiculated>lobular>smooth.
- Growth rate (compare with prior studies):
  - The "doubling time" of lung cancer can range from 30–500 days, median 100 days. This is best assessed using volume measurements.
  - A solid nodule that is stable for 2 years is considered benign.
  - Very fast growing masses (doubling <20 days) are usually infectious/inflammatory.
- Calcification (small calcified nodules rarely malignant).
- Number of masses: multiple small nodules with no history of malignancy elsewhere favors granulomatous disease rather than metastases.
- Patient history of smoking or known non-pulmonary malignancy.

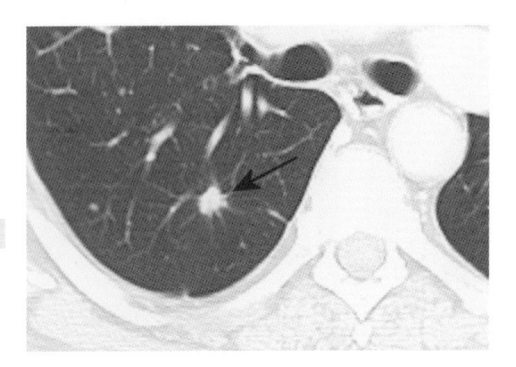

Figure 2.40 Spiculated 12 mm nodule in the RUL on CT. Adenocarcinoma on biopsy.

Management of pulmonary nodules seen on CT

Management options include: ignore (no further follow-up); follow up with serial CT to assess growth; biopsy (CT guided needle biopsy); excision; or further imaging with PET FDG scanning.

For the management of <u>indeterminate</u> (i.e., those nodules that do not have definitely benign or highly suspicious characteristics) solitary pulmonary nodules newly detected in patients > 35, the Fleischner Society developed the following guidelines:
- Low risk patients: Minimal or absent history of smoking and of other known risk factors for lung cancer.
- High risk patients: History of smoking or of other known risk factors for lung cancer.

Table 2.2		
Nodule Size (mm)	Low risk patients	High risk patients
≤4	No follow-up needed.	Follow up at 12 months. If no change, no further imaging needed.
>4–6	Follow up at 12 months. If no change, no further imaging needed.	Initial follow-up CT at 6–12 months and then at 18–24 months if no change.
>6–8	Initial follow-up CT at 6–12 months and then at 18–24 months if no change.	Initial follow-up CT at 3–6 months and then at 9–12 and 24 months if no change.
>8	Follow-up CTs at 3, 9, and 24 months OR dynamic contrast enhanced CT, PET, and/or biopsy.	Same as for low-risk patients.

Note this is a constantly evolving field as new data becomes available from lung cancer screening studies including those using volumetric measurements.

Mediastinal abnormalities
Masses
The differential diagnosis for masses in the mediastinum is the same for that described for chest radiographs on p. 66.

Benefits of CT over radiography:
- Better lesion characterization:
  - Distinction between cystic and solid masses.
  - Identification of fat or calcifications in masses.
  - Assessment of enhancement (CECT).
  - Identification of aneurysms and other vascular masses (CECT).
- Higher sensitivity to detect much smaller masses and nodes.
- Much better anatomical localization of masses.
- Assessment of invasion of mediastinal structures and chest wall (see Figure 2.41).

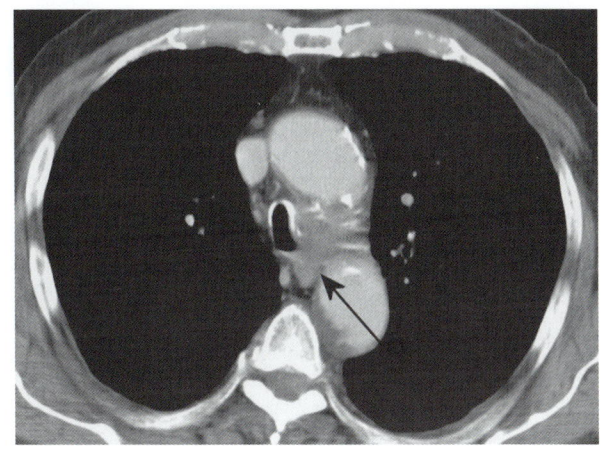

Figure 2.41 Mediastinal mass (small cell lung ca) in a patient who presented with a hoarse throat. The mass is compressing the L recurrent laryngeal nerve and there is loss of the fat plane between the mass and the esophagus due to local invasion (arrow).

Lymph nodes
Normal lymph nodes are seen throughout the mediastinum. Nodes can be enlarged in any metastatic cancer, lymphoma, sarcoidosis, pneumoconiosis and other granulomatous conditions, and a wide variety of infectious and inflammatory processes.

<u>Normal appearance:</u>
- Oval shape, sharp margins with short axis <10 mm.
- Fatty hilum (if large enough to see) – look like tiny kidneys.

CHAPTER 2 Chest Imaging

Common sites of lymphadenopathy:
(numbers indicate sites on Figure 2.42)
- R paratracheal (1).
- Adjacent to azygous vein (2).
- Aorto-pulmonary window (just below aortic arch) (3).
- Pre-carinal (anterior to carina) (4).
- Lung hila (5).
- Sub-carinal (below carina) (6).
- Pre-aortic (anterior to aortic arch).
- Peri-aortic (adjacent to descending aorta).

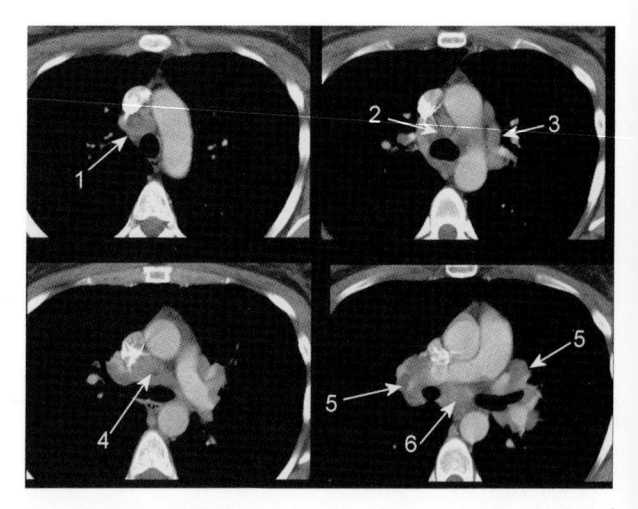

Figure 2.42 Mediastinal adenopathy in a patient with sarcoidosis (see text for legend).

Vascular abnormalities
Vascular abnormalities are best assessed on CT angiograms, with image reconstruction in multiple planes. 3D reconstructions are often useful to show the relationships with adjacent structures and the morphology of the abnormality.

Aneurysms
Vessels can be dilated and tortuous (ectatic) or aneurysmal. Aneurysms can be <u>fusiform</u> or <u>saccular</u> (see Figure 2.59).
- Definition: Maximal transverse diameter >50% larger than normal vessel.
- Ascending aorta should be approximately the same size as the proximal main pulmonary artery (see Figure 2.33).

- Upper limit normal ascending aorta = 40 mm, descending = 30 mm.
- The vessels arising from the aortic arch can also be ectatic/aneurysmal.

Stenoses

Vessels can be diffusely or focally narrowed (stenotic).

- Great vessels: Can be narrowed by atheroma +/− calcification (most commonly involves origin), or vasculitis.
- Aorta: Can be focally narrowed in coarctation, or diffusely or multifocally narrowed in vasculitis, or severe atherosclerosis.
- Coronary arteries: Evaluation requires a dedicated coronary artery CT (see p. 108).

Pleural abnormalities

Normal pleura is a barely visible thin dense line. Abnormalities of the pleura include:

Pleural effusions

- As little as 10 cc of pleural fluid can be seen on CT.
- Simple fluid: Uniformly low attenuation (<20 HU).
- Complex fluid: Dense effusions (>20 HU) suggest blood, pus, or highly proteinaceous fluid (e.g., in malignancy).
  - Thickening and enhancement of the pleura is suspicious for empyema (infected effusion) or malignant involvement.
  - Air-fluid levels or air bubbles in the effusion are suspicious for empyema (if no procedures have been performed and there is no traumatic injury).
- Location: Should be dependent and continuous, crescent shaped.
  - Effusions are loculated when they are not flowing posteriorly.
  - Loculated effusions may be more rounded in shape.

Pneumothorax (see p. 81).

Pleural thickening

Soft tissue attenuation. May be smooth or lobular.

<u>Differential diagnosis:</u>

- Often normal in apices.
- Post-surgical.
- Current or prior infection or inflammation.
- Prior chronic effusions or hemothoraces.
- Malignancy—for example, metastatic adenocarcinoma or mesothelioma—usually has associated pleural effusion (see Figure 2.43).

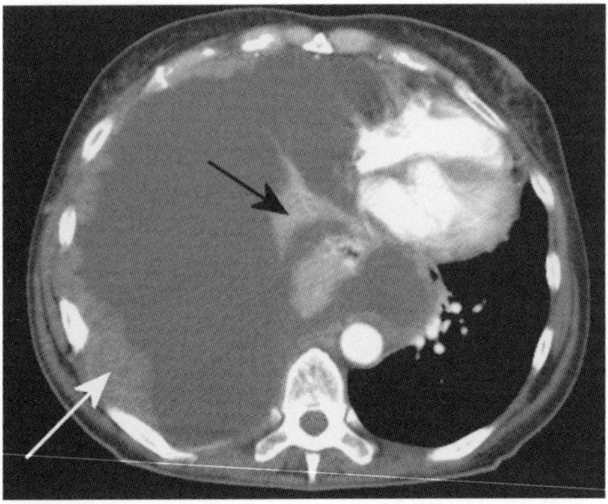

Figure 2.43 Patient with mesothelioma. There is a large R pleural effusion with mass effect and mediastinal shift. Black arrow = collapsed right lung. The pleura has nodular thickening (white arrow).

Pleural masses
- May originate from the pleura (e.g., fibroma, mesothelioma, pleural plaques in asbestos exposure).
- May be metastatic (e.g., adenocarcinoma, malignant thymoma).
- May be within the lung abutting it (e.g., bronchogenic carcinomas).

Pleural calcifications
See p. 76 (pleural calcifications, CXR).

Pericardial abnormalities
The pericardium can be evaluated on both CT and MRI.

Thickening
- > 4 mm is abnormal.
- Benign (e.g., infection—viral, TB, or inflammatory), and malignant causes.

Fluid
A trace amount of fluid is normal (15–50 ml).
- Small effusions layer posteriorly.
- Is there tamponade? (takes 150–250 ml).
  - Dilated SVC, IVC, R atrium, and hepatic veins.
  - Ascites and pleural effusions.
  - Elongated appearance of ventricles.

Calcification
Calcified pericardium can cause constrictive pericarditis.
- Thin or thick line of calcium along the pericardium.
- May be continuous or discontinuous, over RV as well as LV.

Differential diagnosis:
- Infectious: Viral, rheumatic, tuberculous.
- Prior hemopericardium.
- Idiopathic.

About 50% with pericardial calcification will have constrictive physiology, but about 90% of those with constrictive physiology have pericardial calcification.

Common conditions on CXR and CT

This is not intended to be an exhaustive list of conditions, but some of the common abnormalities you will encounter.

Pulmonary edema

Pulmonary edema may be <u>cardiogenic</u>, or <u>non-cardiogenic.</u> The heart is usually enlarged with cardiogenic pulmonary edema, but not always. The enlargement may be global or affect only the LA +/− LV.

The different causes of pulmonary edema are rarely distinguished on the basis of the CXR/CT alone.

Causes of cardiogenic pulmonary edema with cardiomegaly
- Coronary artery disease.
- Aortic valve incompetence.
- Mitral valve disease (incompetence>stenosis).
- Congenital heart disease.
- Cardiomyopathies of all types (e.g., viral, alcoholic).

Causes of cardiogenic pulmonary edema with normal heart size
- Acute myocardial infarct (MI).
- Acute arrhythmias.
- Ruptured papillary muscle after MI producing acute mitral regurgitation.

Causes of non-cardiogenic pulmonary edema
- Fluid overload (e.g., in renal failure).
- Acute respiratory distress syndrome (ARDS), tends to be more patchy and peripheral in distribution rather than bilateral perihilar (see Figure 2.47).
- Neurogenic pulmonary edema due to traumatic and non-traumatic brain injuries (tends to be predominantly upper lobes).
- Rarer causes: Drowning, smoke inhalation, drug overdoses (e.g., heroin).

Signs of pulmonary edema (with increasing severity)
Vascular findings ($\cong$ 15 mm Hg L atrial pressure)
- Cephalization of pulmonary venous flow—in a normal upright CXR, the upper lobe vessels are larger than the lower due to gravity. This is reversed as the L atrial pressure rises.
- Enlargement and blurring of vessels due to perivascular edema.

Interstitium ($\cong$ 20 mm Hg L atrial pressure)
- Peribronchial cuffing due to edema around the bronchi. Normally the bronchi have very thin walls when seen end on, near the hilum. As edema occurs, the bronchi appear thickened and fuzzy (see Figure 2.44).

- Hila are enlarged and "shaggy" looking and the heart may also appear "shaggy".
- Diffusely increased interstitial markings including Kerley lines (see Figures 2.45 and 2.16).

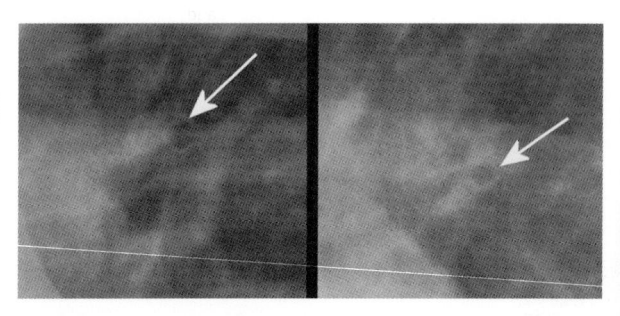

Figure 2.44 Peribronchial cuffing in a patient with interstitial pulmonary edema (R) compared to the normal (L).

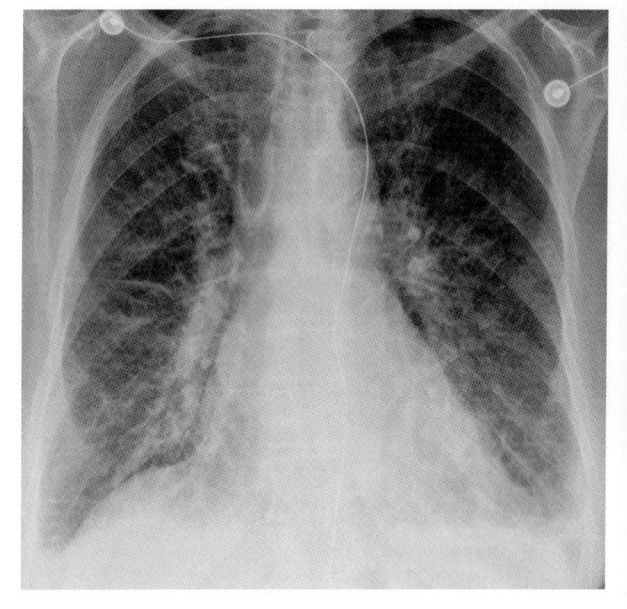

Figure 2.45 Interstitial pulmonary edema and mild cardiomegaly in a patient with left ventricular failure.

Alveoli ($\cong$ 25 mm Hg L atrial pressure)
- Alveolar opacification.
- Typically in cardiogenic pulmonary edema this is symmetrical and perihilar, producing the classic "batwing" pattern, but the distribution is variable and will depend on patient position and underlying lung disease (see Figure 2.46).
- ARDS tends to be more peripheral), but again is very variable (see Figure 2.47).

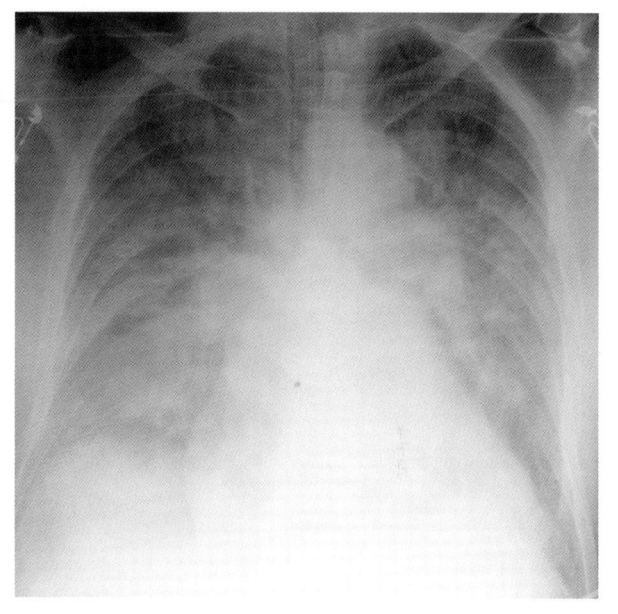

Figure 2.46 Severe alveolar pulmonary edema due to an acute large myocardial infarct.

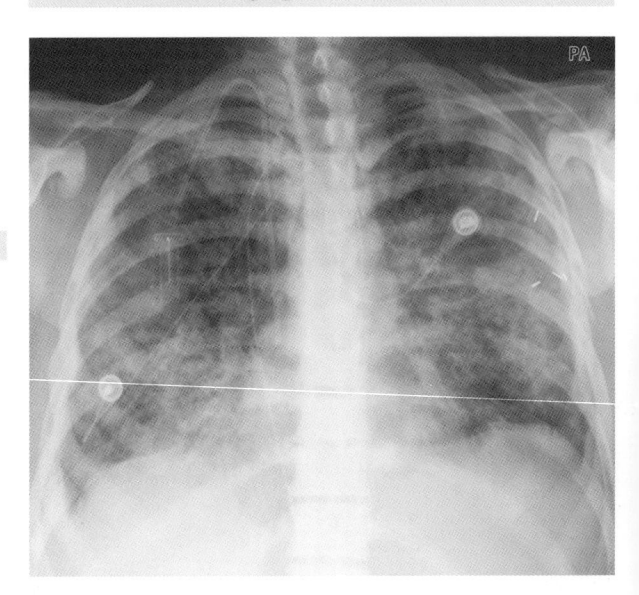

Figure 2.47 Patient with ARDS due to septicaemia. Note the more patchy distribution of the air space opacities.

Pleural effusions:
- Effusions take time to accumulate and clear, so they may lag behind the lung changes.
- Provides a sign of the patient's longer term fluid balance/L atrial pressure changes (both improvement and deterioration).

> Older films when the patient was not in pulmonary edema are helpful in seeing the subtle signs of early interstitial edema

CT findings in pulmonary edema
The findings on CT reflect those of chest radiography with the caveat that the patient is in a supine position for CT, so abnormalities tend to be more posterior (dependent).
- Ventral pulmonary venous distension.
- Thickening of intralobular and interlobular septae.
- Pleural effusions.
- Hazy ("ground-glass") perihilar opacities.
- Consolidation with air bronchograms in bilateral perihilar distribution.

Infection
See also p. 55 air space opacification and the silhouette sign.
The radiographic manifestations are highly variable depending on the severity and the organism involved.

Typical bacterial pneumonia
- Lobar or segmental areas of consolidation (see Figure 2.48).
- Air bronchograms commonly seen.

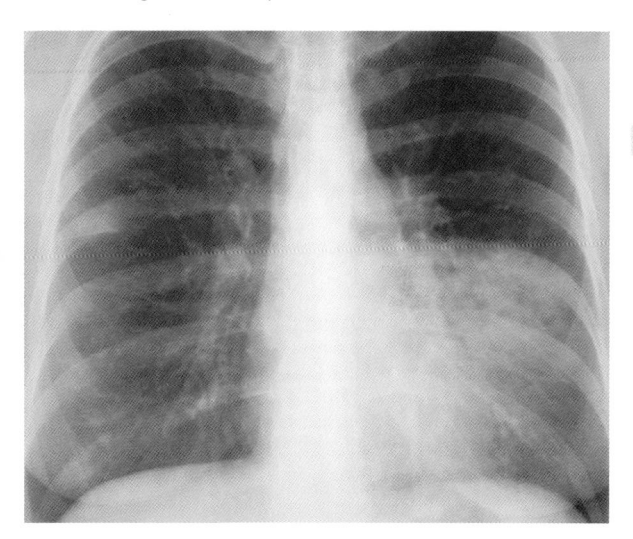

Figure 2.48 Typical community acquired pneumonia involving the lingular segment of the LUL. Notice how the left heart border is obscured (silhouette sign).

Specific findings:
- Staph. aureus pneumonias may cavitate.
- Klebsiella pneumonias may occasionally "expand" the lobe.
- Aspiration pneumonias are typically basilar +/− bilateral.
- Patients who are immunocompromised or have pre-existing lung disease (e.g., COPD, emphysema, cystic fibrosis) can have atypical or more extensive changes even with typical organisms.
- Reactive pleural effusions are common, but they may need to be tapped to exclude empyema.

Typical bacteria pneumonia on CT
Will have many of the same signs as on radiographs.
- Air space opacification with typical pneumonias.
- Air bronchograms (show clearer than on CXR) (see Figure 2.49).
- +/− reactive pleural effusions.

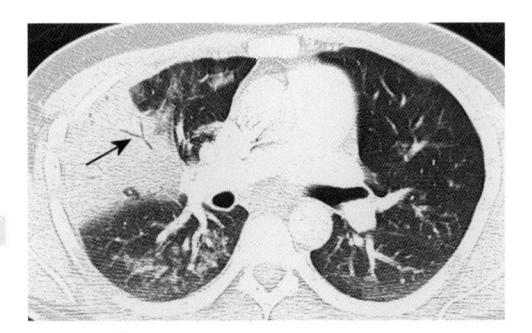

Figure 2.49 RUL pneumonia. Note air bronchograms (black arrow) and extension of airspace opacification to major fissure.

Follow up CXRs are recommended (e.g., 4–8 weeks) after treatment of a pneumonia to ensure there is no underlying lesion producing a post – obstructive pneumonia or a BAC masquerading as pneumonia.
- In high risk patients, e.g., smokers.
- If symptoms do not resolve.
- In elderly (note radiographic clearance may be slow).

Atypical bacterial and viral pneumonias

<u>Atypical</u> bacteria such as mycobacterium, legionella, or mycoplasma; viruses, fungi, or protozoa such as pneumocystis jirovecii tend not to produce lobar patterns of consolidation.
- Consider atypical pneumonias if patient is immunocompromised, e.g., elderly, on chemotherapy or steroids, HIV+ or post-transplant.

The appearance of atypical pneumonias is highly variable, and a full discussion of these entities is beyond the scope of this book.

<u>Key radiographic findings include:</u>
- "Ground-glass" (hazy, less dense) opacities rather than consolidation, e.g., pneumocystis jirovecii (carinii) pneumonia (see Figure 2.50).
- Bilateral, multilobar, patchy opacities.
- Predominantly an interstitial pattern (mycoplasma).
- Tend not to have air bronchograms.
- Cavitation within consolidation—mycobacterium infection (including TB and MAI), fungi (though also seen with Staph. aureus and septic emboli).

<u>CT findings:</u>
All previously mentioned radiographic findings plus atypical pneumonias may have scattered ground-glass opacities, interstitial, airspace, or some combination of all.

Consider CT in symptomatic immunocompromised patients with normal CXRs as it is more sensitive in early infections.

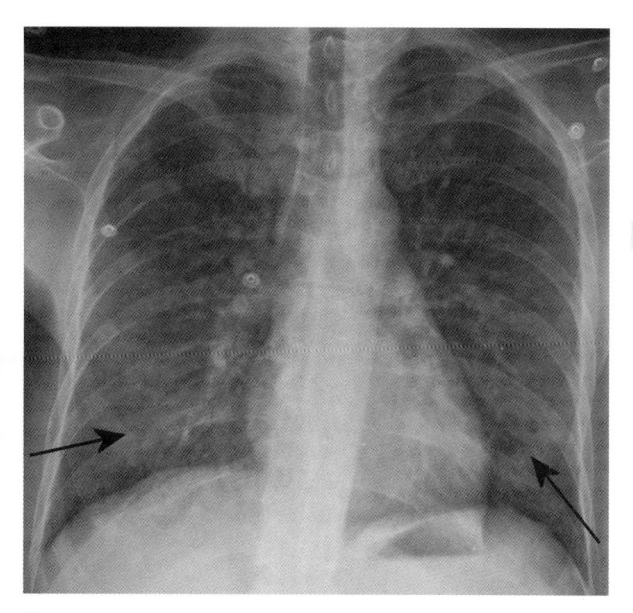

Figure 2.50 Early PCP pneumonia in a patient with AIDS. Diffuse patchy ground glass opacities in both lower lobes R>L.

Mycobacterium tuberculosis
TB can be primary or post-primary (more commonly seen).

Primary TB:
- Most common in children—hilar/mediastinal adenopathy in children.
- Lobar/segment consolidation (any lobe) +/− effusions.
- Cavitation rare.
- Normal CXR in 15%.

Post-primary TB:
- Apical predilection with cavitation within segmental consolidation.
- Adenopathy rare (except in AIDS patients).
- Effusions may progress to empyema.
- Bronchial spread into small airways involvement is described as a "tree in bud" appearance on CT (see Figure 2.51) (also seen with other small airway diseases).
- Progression to fibrosis and volume loss (hilar elevation).

Military TB:
- Hematogenous spread: multiple tiny (2 mm) widespread nodules.

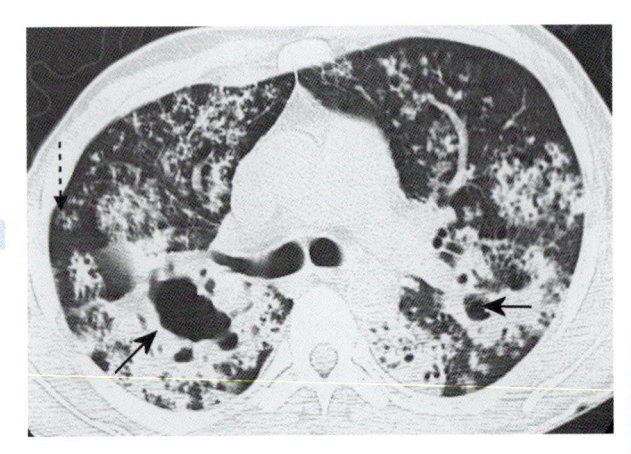

Figure 2.51 Extensive mycobacterium tuberculosis in a patient with AIDS. Combination of air space opacification, cavities (solid arrows) and "tree in bud" appearance (dashed arrow) of small airway opacification.

Lung abscess
Pneumonia may progress to form a lung abscess.
- Most commonly due to Staph. aureus or gram negative organism (in the setting of aspiration).
- Septic emboli (e.g., drug abuse, septic endocarditis) commonly form small abscesses that are better seen on CT as multiple ill-defined nodules with central cavitation +/− air fluid levels (see Figure 2.52).
- Abscess wall is usually thin (in contrast to cavitating neoplasm, where wall is often thick, lobular, and asymmetric) (see Figure 2.53).

Cavitatory masses in the lung
- Abscess
- TB
- Septic emboli
- Lung cancer (squamous)
- Some metastases (squamous—cervical cancer, head and neck cancer)
- Wegener granulomatosis
- Rheumatoid nodules
- Rarely: infarcts

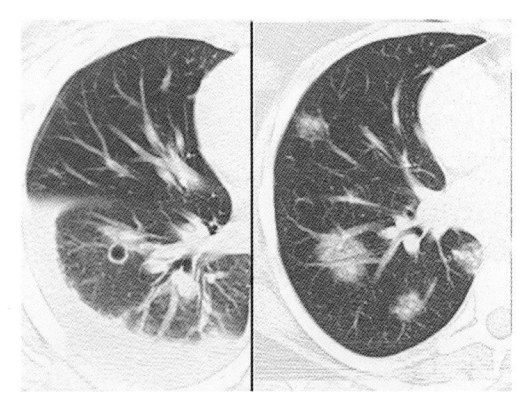

Figure 2.52 Two patients with septic emboli. The left image shows cavitations in RLL and a pleural effusion (patient with tricuspid endocarditis), and the right image shows non-cavitary septic emboli (drug abuser).

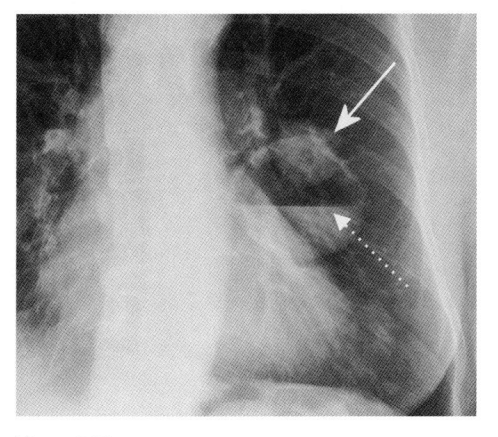

Figure 2.53 Two lung abscesses in the LLL. Note the thin wall and the air fluid level in the larger abscess (dotted arrow).

COPD and emphysema

CXRs are frequently normal in mild to moderate disease. In more severe disease, there are characteristic radiographic findings:
- Hyperinflation—best seen as flattening of hemidiaphragms on the lateral radiograph.
  - Diaphragm dome should be >3 cm above a line from anterior to posterior costophrenic sulcus.

- Increased retrosternal space.
- Narrow heart and mediastinum.
- Sparse/attenuated vascular markings.
- Bullous changes, most common at apices, may depress hila.
- On CT, the attenuated vessels and alveolar destruction are more clearly seen, with large airspaces.

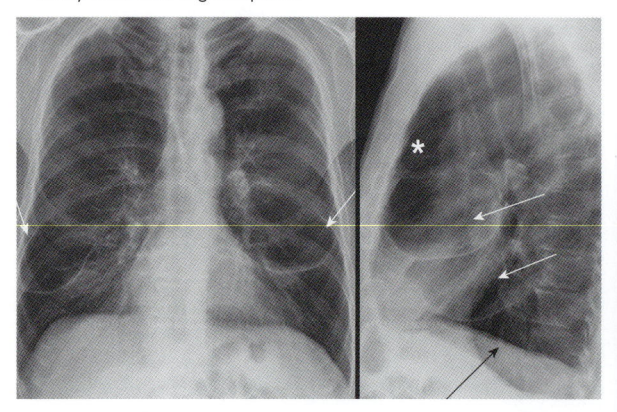

Figure 2.54 Patient with emphysema showing flattened hemidiaphrams (black arrow), increased retrosternal space (*) and bullae (white arrows). Note the attenuated lung markings in the apices.

WARNING:
Large bullae in patients with emphysema can be mistaken for a pneumothorax. Insertion of a chest tube into a bulla can be fatal. Look for the pleural line of a pneumothorax. If in doubt, do a CT.

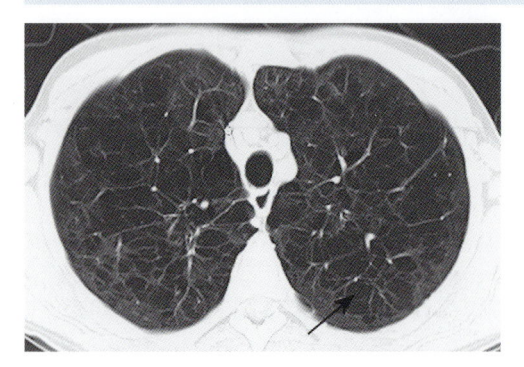

Figure 2.55 CT scan in a patient with emphysema showing lung destruction seen as areas of increased lucency and bullous changes (arrow).

Bronchiectasis

- Bronchial thickening and dilatation with increased interstitial markings. Dilatation may be saccular, cylindrical or cystic (e.g., CF).
- Distribution:
  - Typically basilar if due to recurrent infections.
  - Cystic fibrosis patients typically worst in the apices.
- Best seen on CT (see Figure 2.56 for findings).

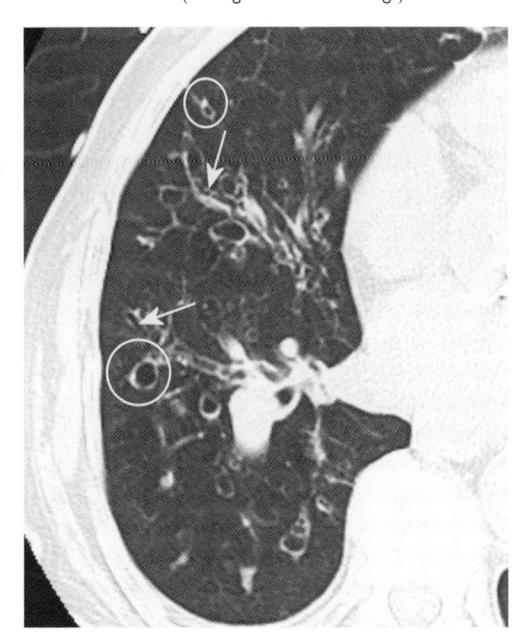

Figure 2.56 Bronchi larger than accompanying pulmonary artery, appears as a "signet ring" (circles), bronchi seen too peripherally (arrows).

Sarcoidosis

Depending on the stage of the disease, radiographic findings can be normal, or there can be adenopathy and/or interstitial changes. CXR is abnormal in about 70% of patients.

<u>Imaging findings:</u>

- Increased reticulo-nodular ("lines and nodules") interstitial markings.
- Mediastinal adenopathy, most common is R paratracheal and bilateral hila (see Figures 2.42 and 2.57).
- Advanced disease may have coarse interstitial changes due to fibrosis, most severe in upper lobes (see Figure 2.57).
- Multiple tiny nodules on CT, tending to follow the bronchovascular tree and pleural surfaces including fissures.

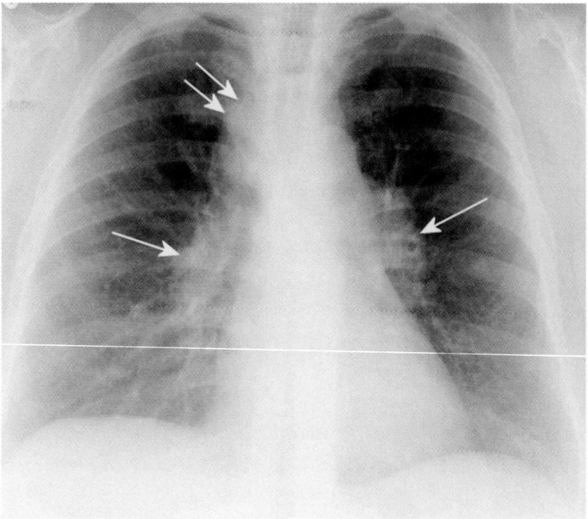

Figure 2.57 Patient with sarcoidosis showing bilateral hilar (single arrows) and R paratracheal (double arrows) adenopathy as well as diffusely increased reticulo-nodular interstitial markings.

Lung cancer
A full discussion of lung-cancer subtypes, staging, and treatment is not possible in this format. Lung cancer is frequently clinically silent until large, unless found as an incidental finding or by screening CXR or CT.

Imaging findings:
- Mass or nodule within the lung parenchyma, usually with ill-defined, lobular or spiculated margins. +/− cavitation (see Figure 2.58).
- Hilar mass.
- Lobar atelectasis or postobstructive pneumonia from a proximal lesion.
- Segmental or lobar consolidation (especially BAC).
- Enlarged hilar/mediastinal nodes from metastasis.
- Distant metastases (e.g., presenting with brain or bone metastases).

Lung cancer subtypes

Non-small cell carcinoma: 85% of lung cancer is non-small cell, which includes squamous cell carcinoma, adenocarcinoma and its subtypes, and large cell carcinoma.
- Squamous cell carcinomas may cavitate and are typically parahilar.
- Adenocarcinomas are usually more peripheral with variable growth rates (includes bronchoalveolar carcinoma).

Small cell carcinoma: and other unusual types such as carcinoid are less common. Small cell cancers are typically central.

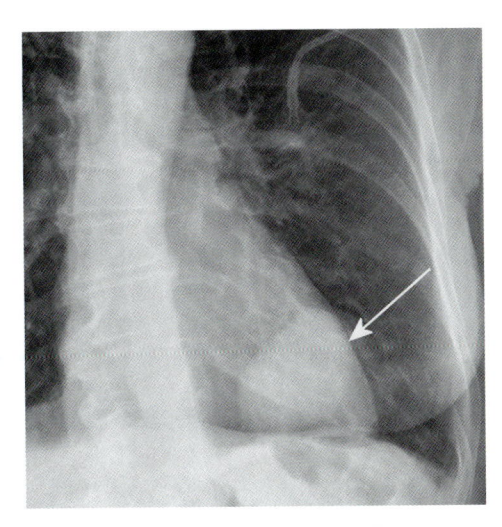

Figure 2.58 Large adenocarcinoma in the LLL. The mass is seen as a double density through the heart.

Bronchoalveolar carcinoma (BAC)
Bronchoalveolar carcinoma has multiple imaging presentations:
- Slow growing SPN (may be PET negative).
- Lobar or segmental chronic air space opacity – can look identical to pneumonia (see Figure 2.36).
- "Ground glass" mixed density mass opacity on CT.
- Multifocal bilateral opacities (the most aggressive form).

> **Bronchoalveolar carcinoma: special considerations**
> - Always consider BAC when treating a patient for a presumed pneumonia when radiographs do not improve and/or symptoms are mild/absent.
> - PET negative lung nodules need to be followed by CT/CXR, depending on size, because they may be slow growing BAC.
> - No consensus guidelines on how long to follow with imaging (2+ years).

Staging of lung cancer
Lung cancer is staged (Stage I–IV) by assessing mass size and location, nodal spread, and distant metastatic disease using the TNM system.
- The most accurate staging uses a combination of PET-FDG scans and CECT.
- PET provides information about both loco-regional lymph node and distant metastases. See p. 423 for further details regarding PET-CT staging.

- Nodal spread progresses in a typical pattern:
  - To ipsilateral hilar nodes → ipsilateral mediastinal nodes → contralateral mediastinal and hilar nodes.
- Gadolinium enhanced brain MRI may be indicated (depending on neurological symptoms, mass size, histology, e.g., small cell cancer).

Lung cancer screening

Lung cancer screening is not indicated in the low risk population, and remains controversial in the high risk population (smokers>50) because of the cost, risk (radiation, biopsies, etc,)/benefit ratio.

<u>The National Lung Cancer Screening Trial (2011) showed:</u>
- A 20% decrease in mortality for high risk patients screened with CT rather than CXR.
- A very high incidence of lung nodules found, requiring follow-up or biopsy, and resulting in low specificity.

Vascular conditions

Aortic dissection

CT angiography is the modality of choice to diagnose aortic dissection and traumatic injury, and assess extent and involvement of branch vessels. (MRA is an alternative in some patients; see "MRA," p. 13).

<u>Aortic dissection:</u>

A tear in the intima allows blood to track into the media layer of the vessel wall, creating a "false lumen."
- A flap is seen as a thin hypodense line across the lumen of the vessel, separating the true lumen (TL) and false lumen (FL).
- The TL and FL may have equal or different densities depending on the flow through them (see Figure 2.59).
- If flap extends into branch vessels; vessels may originate from either lumen.
- Categorized into Stanford A (involves ascending aorta +/− descending) or B (descending only).
  - Stanford A requires open surgical repair.
  - Stanford B may be medical or endovascular treatment.

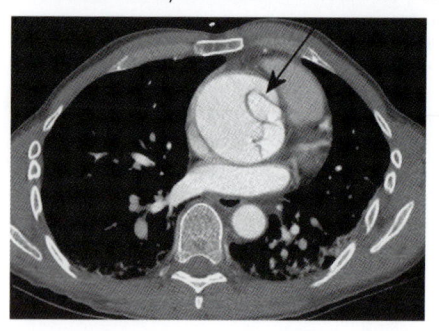

Figure 2.59 Large ascending aortic aneurysm with a non-ruptured dissection. Note the serpiginous intimal flap (arrow) and the different densities of the TL and FL, indicating different flow rates.

CHEST CT

<u>Leaks:</u>
Leaks from vessels (usually aorta)—either due to trauma or dissection—are seen as focal irregularities in the aortic wall, with contrast extending outside of the normal lumen (see Figure 2.61).
- May be contained (e.g., pseudoaneurysm).
- Associated peri-aortic mediastinal hematoma.
- May rupture freely into mediastinum, +/− associated L hemothorax.

Blunt traumatic aortic injury (BTAI)
Traumatic rupture of the aorta is a highly fatal injury that requires urgent treatment (usually endovascular stenting). The CXR findings are neither sensitive nor specific and CT angiography should be performed in all patients at significant risk (e.g., high speed MVA).

Radiographic findings (supine trauma AP CXR):
Any of the following may be present (see Figure 2.60).
- Widening of the mediastinum at the level of the aortic arch (on L or bilateral (white solid arrows).
- Loss of the normal contour of the aortic arch (white dotted arrow).
- Loss of the paraortic stripe of the descending aorta (black solid arrow).
- "Left apical capping"—curved opacity in the left apex due to blood flowing up over apex (black dotted arrow).
- Deviation of nasogastric tube, if present, to right.
- Pleural effusions.

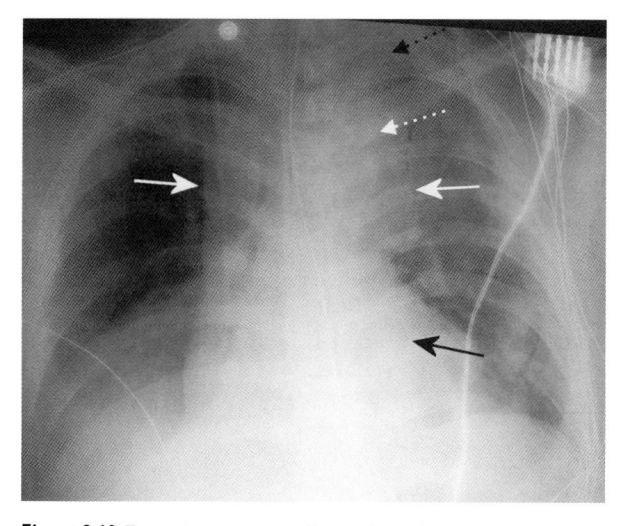

Figure 2.60 Traumatic aortic rupture. See text for explanation.

Findings on CTA (see Figure 2.61):
- Irregularity of the internal or external aortic contour (black arrow), or intimal flap
- Peri-aortic hematoma (soft tissue density material) contiguous with the aortic wall.
- Blood in the mediastinum (white arrow).
- Contrast extending beyond the aortic wall (black arrow).
  - Pseudoaneurysm.
  - Free extravasation into mediastinum or pleural space.
- Hemothorax (*).

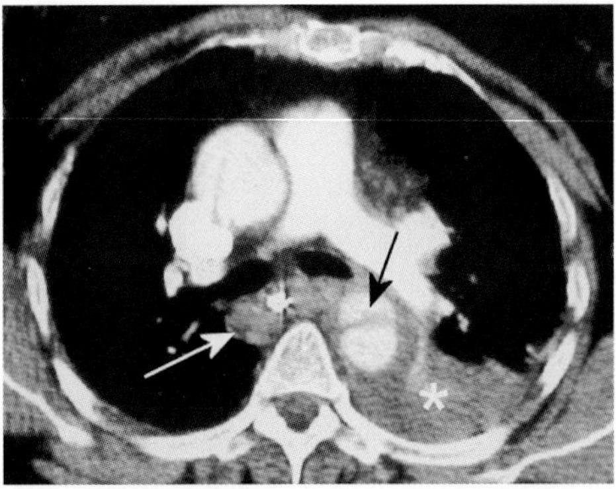

Figure 2.61 Traumatic aortic rupture on CT. See text for explanation.

Pulmonary emboli

CXR is important to perform to exclude other cause of patient's symptoms before a CT is requested (e.g., pneumonia, pneumothorax).

Radiographic findings:
- Often normal; when abnormal, usually non-specific findings such as pleural effusions or linear atelectasis.
- Decreased perfusion to one or more areas of the lung, creating a hyperlucency or attenuated vessels (Westermark's sign)—rare.
- Focal wedge shaped pleural based opacity (Hampton's hump) from a pulmonary infarct—rare.
- Enlarged pulmonary arteries.

CT is the gold standard for the diagnosis of PE with a negative predictive value of 99% for emboli in first- and second-order vessels.
Accuracy will depend on the quality of the study (patient size, respiratory artifact, bolus quality, and timing). The majority of the contrast should be in the pulmonary arteries.

CT findings:
- Low-attenuation-filling defects in the pulmonary arteries, usually surrounded by contrast if acute.
  - Thrombi should be seen on > 1 slice.
- Chronic emboli may adhere to walls of pulmonary arteries.
- Signs of right heart strain: enlargement of RV +/− RA, deviation of intraventricular septum to L (poor prognostic factor).
- Pleural effusions.
- Pulmonary infarcts—wedge-shaped, pleural based consolidation.

Patients who are allergic to contrast, have renal insufficiency, or some other contraindication to IV contrast should be referred for a V/Q scan (p. 444). See p. 29 for management of pregnant patients.

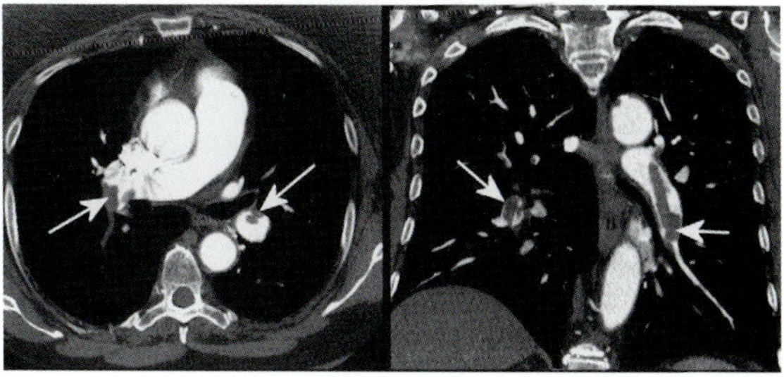

Figure 2.62 Patient with multiple large filling defects bilaterally in the pulmonary arteries due to acute pulmonary emboli

Cardiac imaging

Cardiac CT/Coronary CTA

Currently, the chief use of cardiac CT is for the non-invasive evaluation of coronary arterial atherosclerotic plaque and stenosis. The heart can be imaged in different ways by CT depending on the indication. All studies need to be ECG-gated (synchronized with the heart beat). Patients may need medications to slow their heart rates and/or vasodilate their coronary arteries.
- Non-contrast studies are used to evaluate for coronary artery calcium scoring with a single image acquired in end-diastole.
- Contrast is given for coronary artery CT angiography (contrast in the coronary arteries) and when morphological and functional information is needed (contrast in the ventricles/myocardium).
  - Coronary CTA acquires a single image usually in end-diastole.
  - Contrast cardiac CT acquires images throughout the cardiac cycle.

Applications for cardiac CT imaging	
Noncontrast cardiac CT	Coronary calcium scoring for risk stratification
	Anomalous coronary arteries (modality of choice)
Coronary CTA	Coronary artery stenotic/occlusive disease
	Coronary artery bypass graft evaluation
Contrast cardiac CT	Cardiac morphology and quantitative systolic function
	Pulmonary-vein mapping for radiofrequency ablation of atrial arrhythmias
	Congenital-heart-disease evaluation
	Cardiac masses and pericardial disease
	Valve evaluation (stenosis)

Coronary calcium scoring
Screening study in asymptomatic individuals with intermediate risk for a major coronary event (clinical risk stratification, e.g., Framingham risk score):
- No intravenous contrast or patient preparation necessary.
- Relatively low radiation dose compared to contrast CT evaluation of the heart and coronary arteries.

<u>Imaging findings:</u>
The amount of calcium in the coronary arteries is given a score ("Agatston score") dependent on the amount of calcium present and the density of the calcium (in Houndsfield units).
- The risk of coronary artery disease increases with a higher score.
- Scores >100 are associated with increased risk of a cardiac event (>2% annually over next 5 years).
- Scores >1,000 have a 20% risk of a cardiac event within the next year.
- These scores identify overall risk and do not identify which vessels are stenotic. For that you need CTA or conventional coronal angiography.

Coronary CTA
The gold standard for imaging coronary stenosis is catheter angiography. Symptomatic patients with high pre-test probability should proceed directly to diagnostic catheterization, because they may also need revascularization with percutaneous balloon angioplasty and stenting.

<u>Indications for CTA:</u>
- Symptomatic patients (angina) with intermediate pre-test probability for coronary stenosis.
- Patients with coronary anomalies.

<u>CTA technique:</u>
- High volume, high injection rate IV contrast administration with rapid helical image acquisition. ECG gating is performed.
- The volumetric imaging data is often reconstructed in multiple cross-sectional and 3D formats (see Color Plate 1, Figure 2.64).

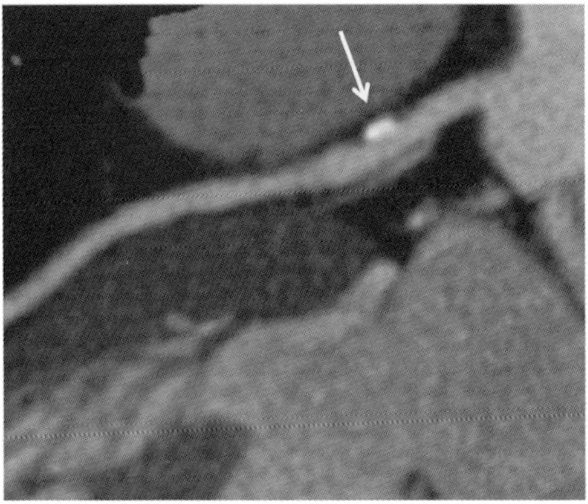

Figure 2.63 Mixed calcific and noncalcific plaque (arrow) producing <50% stenosis in the proximal left anterior descending coronary artery.

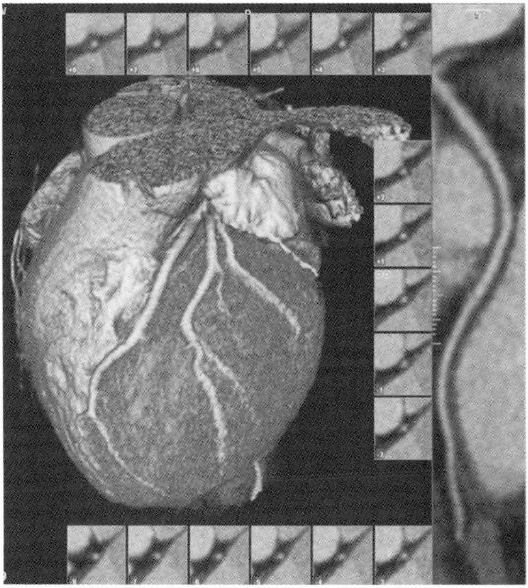

Figure 2.64 3D volumetric depiction of the heart in color, as well as reformatted images along the long axis and short axis of one coronary artery. See Color Plate 1.

CTA findings and performance:
- Stenoses can be quantitatively measured by software.
- High negative predictive value (>97%) for excluding a potentially hemodynamically stenosis (>50% diameter stenosis).
- Positive predictive value is somewhat less, particularly in patients with heavily calcified coronary arteries.

> Radiation dose for coronary CTA is comparable to radionuclide stress imaging and catheter angiography.
> - Newer CT technologies that reduce radiation dose by over half are becoming available.

Cardiac MRI

Cardiac MRI allows noninvasive evaluation of cardiac morphology and function. Like cardiac CT, MR imaging uses ECG-gating and breath holding. Both static and cine (movie-loop) images can be obtained. Gadolinium is required to evaluate cardiomyopathies and for MR angiography (MRA).

Indications
- Ischemic cardiomyopathy (assessing extent of infarction and viable myocardium and to determine areas that may benefit from revascularization).
- Non-ischemic cardiomyopathy (evaluation of abnormal myocardial deposits such as fat or amyloid).
- Valvular heart disease (valve thickening and size, abnormal movement, regurgitant volume).
- Pericardial thickening and effusion, constrictive physiology.
- Comprehensive congenital-heart-disease evaluation including MRA of the great vessels.
- Contrast-enhanced studies are often performed dynamically (i.e., multiiple images are obtained during the cardiac cycle gated to the ECG).

Technique
By exploiting flow phenomenon and inherent tissue differences between myocardium and blood, non-contrast cardiac MR specific sequences can be performed. These make the blood pool (chamber and vessel lumens) appear:
- Dark (called "black blood").
- Bright (called "bright blood").
- Static image slices are obtained during diastole to see fine structural details, such as the "black blood" technique called Double Inversion Recovery.
- Imaging throughout the cardiac cycle allows visual evaluation of motion, as well as quantitative analysis of cardiac chamber function and of vascular flow.

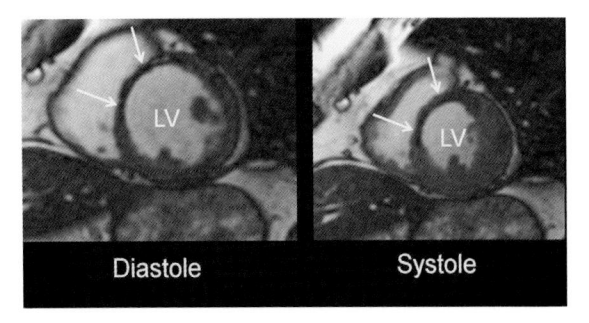

Figure 2.65 Non-contrast short axis images of the heart ('bright blood' technique, see chapter 1, Radiology Essentials, p. 13) in diastole (left) and systole (right) showing the lack of thickening of the anteroseptum (arrows) in systole in a patient with an anteroseptal infarct.

Table 2.3 Cardiac CT versus Cardiac MR

STRENGTHS	LIMITATIONS
Cardiac CT	
Fast volumetric imaging (one breath-hold)	Uses ionizing radiation
Requires contrast (except Ca scoring)	Contrast allergies and renal failure
Higher spatial resolution	Patient preparation/drugs for heart rate reduction
Safe with implantable devices	Ectopy and arrhythmias impair or preclude study
Evaluation of extracardiac structures	Lower temporal resolution limits the dynamic information
Cardiac MR	
No radiation	Slice-by-slice imaging; studies may take 1 or more hrs (many breath holds)
Flow quantification and soft-tissue characterization better	Safety issues with many medical devices
Structure and function does not require contrast	Lower spatial resolution limits use for coronary artery evaluation
No patient preparation/drugs	Claustrophobia
	Noisy, heating potential
	Artifacts with ferrous clips, etc.

Vascular MRA
See chapter 1, Radiology Essentials p. 13 for technique.

Aortic dissection and aneurysm
Acute thoracic aortic dissection is most appropriately evaluated by aortic CTA. In unstable patients or patients who cannot receive radiographic contrast secondary to prior severe allergic reaction, transesophageal echo is the best alternative.

<u>Indications for MRA of the aorta:</u>
- Patient's with IV contrast allergy or renal failure.
  - Gadolinium is not always required, as "bright blood" sequences can be used.
- Young patients who may require serial imaging follow-up (e.g., Marfan syndrome).

<u>MRA findings:</u>
- The intimal flap is seen as a dark line between the true and false lumens. Different flow velocities in the two lumens may appear as different signal intensities (see Figure 2.66).
- Thoracic aortic aneurysms can be monitored for progressive dilatation versus stability with CTA or MRA.

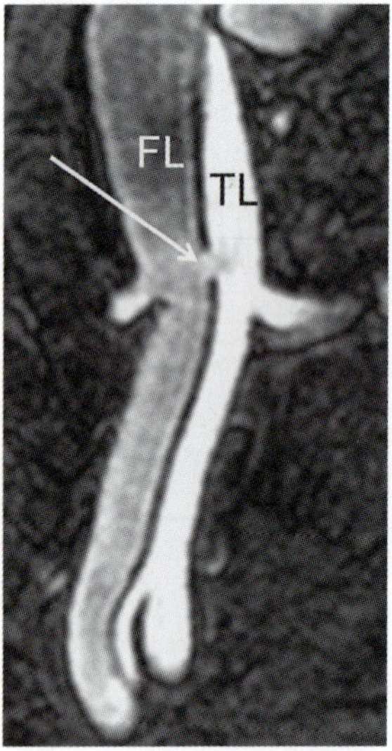

Figure 2.66 Coronal thick-slice MIP image of an abdominal aortic dissection. The true lumen (TL) appears brighter than the false lumen (FL) due to more flow. The two lumens are separated by the dark line of the intimal flap. A communication (arrow) is present between the two lumens, a "reentry" tear.

CARDIAC IMAGING

Pulmonary emboli
Rarely evaluated with MRA, given the more rapid acquisition and greater spatial resolution of CT pulmonary angiography. Ventilation-perfusion scintigraphy (V/Q scan) is the recommended alternative to CT.

Don't miss diagnoses
Foreign body aspiration p. 307
- Mediastinal shift.
- Unilateral hyperlucent lung.

Traumatic aortic injury p. 105
<u>CXR:</u>
- Widened mediastinum, loss aortic stripe/arch.
- Deviation of nasogastric tube to right, left apical cap.

<u>CT:</u>
- Blood around aorta, focal irregularity to wall or contrast extravasation.

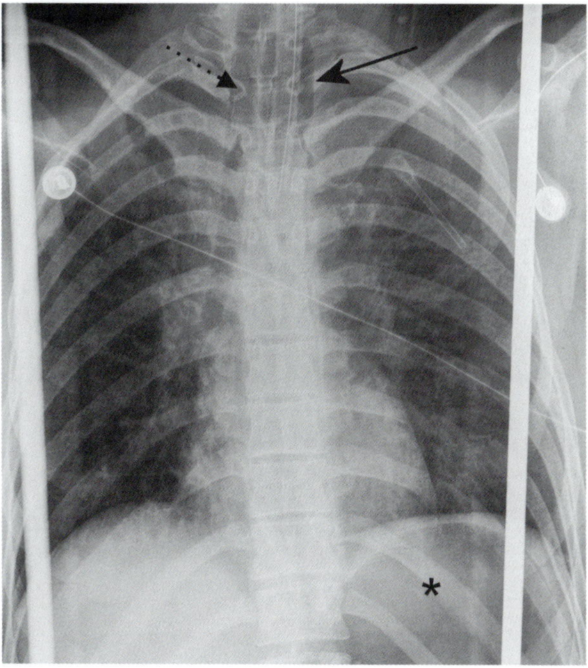

Figure 2.67 Endotracheal tube malpositioned in esophagus. You should NOT see the balloon (black solid arrow) on an ETT if in the trachea. Note the trachea displaced lateral to the balloon (black dotted arrow) and the distended stomach(*).

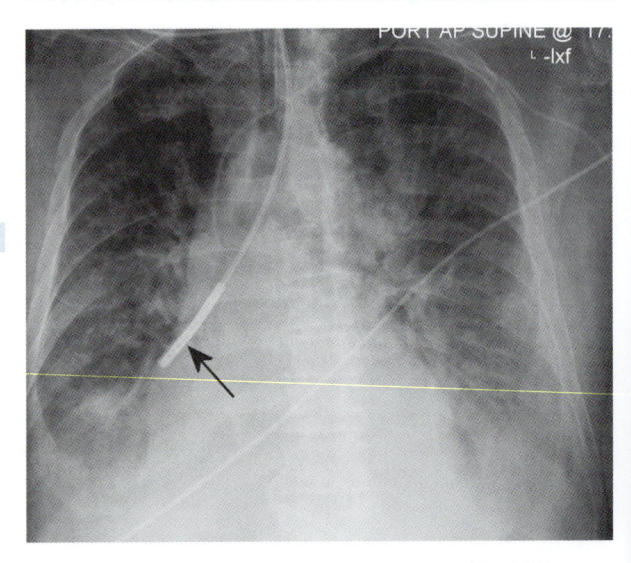

Figure 2.68 Dobhoff tube in the RLL bronchus (arrow). L PICC and ETT correctly positioned.

Tension pneumothorax p. 70
- Pneumothorax with variable degree collapse.
- Mediastinal shift +/− diaphragmatic depression.

Malpositioned tubes and lines p. 52
- ETT in esophagus.
- ETT in RMB.
- NGT or Dobhoff in airway.

References

Cho J, Lewis P, "Lines and Tubes Radiology Learning Module." Available from: https://www.mededportal.org/publication/8399.

Collins J, Stern EJ. *Chest Radiology: The Essentials*. New York: Lippincott Williams & Wilkins, 2007. 340 pp.

Goodman LR. *Felson's Principles of Chest Roentgenology: A Programmed Text*. 2nd ed. Philadelphia, PA: Saunders, 1999.

Hansell DM, Bankier AA, MacMahon H, "Fleischner Society: Glossary of Terms for Thoracic Imaging." *Radiology* 2008, 246(3):697–722.

Heber MacMahon JHM,, Austin JHM, Gamsu G, Herold CJ, Jett JR, Naidich DP, Patz, EF Jr, and Swensen SJ. "Guidelines for Management of Small Pulmonary Nodules Detected on CT Scans: A Statement from the Fleischner Society." *Radiology* 2005, 237: 395–400.

University of Virginia website CT and CXR anatomy: http://www.med-ed.virginia.edu/courses/rad/

Chapter 3

Abdomen/Pelvis Imaging

Nancy McNulty, MD and Anne M. Silas, MD

Radiographs *116*
  Normal anatomy *116*
  How do I read a radiograph of the abdomen? *117*
  Patterns of disease *120*
  Common conditions evaluable with radiography *130*
CT *136*
  How are images acquired and reviewed? *136*
  Normal anatomy *140*
  How do I read a CT of the abdomen? *141*
  Patterns of disease *142*
MRI *151*
  How are images acquired? *151*
  What do normal structures look like on MRI? *153*
  Patterns of disease *153*
Common conditions evaluated with CT and MRI *154*
  Trauma *154*
  Appendicitis *160*
  Diverticulitis *161*
  Crohn disease *162*
  Pancreatitis *163*
  Aortic aneurysms and dissection *163*
  Cirrhosis *166*
  Liver masses *166*
  Pancreatic masses *171*
  Choledocholithiasis and pancreatico-biliary abnormalities *172*
  Urolithiasis and hydronephrosis *173*
  Renal masses and hematuria *175*
  Adrenal masses *176*
Common conditions best evaluated with MRI *178*
  Acute abdomen in the pregnant and young patient *178*
  Uterus *179*
  Ovary *179*
Don't miss diagnoses *180*
References *182*

Radiographs

Abdominal radiographs are also known as "KUBs" (Kidneys, Ureters, Bladder). In this book, the term abdominal radiographs will be used.

How are images acquired?

No special patient preparation is necessary. Images can be acquired portably or in the radiology department. The views obtained will depend on both the clinical question and the mobility of the patient.

Views

Supine
AP image including the diaphragms through the pubic symphysis in the field of view.

Supine and upright
- AP images, again including diaphragms through pubic symphysis in the field of view.
- The upright image allows assessment of air-fluid levels in the stomach and bowel in patients with suspected ileus or bowel obstruction.

Decubitus
- Obtained with the patient lying with their right side (right lateral decubitus) or left side (left lateral decubitus) down.
- Performed in patients who are unable to stand for upright images, but are suspected of having free air, bowel obstruction, or ileus.
- A left lateral decubitus is more sensitive for free air (it layers lateral to the liver) and is performed more often than right lateral decubitus.

Acute abdominal series
- Includes AP, upright or decubitus, and upright CXR.
- This series optimally detects pneumoperitoneum, and also allows assessment for chest pathology that may present as abdominal pain.

Indications
- Initial evaluation of abdominal pain.
  - Especially if initial concern is for obstruction or free air.
- Initial evaluation of nausea/vomiting.
- Assess enteric tube positioning.
- Assess amount of stool.
- Follow up of ileus, obstruction, and other pathologies.

Normal anatomy

Hollow viscera
The stomach and intestines are visible primarily when they contain air.
- Most air seen in the bowel is swallowed.
- Air-fluid levels in the stomach are normal.
- In the small bowel, it is normal to see a few air fluid levels, however numerous air fluid levels are abnormal.
- Air fluid levels generally should not be present in the colon.

Where is the air?
Stomach
- Recognizable by the rugal folds and sub-diaphragmatic position.
- Can be quite large and extend toward pelvis.

Small intestine
- Recognizable by the plicae circularis (aka: valvulae conniventes). These are thin, uniform folds extending circumferentially across the entire diameter of the bowel loop.
- In the jejunum, there are many plica packed close together, whereas in the ileum, they are shorter, less numerous, and more widely spaced.
- Normally < 2.5 cm in transverse diameter.

Large intestine
- Recognizable by the semilunar folds that create the haustra (saccular appearing).
- Semilunar folds are thicker than small bowel folds, and do not extend across the circumference of the loop.
- Large intestine contains stool, which appears as tiny air bubbles inter-mixed with soft tissue material.
- Normal cecum is < 8 cm, and normal transverse colon is < 6 cm; the descending and sigmoid colon are smaller.

(see Figure 3.1)

Solid viscera

Liver, spleen, kidneys, adrenal glands, and pancreas.
- Not readily identifiable on radiography because:
  - They are all similar soft tissue density; there is no contrast between them.
  - They are superimposed on 2D images (i.e., radiographs).
- If adequate fat surrounds the organ, there may be enough contrast in density to render them visible on x-rays. Most commonly seen:
  - Inferior liver edge, inferior spleen edge, and renal outlines (see Figure 3.2).

Intraperitoneal compartment
- A potential space, rendered visible only by the pathologic presence of air within it ("free air").
- Extends from the diaphragms to the pelvic cul-de-sac.

Retroperitoneal compartment
- Occupied by the second to fourth portions of the duodenum, parts of ascending and descending colon, pancreas, adrenal glands, kidneys, aorta, IVC, and fat.
- The low density fat intervening between the retroperitoneal structures allows them to be visible in some patients (see Figure 3.2).

How do I read a radiograph of the abdomen?
A search pattern is essential. Remember "stones, bones, mass and gas," and you won't forget to look at any structures. Leave the gas for last, because it is doubtful you will forget to look at the bowel!

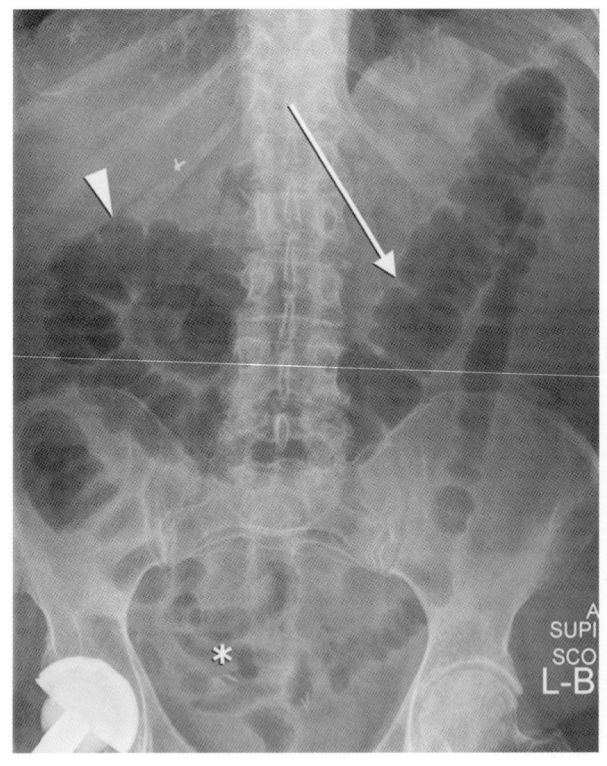

Figure 3.1 Supine abdomen shows normal haustra (arrowhead) and semilunar folds (arrow) of colon, and normal air filled loops of distal small bowel (*).

Search strategies

Stones

Most contain calcium and are radioopaque.
- Look in the expected location of the gallbladder (although most gallstones are not radio-opaque), kidneys, ureter, and bladder.
- Small stones may be obscured by stool.
- Also look for linear or parallel calcifications, which are seen with atherosclerosis, in the arterial walls.

Bones

Look at the spine, pelvis, and lower ribs for unexpected lytic or sclerotic bone lesions.

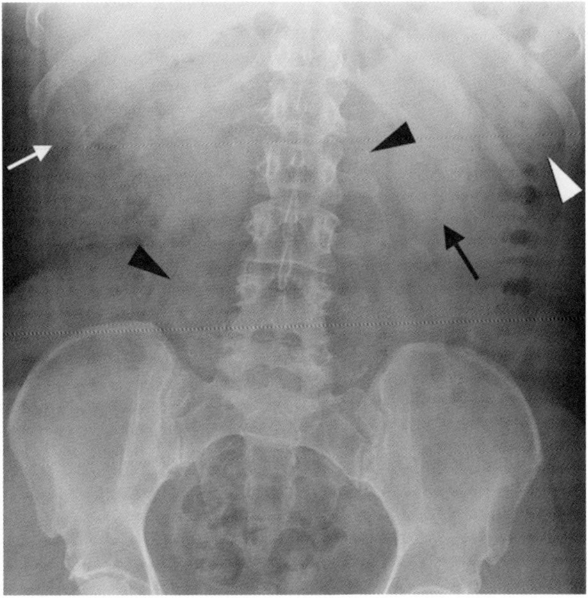

Figure 3.2 The inferior edge of the liver (white arrow), inferior left kidney (black arrow), inferior edge of spleen (white arrowhead), and lateral borders of the psoas muscles (black arrowheads) are visible due to the contrast in density between them and the adjacent fat.

Mass

Abdominal masses are hard to identify on radiography, however, there may be subtle clues that one is present:
- Look for displacement of bowel, such as superiorly out of the pelvis due to a large pelvic mass, peripherally from an aortic aneurysm, or medial displacement of the stomach from splenomegaly (see Figure 3.12, p. 129.)
- The bladder may be displaced by pelvic masses/hematomas.
- Look for an area of diffusely increased density; sometimes seen with large masses.

Gas

Evaluate the pattern of intestinal gas:
- Is it evenly distributed in small and large bowel?
- Is the small or large bowel dilated?
- Is there wall or fold thickening?

Look for extra-luminal air and for air within the bowel wall:
- Is the gas located anatomically where bowel loops should be?
- Look under hemidiaphragms (or liver edge on decub study)
- Look for gas over the obturator foramen, which could indicate an inguinal hernia.

CHAPTER 3 Abdomen/Pelvis Imaging

Lines and tubes
Nasogastric or orogastric tube (NGT)
Have a radio-opaque line that is discontinuous at the proximal side port. Both the tube tip and side port should be in the stomach.

Feeding tube (aka Dobhoff tube-DHT)
- Have a weighted radio-opaque tip that aids in placement, helping the bowel peristalsis to carry it into the duodenum.
- The tip should be positioned beyond the pylorus.

> If a requisition says "check NGT/DHT placement" and you don't see a tube on the KUB, you must suspect that the tube is in the thorax, either in the esophagus or mal-positioned elsewhere.
> **Ideally, these "check tube" studies should include the lower chest.**

Femoral vascular catheters
- Tip should be in the external or common iliac vein.
- Make sure that catheter follows the expected course of the vein and isn't in a side branch such as the circumflex iliac.

Drainage catheters
- These may be surgically placed (typically straight catheters), or percutaneously placed (typically pigtail catheters).
- Look for change in position from prior films, or for retraction or unwinding of the pigtail.

Patterns of disease

Air that shouldn't be there
A collection of air that is not within the stomach or intestine is abnormal, except in the recent post-operative patient. Abnormal air can reside in the peritoneal cavity, retroperitoneum, bowel wall, biliary tree, and portal veins. Each has a characteristic appearance.

Pneumoperitoneum
Upright CXR:
- Is the most sensitive radiograph to detect free air.
- Visible as lucency outlining the undersurface of the hemidiaphragms.
- Can demonstrate small amounts, although less sensitive than CT (see Figure 3.3).

Decubitus abdomen:
- Obtain when upright CXR is not possible: patient cannot stand.
- Free air will accumulate non-dependently, creating a crescent of lucency between the lateral liver edge and abdominal wall.

Supine abdomen:
Large amounts of free air may be visible, but insensitive for small volumes.
- *Falciform ligament*: may be outlined by non-dependent air (see Figure 3.4).
- *Football sign*: a central lucency over the abdomen, seen with large amounts of free air, the falciform ligament is seen as the "laces."

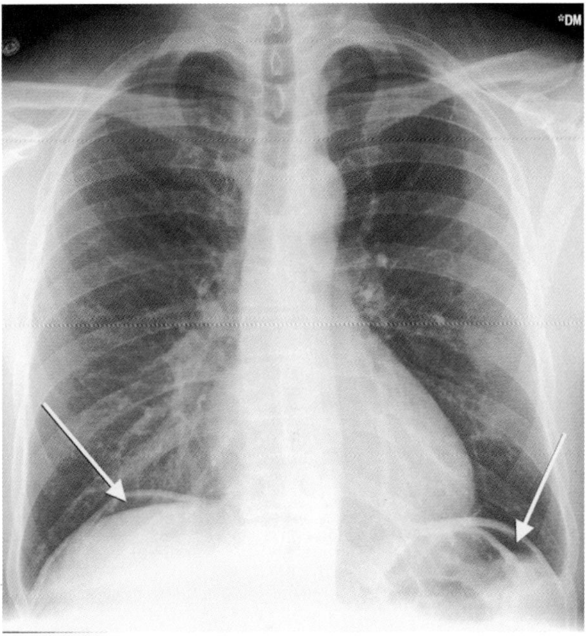

Figure 3.3 Free air collects under the right and left hemidiaphragms on this upright CXR (arrows).

- *Rigler's sign*: free air outside small bowel loops/stomach, adjacent to intraluminal air renders both sides of the bowel wall visible (see Figure 3.5).

Retroperitoneal air

<u>In the upper abdomen:</u>
- Outlines and parallels the psoas muscles—the lucent air looks streaky, linear, and vertically oriented.
- Outlines the retroperitoneal organs—borders of kidneys may appear much more distinct.

<u>In the lower abdomen</u>
Retroperitoneal air is more difficult to identify, as it is more irregular in configuration (see Figure 3.6).

Pneumatosis intestinalis
Air located in the bowel wall. Can occur in the stomach, small or large bowel (see Figure 3.13, p. 130).
- Streaky or linear lucencies, occasionally are circular or ovoid.
- Air parallels the wall and is in both dependent and non-dependent wall.
- Does not change with position (as intraluminal air should).

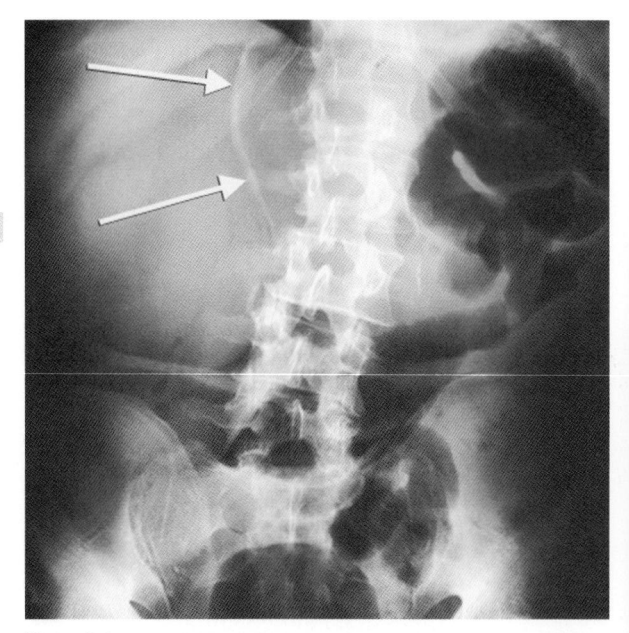

Figure 3.4 Free air. Supine abdomen shows an ovoid lucency over the right upper abdomen due to layering free air. The falciform ligament is rendered visible by the surrounding air (arrows).

Although there are known benign causes of pneumatosis, it is more commonly caused by bowel ischemia.

Pneumobilia
Air in the bile ducts can be normal post-operatively/post-intervention from surgical choledocho-jejunostomy, bililary sphincterotomy, and biliary stent placement. It can also occur with intestinal-biliary fistulas.
- Branching lucencies in the right upper quadrant over the expected location of the central liver (see Figure 3.7).

Portal venous gas
An ominous sign indicating intestinal ischemia.
- Linear, branching lucencies over the liver.
- Can be confused with pneumobilia, however biliary air collects more centrally and portal venous gas more peripherally, corresponding to the direction of flow of fluid (bile versus blood).

Bowel wall thickening
Mural thickening is a non-specific finding, and can be seen with diverse etiologies such as infection, neoplasm, hemorrhage, ischemia, and inflammation. It manifests with the following radiographic findings:

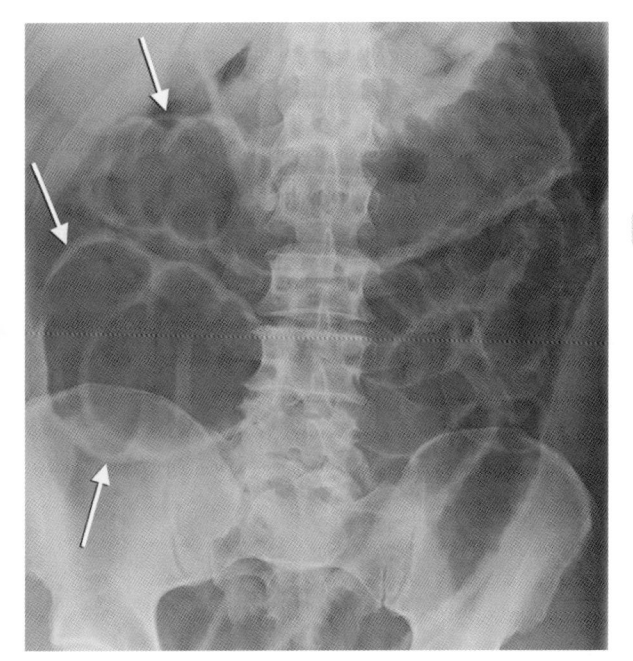

Figure 3.5 Free air. Both sides of the wall of a loop of bowel are visible (arrows). This can only occur if there is air on both sides of the wall; intraluminal and intraperitoneal.

Small bowel
- Plicae circulares > 3 mm thick.
- Wall also thickens, however, this is not readily apparent on radiography. Thickened folds may be smooth or nodular, regular or irregular, depending on the etiology.

Colon
- Wall and folds >3 mm thick.
- Severe thickening is easily identified as thickened semilunar folds (see Figure 3.8).
- "Thumbprinting": it looks as though someone has pressed their thumb from outside the wall into the bowel lumen (see Figure 3.9). This is seen with:
  - Infectious colitis (e.g., pseudomembranous colitis).
  - Inflammatory colitis (e.g., inflammatory bowel disease).
  - Ischemia.

The length of bowel affected, distribution, severity, and presence or absence of air in the bowel wall will aid in the differential diagnosis.

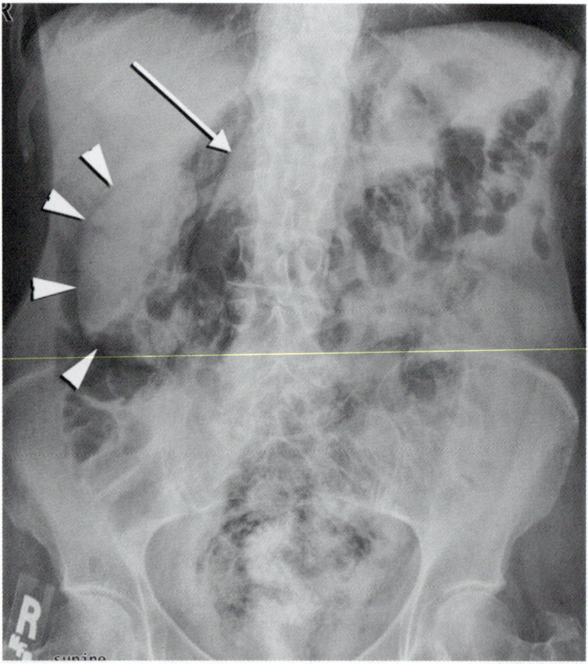

Figure 3.6 Retroperitoneal air. The right psoas margin (arrow) and right renal outline (arrowheads) are sharply demarcated by the air surrounding them. In the lower abdomen, it is more difficult to determine what air is intraluminal versus extraluminal.

Dilated bowel
Small bowel –transverse dimension > 2.5 cm.
Large bowel – transverse dimension >6 cm, cecum >8 cm.
Bowel may be filled with fluid, air, or stool (colon).
- Air filled dilated bowel is readily identified on radiography.
- Since fluid is soft tissue attenuation, fluid filled loops are usually not apparent on radiographs. In some cases, fluid filled, dilated loops of bowel are identifiable as tubular, "sausage" shaped soft tissue densities.
- Concomitant air and fluid in dilated bowel produces air-fluid levels on upright or decubitus films. The pattern of air-fluid levels can aid in the differential diagnosis (see Common Conditions—Ileus, p. 132).

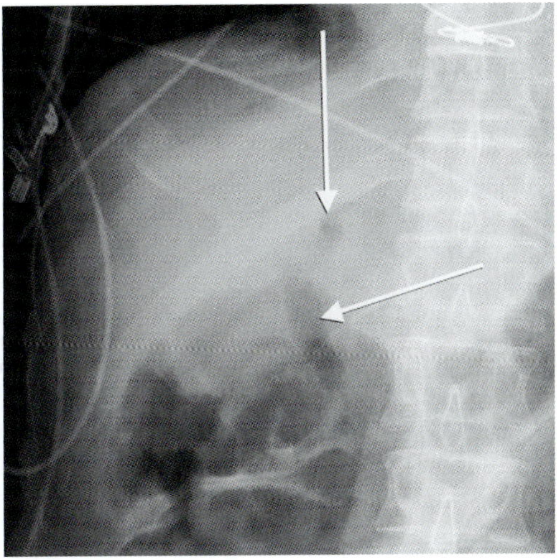

Figure 3.7 Arrow indicates branching lucencies in the right upper quadrant corresponding to air in the biliary tree.

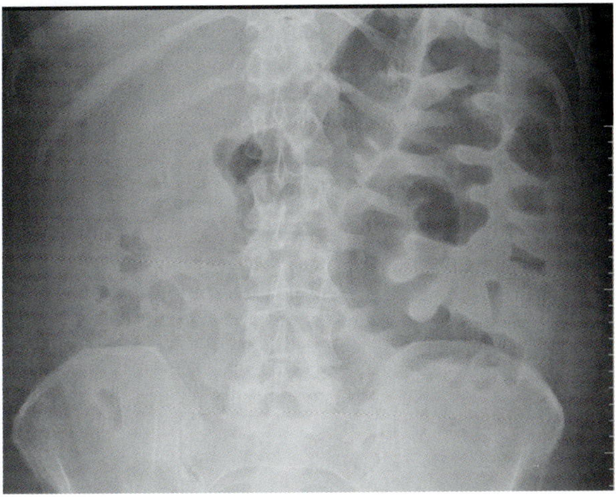

Figure 3.8 Colon wall edema. Supine radiograph of a patient with *e. coli* colitis shows thickened semilunar folds.

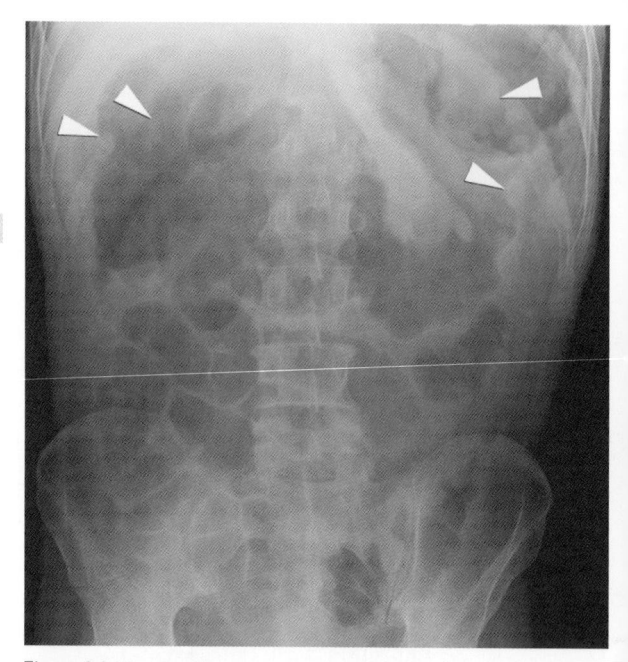

Figure 3.9 Thumbprinting. Supine abdominal radiograph shows air filled, dilated transverse colon with lobular areas of soft tissue density protruding into the lumen of the transverse and descending colon (arrowheads). Marked colon dilatation is consistent with toxic megacolon.

Calcifications
To be visible on radiography, calcifications must have sufficient density to stand out from the soft tissues; not all abdominal calcifications are dense enough to be discretely visible.
- The size of the calcification and the amount of calcium/unit volume influence the conspicuity on radiography.
- The location, morphology, and mobility of calcifications can be used to determine their origins.

Patterns of calcifications

<u>Tubular:</u>
- Linear, discontinuous, parallel tubular calcifications with lucent centers.
- "Tram-track" appearing when the wall is circumferentially calcified.
- Found primarily within blood vessel walls, vas deferens, less commonly the pancreatic or biliary ductal system.

<u>Cystic or egg shell (see Figure 3.10):</u>
- Smooth peripheral rim calcification of a round or ovoid shape.
- Only a portion of the wall may be calcified.
- No internal calcifications.
- Can be anywhere in the abdomen. Aneurysms may have this pattern.

<u>Stones/concretions:</u>
- Round, oval, or faceted. Solid or peripherally densely calcified with lucent center (see Figure 3.11).
- Found in gallbladder, renal collecting system, ureter, and bladder, GI tract lumen, and veins (phleboliths).

<u>Solid mass associated calcifications:</u>
- Irregular, heterogeneous, complex inner density.
- Lymph nodes, uterine leiomyomata, and malignant neoplasms demonstrate this pattern.

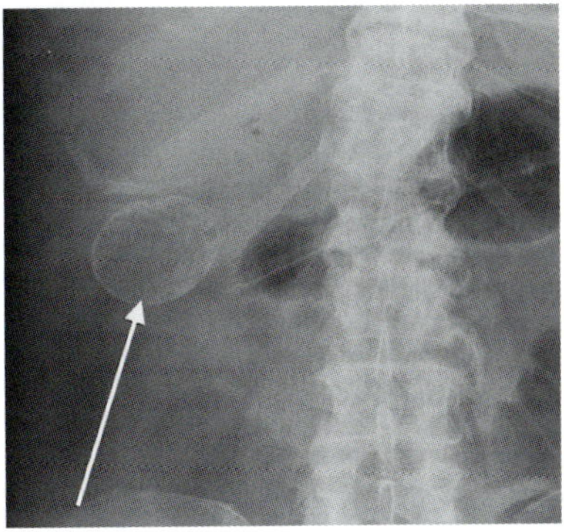

Figure 3.10 Cystic pattern of calcification. Peripheral, continuous rim calcification in the RUQ (arrow) represents calcification within the gallbladder wall, termed "porcelain gallbladder." Just superior to this is a calcified costal cartilage.

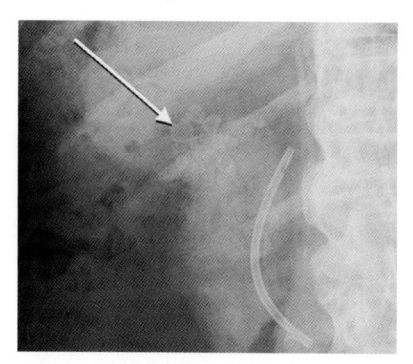

Figure 3.11 Cholelisthiasis. Multiple faceted calculi in the RUQ have peripheral continuous calcification with lucent centers (arrow). They conform to the expected shape of the gallbladder. A common-bile-duct stent is also present.

> Beware of the non-calcified stone! Only 30% of gallstones are calcified, and not all of these contain *enough* calcium to be visible. Therefore, cholelisthiasis cannot be excluded on radiography. Conversely, 90% of renal calculi are radio-opaque.

Masses
- Masses are only "visible" on radiography if they are large enough to cause a focally increased density, or by their displacement of adjacent structures. See "Search Strategies" p. 118.
- If displacement is present, the direction of displacement helps to determine the organ of origin.
- Some masses are rendered visible by intra-lesional air or calcifications

Organomegaly
An enlarged organ is denser on a radiograph, and can displace adjacent structures (see Figure 3.12).

Hepatomegaly
- Soft tissue density extending from RUQ, can extend into the pelvis.
- Bowel loops are displaced infero-medially.
- Enlarged left lobe can displace the stomach inferiorly.

Splenomegaly
- Soft tissue density LUQ, extending inferiorly and medially. May extend to the level of the iliac crest.
- Splenic flexure of the colon displaced inferiorly.
- Fundus of the stomach displaced medially.

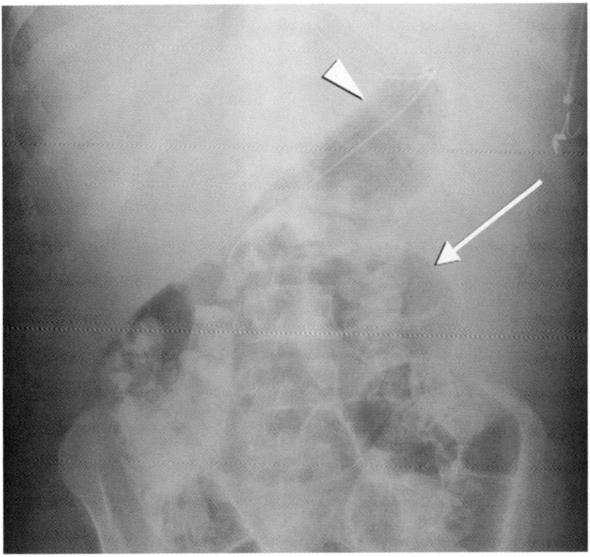

Figure 3.12 Hepatosplenomegaly. The enlarged liver displaces both the hepatic flexure and stomach (with its NGT) inferiorly, flattening the superior surface of the stomach (arrowhead). The markedly enlarged spleen extends beyond the iliac crest and displaces the splenic flexure of the colon medially and inferiorly (arrow).

Common pitfalls
Not obtaining the correct view
If an upright CXR or a left lateral decubitus view is not obtained, free air may be missed.

The "gasless abdomen"
In the absence of intraluminal air, the stomach/intestines may not be visible.
Fluid filled, dilated loops of bowel, and, therefore, bowel obstruction, cannot be excluded.

Is it pneumatosis or stool?
Air in the bowel wall can be difficult to differentiate from air within stool or diverticula.
- Stool typically has a bubbly appearance with small rounded foci of air conforming to the expected shape and position of colon.
- Air within diverticula is usually round or ovoid.
- Pneumatosis is linear and will be seen at the periphery of a loop of bowel. It will be present on supine and upright image in both the dependent and non-dependent walls (intraluminal air should layer non-dependently) (see Figure 3.13).

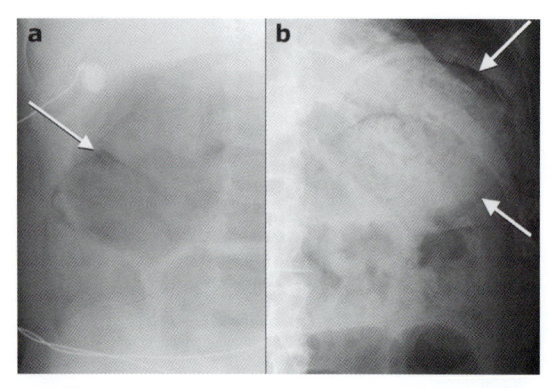

Figure 3.13 Supine KUB images demonstrate pneumatosis in two different patients. (a) Air in the ascending colon wall is linear and streaky, and is visible extending into the semilunar folds (arrows). (b) Pneumatosis in the stomach is linear and involves both sides of the wall (arrows), whereas air within stool in the descending colon is bubbly and round.

Common conditions evaluable with radiography

Radiography is usually the first imaging test obtained in patients with abdominal pain, nausea, and/or vomiting.

Bowel obstruction

The clinical presentation of obstruction and ileus are similar (abdominal pain, distension, nausea, and vomiting), and some radiographic findings such as bowel dilatation and air fluid levels are present in both. There are several imaging features that can help to differentiate them.

Small bowel obstruction

75% of cases are caused by adhesions. Although often discussed as "partial" or "complete," in truth, most small bowel obstructions are partial and can be categorized as high grade or low grade.

Key findings:
- Dilated small bowel.
- Dilatation out of proportion to the colon.
- Multiple small bowel air fluid levels at different heights within same loop.* (see Figures 3.14 and 3.15)
- "String of pearls" sign (see Figure 3.16).

Small bowel loops proximal to the point of obstruction will dilate, thus the number of loops dilated can help to localize the site of obstruction as proximal or distal.

*Air fluid levels at differing heights within the same loop are highly suggestive of obstruction due to the to and fro peristalsis that occurs.

RADIOGRAPHS   131

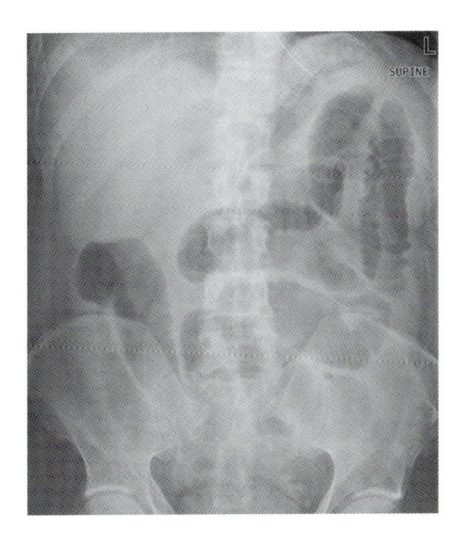

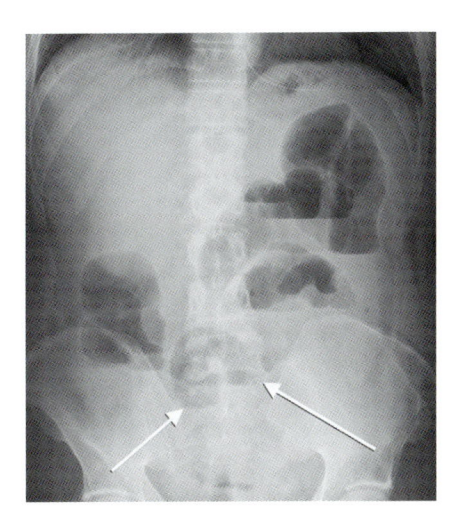

Figures 3.14 and 3.15 Small bowel obstruction. The supine image (3.14) top shows multiple loops of dilated small bowel and little to no air within the colon. NGT has decompressed the stomach. Upright image (3.15) bottom shows multiple air- fluid levels in dilated small bowel. Note the air-fluid levels are at different heights in the central upper pelvis (arrows), highly suggestive of obstruction.

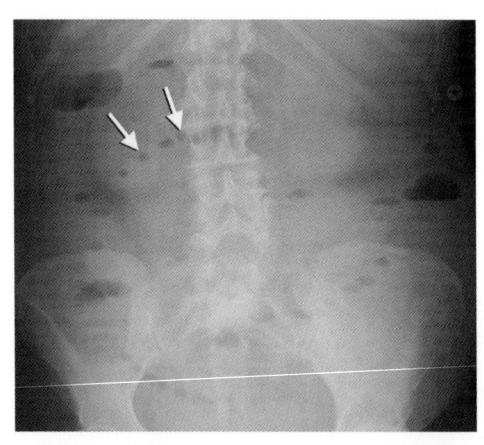

Figure 3.16 String of pearls sign. In the upright position, small amounts of air within filled, dilated small bowel become trapped between the plicae circulares (arrows), causing evenly spaced round lucencies resembling a string of pearls.

Be careful of the presence of an NGT! It can decompress the proximal small bowel, and in cases of proximal small bowel obstruction, can cause a false negative abdominal radiograph.

Colon obstruction
Both benign (stricture) and malignant causes exist. Clinical presentation varies depending on location.

Key findings:
- Colon proximal to the point of obstruction dilates.
- Incompetent ileo-cecal valve can result in distal small bowel dilatation.
- Air fluid levels distal to the hepatic flexure are highly suggestive of obstruction; air fluid levels should *not* be seen in the normal colon.

In colonic obstruction, the cecum is always the most dilated, and when the cecum is > 10 cm in diameter, it is at risk for perforation.

Ileus
Also called "paralytic" or "adynamic," ileus is due to impaired bowel motility. The most common cause is post-operative, and this usually resolves in 4–7 days. Other causes include hypokalemia, gastroenteritis, and medication related.

Never forget to listen to your patient's abdomen! Lack of bowel sounds is much more suggestive of ileus than obstruction (unless its a long term obstruction and resultant ileus has occurred).

Key findings:
- Absent peristalsis; bowel loops accumulate air and fluid and gradually dilate.
- Both colon and small bowel are dilated to a similar degree.
- Air-fluid levels may or may not be present; more common with prolonged ileus (see Figure 3.17).

Focal ileus
A focal ileus can develop adjacent to an inflammatory process such as pancreatitis or diverticulitis. In this case, bowel dilatation is focal instead of diffuse.

Volvulus
Torsion of a loop of bowel, most commonly affecting the colon. The bowel twists upon its mesentery and causes a closed loop obstruction, which may lead to ischemia of the involved loop. The radiographic manifestation of gastric or colonic volvulus is a single, extremely dilated loop of bowel.

Sigmoid volvulus
An elongated, redundant sigmoid colon predisposes to volvulus. Other risk factors include long term high fiber diets, chronic constipation, elderly, bed bound, immobile, or severely handicapped patients.

Key findings:
- Dilated loop assumes an inverted U configuration, extends from the left lower quadrant obliquely into the right upper quadrant or mid-abdomen.
- Dilated loop usually extends higher than the transverse colon.
- Dilatation of the descending and transverse colon may occur, depending on the time course of the patient's presentation. This can make it difficult to distinguish from Ogilvie syndrome.
- Haustra are generally effaced (see Figure 3.18).

Cecal volvulus
Uncommon (1–2% of bowel obstruction in adults). Generally, a mobile cecal mesentery predisposes to this condition.

Key findings:
- Cecum is markedly dilated with air.
- Extends from the RLQ toward the LUQ, or horizontally across the mid-abdomen.
- Dilatation of the small bowel may occur (see Figure 3.19).

The diagnosis of both sigmoid and cecal volvulus can be confirmed with a contrast enema (usually water soluble contrast, such as Gastrograffin). In RARE instances, a barium enema can reduce a sigmoid (but not a cecal) volvulus.

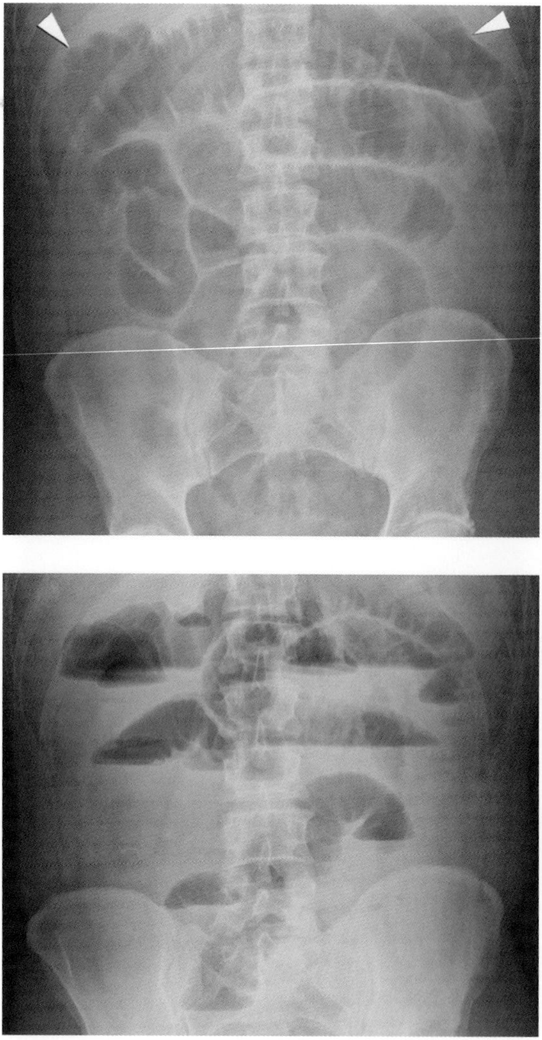

Figure 3.17 Supine image (a) demonstrates multiple dilated loops of small bowel and dilated transverse colon (arrowheads). A surgical suture line is visible in the right mid-abdomen. The upright image (b) shows numerous air fluid levels in *both* the small and large intestine, characteristic of ileus.

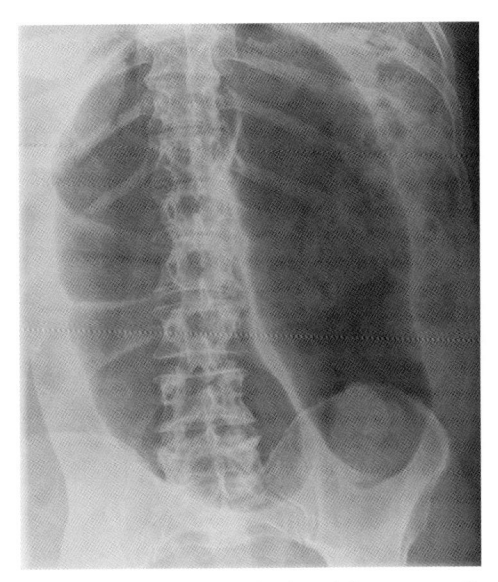

Figure 3.18 Sigmoid volvulus. Abdominal radiograph demonstrates a dilated loop of bowel in an inverted U shape, which begins and ends in the LLQ. Stool is seen in the proximal left colon and splenic flexure.

Gastric volvulus
Please see Fluoroscopy, chapter 7, p. 348.

Toxic Megacolon
This emergency condition is most commonly caused by acute ulcerative colitis. There is loss of bowel muscle tone, absent peristalsis, and progressive bowel dilatation. There is a high risk of colonic perforation, and enemas are contraindicated.

Key findings:
- Extreme dilatation of the transverse colon; > 6.5 cm transversely.
- Absent haustra & loss of normal fold pattern.

Thumbprinting or pseudopolyps may be seen (also known as cobblestoning, these are heaped up areas of mucosa intervening between ulcerations) (see Figure 3.9).

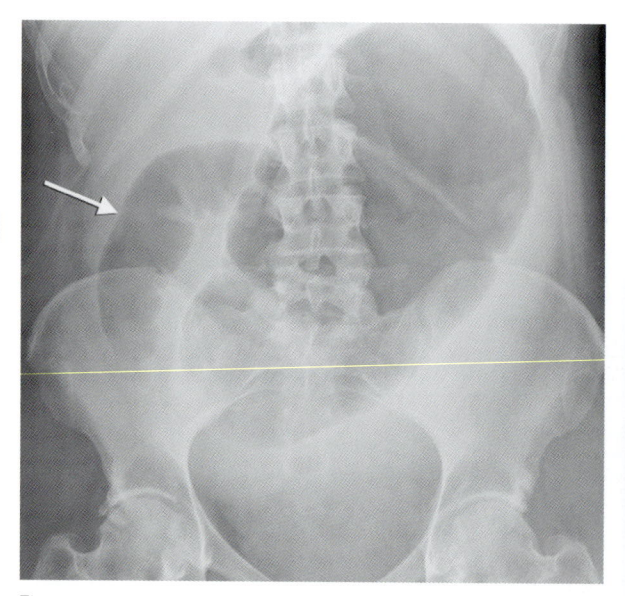

Figure 3.19 Cecal volvulus. Abdominal radiograph demonstrates a markedly dilated loop of bowel extending from the RLQ to LUQ. Note the dilated loop of distal small bowel (arrow) indicative of obstruction from the torsed colon.

CT

Computed tomography is widely used in the evaluation of abdominal pain, masses, and suspected inflammatory or neoplastic processes. CT of the abdomen is one of the most common imaging tests ordered from the Emergency Room.

How are images acquired and viewed?
See chapter 1, Radiology Essentials, p. 6.

Acquisition and reconstructions parameters used in the abdomen and pelvis
Slice thickness

Thin sections (0.5–1.25 mm):
- Useful for evaluating small structures, such as the ostia of small branch vessels from the aorta.
- Often used for problem solving and characterizing small lesions.

Thick sections (3–5 mm):
- Appear smoother and are "more pleasing" to look at.
- Used for most general diagnostic purposes.

Reformats

See chapter 1, Radiology Essentials, p. 8 for more details on technique.

<u>Multiplanar reformats:</u>
Coronal reformats now common, useful for evaluating mesenteric lymphadenopathy and spatial relationships.

<u>Curved reformats:</u>
- Commonly used to view the course of the pancreatic duct.
- Frequently used in CTA to "lay out" tortuous vessels.

<u>Maximum intensity projection (MIP)</u>
- Standard use in CT angiography of the abdomen.
- Used to demonstrate renal collecting systems in CT or MR urography

<u>3D.</u>
- Commonly used in CTA, CTU, and MRCP.
- Less useful in the evaluation of stenosis in heavily calcified vessels, as the stenosis can be obscured by the dense calcium.

Protocols

Variables in CT protocols of the abdomen and pelvis include the following:

Oral contrast

The choice is based on the clinical question in conjunction with cost and convenience. For more information on contrast, see chapter 1, Radiiology Essentials, p. 16.

<u>Acute abdominal pain:</u> positive contrast used to differentiate abscesses and fluid collections from bowel.

<u>CT enterography:</u> VoLumen™ or similar agents typically used in lieu of water to maintain adequate distension of the entirety of the small bowel.

<u>Other:</u> choice of contrast for studies looking for masses or metastasis is operator dependent.

Rectal contrast

Used PRN for problem solving when good colonic opacification required (e.g., suspected colon fistulas, diverticulitis).

Intravenous contrast

(See chapter 1 Radiology Essentials, p. 16.)

<u>Injection rate:</u>
- Rapid contrast injections (4–5 cc/sec) are needed to obtain dense opacification of the arteries and brisk peak enhancement of the organs, necessary for many of the protocols used in the abdomen.
- A large caliber IV is required for this (18g).

Phases and timing of scanning

The scan delay is that time between the start of the contrast injection and the start of scanning.

- A short scan delay results in "arterial dominant" images, used for CTA and for detection of hypervascular tumors.
- Longer scan delays are needed to evaluate the solid abdominal organs, to allow adequate time for peak organ enhancement.
  - Each organ enhances at a different rate and to a different degree.

Multiphase imaging protocols are now common in the abdomen and pelvis.
- Each phase has a different scan delay.
- The phases that should be performed depend upon the clinical question.

Phases of imaging in abdominal CT scans (see Figure 3.20)
(numbers in parenthesis refer to the scan delay, in seconds)

Early (true) arterial phase (25 s):
Contrast is in arteries. Used for CTA when 3D reformats are planned.

Late arterial phase (35–40 s):
Contrast is still arterial dominant, but some enhancement of the portal vein and kidneys is occurring. This is the time of peak pancreatic enhancement. Optimal time to detect most hypervascular liver tumors, as well as pancreatic tumors.

Portal venous phase (60–70 s):
The time of peak hepatic enhancement. Both portal and hepatic veins are opacified. Optimal time to detect hypovascular hepatic tumors and to evaluate venous patency.

Nephrographic phase (90–120 s):
Uniform enhancement of the renal cortex and medulla occurs. Optimal time to detect renal masses.

Excretory phase (> 180 s):
Kidneys excreting contrast such that renal collecting system and ureters are opacified. Used in CT urography and for problem solving.

Delay Phase (5–15 min):
Timing is variable, depending on the clinical problem being evaluated.

Special techniques

CT Enterography

Used for diagnosis of Crohn disease and detection of small bowel masses.
- Requires ingestion of a large volume of oral contrast to distend the bowel: 750–1000 cc over ~ 1 hour.
- Negative contrast agents are used to accentuate appearance of mural enhancement. Volumen™ is one agent commonly used.
- Scans are acquired prior to and following IV contrast enhancement.
- Spasmolytics may be administered to reduce peristalsis and artifacts that result from bowel motion.

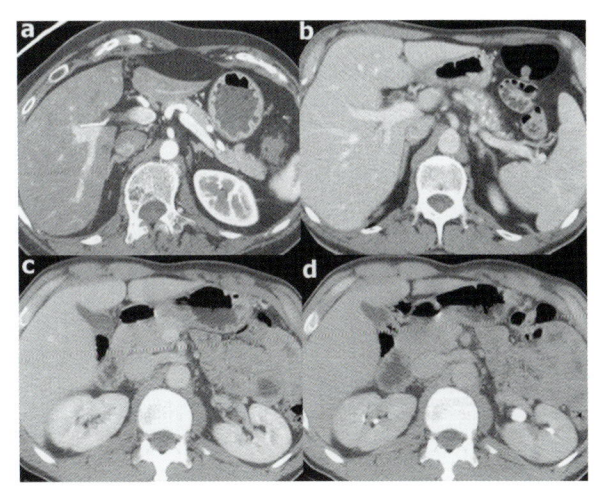

Figure 3.20 Late arterial phase (a), portal venous phase (b), nephrographic phase (c), excretory phase (d). In the late arterial phase, the pancreas and arteries are brightly enhancing, the portal vein is just starting to enhance, but notice the liver is not at peak enhancement, as it is in b. In the nephrographic phase, the kidneys are uniformly enhanced, however the liver is becoming less enhanced, and the pancreas is no longer brightly enhancing.

CT Urography

CT urography protocol is "one stop shopping" for evaluation of hematuria.

Technique:
- Non-contrast: to look for urolithiasis.
- Nephrographic phase: renal mass detection and determination of lesional enhancement.
- Excretory phase: ~ 8 minute delayed phase images are obtained to look for collecting system abnormalities. In some institutions, patients are hydrated to promote robust excretion of contrast and distension of the collecting systems.

3D images of the collecting systems are created: useful for depicting anatomy, congenital abnormalities.

CT Colonography

Also known as "virtual colonoscopy." Unlike colonoscopy, it provides some information about the colon wall and structures *outside* the colon.

Indications:
- Screening for colorectal carcinoma.
- Incomplete or failed colonoscopy.
- Contra-indication to sedation (required for colonoscopy).

Patient preparation and technique:
- Bowel preparation required—same as for colonoscopy.
- Small volume oral contrast given to "tag" any residual stool.
- Carbon dioxide is insufflated into the colon via rectal tube, most commonly by automated device to monitor volume and pressure.
- Non-contrast, low dose CT performed. 2 acquisitions:
  - Supine.
  - Prone.

Image interpretation:

2D images
- Assess degree of distention, adequacy of bowel prep, polyps that may be obscured by residual fluid. Look for incidental findings.

3D images
- Endoluminal view, "Fly Through" the colon with view and perspective similar to colonoscopy.

Normal anatomy on CT

A discussion of normal CT anatomy of the abdomen and pelvis is beyond the scope of this book. See references for suggested resources.

Abdominal compartments

A brief review of the compartments of the abdomen will be provided, as they impact how disease processes appear and spread within the abdomen.

Peritoneal cavity

A potential space between the visceral and parietal peritoneum.
- Fluid, air, blood, and other contents can accumulate in the peritoneal cavity and move freely throughout this potential space, surrounding any of the intra-peritoneal structures.

Intraperitoneal contents:
- Stomach, first portion of the duodenum, jejunum, ileum, cecum, transverse, and sigmoid colon.
- Liver and spleen (see Figure 3.21).

Retroperitoneal space

Located behind the peritoneal cavity, posterior to the posterior parietal peritoneum. Contents are surrounded by fat.

Retroperitoneal contents:
- Kidneys, adrenal glands, pancreas.
- Aorta and IVC.
- Second through fourth portions of the duodenum, ascending and descending colon (see Figure 3.21).

Extraperitoneal space

Continuous with the retroperitoneal space, but generally refers to structures *in the pelvis* outside the peritoneal compartment.

Extraperitoneal contents:

Rectum, bladder, uterus, ovaries, vagina, prostate, seminal vesicles, lymphatics, and blood vessels.

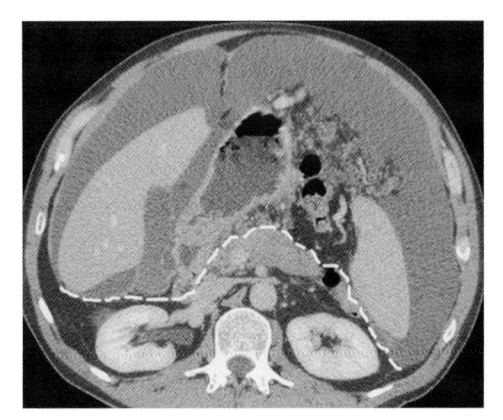

Figure 3.21 Large volume of ascites demonstrates the extent of the peritoneal cavity. The dotted white line demarcates the anterior boundry of the retroperitoneum. Note the pancreas, aorta, IVC, kidneys, and fat are all in the retroperitoneum, and thus are not surround by the ascites fluid.

How do I read an abdominal/pelvic CT

Search strategies

Follow the same method each time to systematically evaluate all structures. Use soft tissue windows (approximate settings: W400 L40). Start with a structure and look at it on each successive image until the entire structure has been seen, then move onto the next.

> Suggested search order:
> - Solid organs—liver, spleen, pancreas, adrenal glands, kidneys
> - Lymph nodes/other non-organ masses
> - Vasculature
> - Bowel and mesentery
> - GYN organs and extraperitoneal pelvis
> - Fluid/fluid collections/blood (look in pelvic cul-de-sac)
> - Free air (use lung window)
> - Bones (use bone window)

What do I look for?
Solid organs

- Organ size—Look for atrophy, enlargement.
- Organ contour—Are there signs of nodularity, masses, scars?
- Uniformity of attenuation and enhancement.
- Focal areas of altered attenuation—increased or decreased?
  - Round (lesion) or wedge shaped (infarct)?
  - Calcifications.
- Patency and adequacy of arterial inflow and venous outflow.

Peritoneal compartment
- Free fluid
  - Collects in the dependent areas such as the pelvic cul-de-sac, para-colic gutters, and Morrison's pouch.
- Free air:
  - Usually non-dependent.
- Peritoneal thickening, enhancement, and nodularity.

Retroperitoneal compartment
- Organs are surrounded by fat, which should be uniformly low attenuation.
- Abnormal fluid (e.g., inflammation) or blood will infiltrate or replace the fat, increasing its attenuation.

Bowel and mesentery
- Look at the bowel diameter and wall thickness.
- Assess the adjacent mesenteric fat; it should be dark gray and uniform in attenuation.

Lymph nodes:
Know where normal nodes reside, look in these areas for enlargement.

Common pitfalls
Not looking
The most common error in abdominal CT is forgetting to look at *every* structure, or not looking at the entire structure on each image.

Missing free air
- It doesn't always layer non-dependently, and it can easily be missed if it is scattered about the abdomen as tiny bubbles. Make sure you look specifically for it each time you read a CT scan.
- Scroll through on lung or bone windows. Are all small gas collections intra-luminal?

Accurately assessing the bowel wall
- Undistended bowel with collapse of the walls can mimic bowel wall thickening. Always evaluate the degree of bowel distension when trying to determine if there is wall thickening.

Not thinking about the clinical problem
Think about the patient's symptoms and potential causes, then look for these on CT.
- For example, on CT for "RLQ pain, rule out appendicitis": if the appendix is normal, look at other structures that can mimic appendicitis (ovarian pathology, ileo-cecal inflammatory processes or lymphadenitis).

Patterns of disease
Extra-luminal air
A collection of air that is not intra-luminal is abnormal, except in the recent post-operative patient. A strict time limit for how long free air should be seen in the post-operative patient has not been established.

- The time since the operation, the type of operation (laparoscopic using CO_2 versus open surgery), and the volume of air should be considered.

Free intraperitoneal air
- Typically non-dependent, often anterior to liver.
- Distributed throughout the peritoneal compartment as tiny gas bubbles.

Retroperitoneal air
- Usually linear or streaky.
- Usually collects adjacent to the site of pathology; such as adjacent to the duodenum in cases of perforated duodenal ulcers.

Mesenteric air
- Air within mesenteric fat is considered extra-peritoneal.
- This occurs with contained perforations of bowel; commonly from contained perforated sigmoid diverticulitis.

Abnormal intraluminal air
Pneumobilia
- Air in the intra- or extrahepatic bile ducts.
- May be expected (e.g., post choledocho-jejunostomy or biliary sphincterotomy).
- Rarely can be seen in cholangitis with gas-forming organisms or a spontaneous biliary-enteric fistula.

Portal venous gas
- Air in the mesenteric or portal veins.
- Always abnormal. Associated most commonly with ischemic bowel.

Inflammation
Inflammation, whether due to infection, trauma, or other causes, results in accumulation of fluid and inflammatory cells. On CT, this changes the attenuation of the structure that is inflamed:
- The density of fat will increase.
- The density of contrast enhanced solid organs may decrease.

Mesenteric
- Fine, smudgy, or hazy increased density of the mesenteric fat.
- This is known as "fat stranding" and is a useful marker to indicate the site of pathology.

Retroperitoneal
- Increased density of fat, with stranding around the inflamed structure.
- Fat stranding is usually localized to one compartment of the retroperitoneum (e.g., anterior pararenal space in acute pancreatitis); however, it can spread with more severe disease (see Figure 3.22).

Bowel wall
- See 'bowel wall thickening', next page. .
- Transmural inflammation is bowel wall thickening accompanied by adjacent mesenteric inflammation.

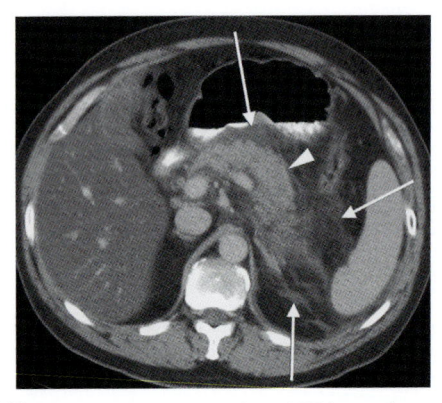

Figure 3.22 Pancreatitis. Axial contrast enhanced CT shows enlargement of the pancreatic body (arrowhead) from inflammation and edema, and extensive peripancreatic fat stranding and fluid secondary to inflammation (arrows).

Solid organ
- As inflammation progresses, fluid accumulation within the organ can cause organomegaly and decreased attenuation (see Figure 3.22).

Bowel wall thickening
Definition:
- Small bowel wall measuring > 1–1.5 mm thick.
- Colon wall measuring > 3 mm thick.
- The plicae circulares (small bowel) or semilunar folds (colon) may be preserved but thickened, or may be effaced and less apparent, depending on the etiology.

> **Causes of bowel wall thickening:**
> - Infection e.g., pseudomembraneous colitis
> - Inflammation e.g., ulcerative colitis, Crohn disease, typhlitis
> - Hemorrhage including traumatic
> - Neoplastic infiltration e.g., lymphoma, colorectal carcinoma
> - Ischemia
> - Shock bowel
> - Hypoalbuminia
> - Graft versus host disease

The distribution and pattern of wall thickening and the presence or absence of adjacent transmural inflammatory changes will help to narrow the differential diagnosis.
- Certain diseases have a predilection for small versus large bowel.
- Some are associated with inflammation in the adjacent fat.

- Some cause luminal narrowing and obstruction, whereas others cause cavitation.

See Figure 3.23.

Bowel wall thickening—diagnostic clues:
- Length of bowel affected.
  - Are there skip areas? (Crohn disease)
  - Is it a focal (neoplasm) or diffuse process?
- Distribution
  - Small bowel, large bowel, or both?
  - Large bowel in isolation? (colitis, UC, pseudomembraneous colitis)
- Does it correspond to a vascular supply? (ischemia)
- Co-existent air in the bowel wall?
  - Ischemia.
- Adjacent inflammatory changes?
  - Indicates a transmural process (Crohn disease, some infections).
- Luminal narrowing and obstruction?
  - Benign stricture (post inflammatory, Crohn disease).
  - Malignant stricture (adenocarcinoma).
- Cavitation or ulceration?
  - Malignancies such as lymphoma, GIST.

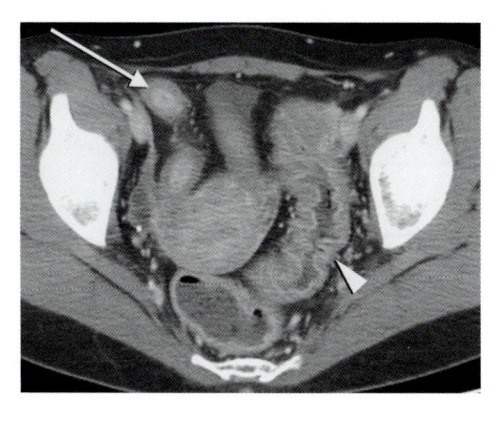

Figure 3.23 Crohns enteritis and colitis. Axial contrast enhanced CT shows marked thickening of a loop of small bowel (arrow) and of the sigmoid colon (arrowhead). Note mucosal hyper-enhancement in both segments, a sign of active inflammation.

Fluid, blood, and pus
Is it blood, pus, or fluid?
Fluid: Should measure low density (<20 HU) and appear homogenous.
Pus: Cannot be differentiated from fluid based on HU measurements.
Blood: Higher in density, and may be heterogeneous. The specific HU value depends on the age of the blood.
- Acute clot is higher attenuation.
- Older blood is lower attenuation.
- Large volumes of blood may layer, giving a "hematocrit" level, with higher attenuation dependently, and lower attenuation non-dependently (see Figure 3.24).

Abscess
Contained, infected fluid collection (see Figure 3.25).
- Thick, enhancing wall around a fluid collection is suggestive of abscess.
- Air bubbles within a fluid collection indicate infection (or a fistula to bowel) provided the patient has not had recent surgery.

Intraperitoneal fluid/blood
- Layers dependently in Morrison's pouch, the para-colic gutters, or the pouch of Douglas (pelvic cul-de-sac).
- As volume increases, it flows throughout the peritoneal cavity.
- Large volumes may displace gas filled bowel loops centrally.

Retroperitoneal/extraperitoneal fluid/blood
- Does not flow freely, as intraperitoneal fluid does.
- Usually is more localized to the area of pathology; for example, hemorrhage after a femoral catheterization may track up the ipsilateral psoas muscle.

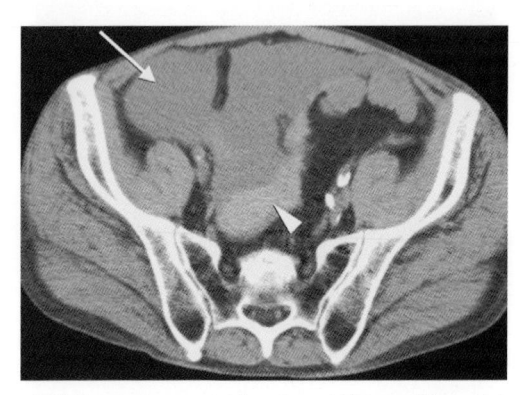

Figure 3.24 Hemoperitoneum. Axial unenhanced CT image of the pelvis in a patient with splenic trauma demonstrates a large amount peritoneal fluid in the pelvis (arrow). Dependently, the fluid is much higher in attenuation, consistent with clotted blood (arrowhead). Simple fluid should be homogeneous throughout the abdomen, and lower in attenuation.

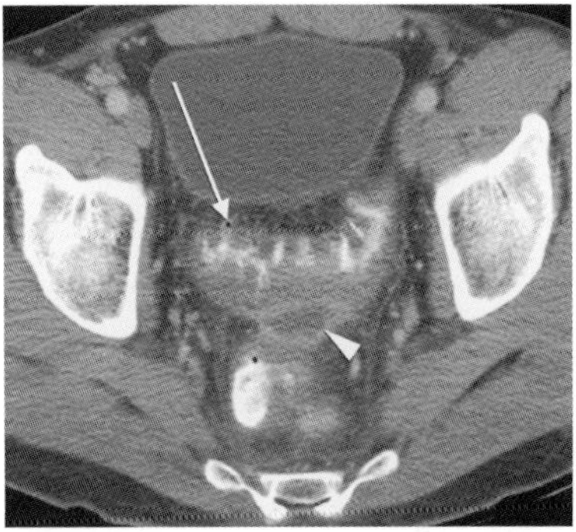

Figure 3.25 Acute diverticulitis with peri-diverticular abscess. The sigmoid colon wall is markedly thickened and diverticula are evident (arrow). A small fluid collection with peripheral enhancement (arrowhead) is consistent with abscess from a contained perforation.

Masses

Solid organ masses

To be visible on CT, the density of the mass must be sufficiently different than the density of the organ parenchyma. This difference is accentuated by the administration of IV contrast.

<u>Hypovascular</u> masses enhance less avidly than the organ. They are lower in attenuation than the enhanced organ (see Figure 3.26).

<u>Hypervascular</u> masses enhance more avidly and rapidly than the organ. They are higher in attenuation than the organ.

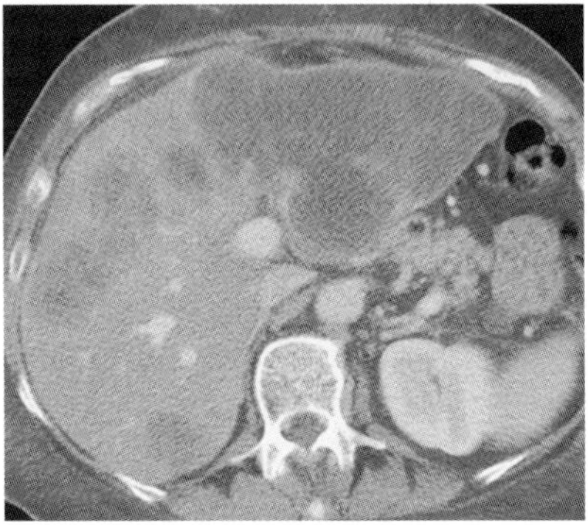

Figure 3.26 Hypovascular liver masses. Axial contrast enhanced abdominal CT obtained in the portal venous phase of imaging shows multiple low attenuation masses within the enhanced liver; metastasis from esophageal adenocarcinoma.

> **What CT protocol do I use to find a mass?**
> It is imperative to know what type of mass is suspected or what type of cancer the patient has so that the CT is performed correctly.
> - Some tumors need arterial phase imaging for best visualization.
>   - E.g. hepatocellular carcinomas, pancreatic endocrine tumors.
> - To minimize radiation exposure to the patient, only the required phases should be acquired.

Identifying the organ of origin:
When abdominal or pelvic masses are large, it can be difficult to determine the organ of origin. Identifying the center of the mass and analyzing which organs are displaced and in which direction can help to pinpoint the origin.

Mesenteric masses
Soft tissue masses are easily seen contrasting with the mesenteric fat.
- Some pathologies (e.g., carcinoid tumors) induce a desmoplastic reaction that causes spiculation and tethering of bowel loops (see Figure 3.27).
- Other large masses (e.g., lymphoma) may displace bowel loops, or surround and encase vascular structures.
- Masses can be cystic (e.g., congenital duplication cysts, lymphangioma).

> **Specific features of common mesenteric masses:**
> Carcinoid tumors: spiculated, bowel tethering, calcifications.
> Lymphadenopathy/lymphadenitis: multiple enlarged ovoid soft tissue nodules, measure > 1 cm in short axis.
> Lymphoma: confluent, homogeneous lobular soft tissue density. May "sandwich" intervening blood vessels without compressing them.

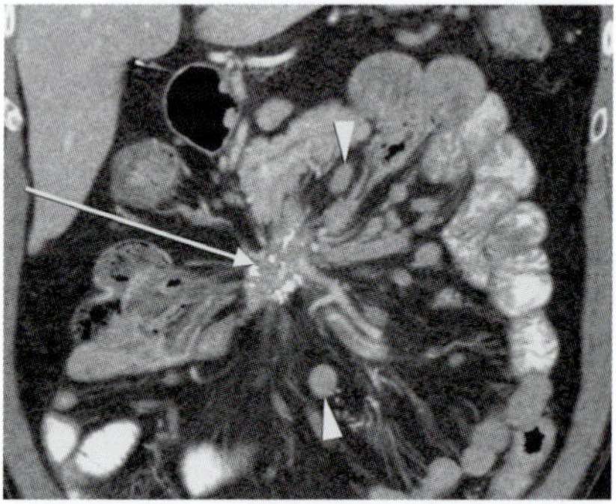

Figure 3.27 Mesenteric mass. Coronal contrast enhanced CT shows a typical calcified carcinoid tumor in the mesentery (arrow). Tumor induces a desmoplastic reaction causing radiating strands of soft tissue. Several discrete enlarged lymph nodes are also present (arrowheads).

Omental

Metastatic disease from ovarian, stomach, and colon cancer is the most common malignancy to involve the omentum. This may be quite subtle initially.
- Tumor deposits are nodular foci of increased density in the normally low attenuation omental fat that gradually become confluent = "Omental caking."
- Often accompanied by ascites (see Figure 3.28).

Lymph nodes

Identification and interpretation of lymph nodes is difficult, particularly for the beginner. Knowledge of the normal distribution of lymph nodes and the patterns of lymphatic drainage are of paramount importance in the correct interpretation of CT scans. It is normal to see small scattered lymph nodes in the abdomen and pelvis. Common sites of lymph nodes on CT of the abdomen and pelvis are shown in Figure 3.29.

Normal lymph nodes

As a general rule, normal nodes in the abdomen and pelvis should be:
- < 1 cm in short axis measurement.
- Uniform in density.
- Contain a fatty hilum.

Enlarged lymph nodes

Lymph nodes may enlarge secondary to infection, inflammation, or neoplastic infiltration. Enlarged nodes in the abdomen and pelvis:
- Generally > 1 cm in short axis measurement.
- Lack a fatty hilum.

Reactive lymphadenitis (non-neoplastic):
Lymph nodes can enlarge due to microbes, cellular debris, and foreign material (e.g., infection and inflammation), termed reactive lymph nodes.
- There may also be inflammation in the peri-nodal tissues.

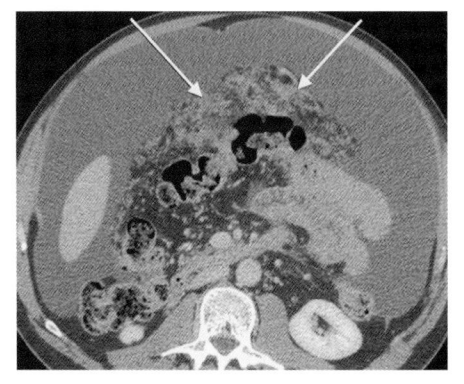

Figure 3.28 Omental metastasis. Axial contrast enhanced CT reveals a large volume of ascites, and soft tissue nodularity of the omentum (arrows).

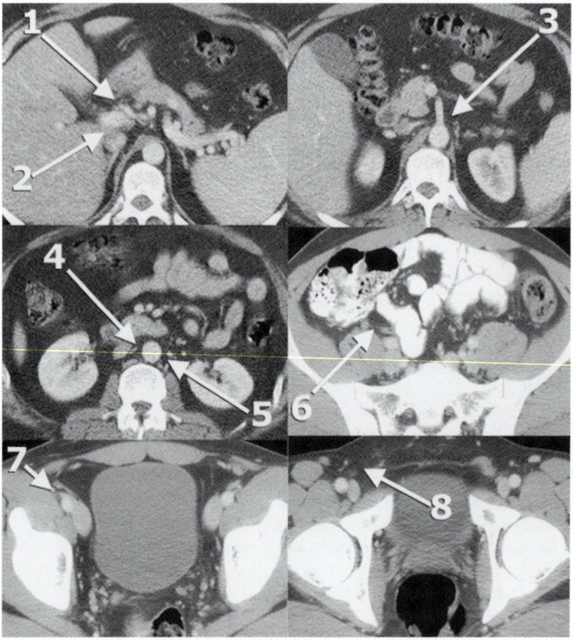

Figure 3.29 Locations of lymph nodes on CT. 1. porta hepatis, 2. porto-caval, 3. para-SMA, 4. aorto-caval, 5. para-aortic, 6. common iliac, 7. external iliac, 8. inguinal.

<u>Neoplastic lymph nodes:</u>
- Nodes may remain discrete or may merge together and become "confluent," as in lymphoma.
- CT is neither sensitive nor specific for the detection of pathologic lymph nodes, since:
  - < 1 cm in short axis may be infiltrated with tumor.
  - > 1 cm in short axis may be reactive.

Features of pathologic lymph nodes on CT (not all need be present) (see Figure 3.30).
- Short axis measurement > 1 cm.
- Clustered nodes in drainage bed of primary tumor.
- Heterogeneous attenuation or abnormal enhancement.
- Central necrosis.
- Loss of fatty hilum.
- Round rather than oval shape.
- Irregular margins/ill defined borders.

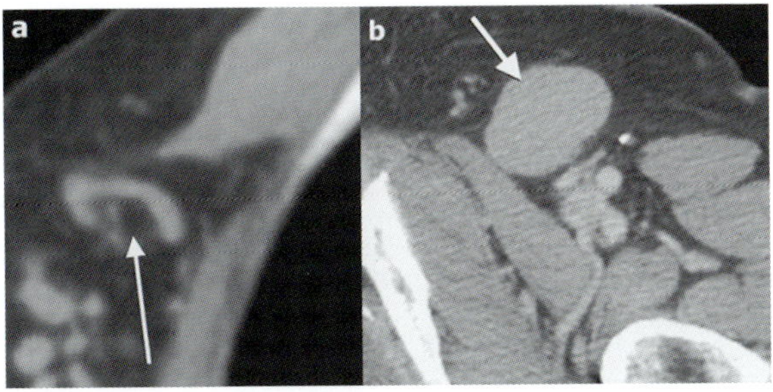

Figure 3.30 Normal axillary lymph node (a) has a thin cortex and fatty hilum (arrow). Neoplastic inguinal lymph node (b) is enlarged, round, and lacks a fatty hilum (arrow).

Interpretating CT scans in oncology patients
Performing accurate, reproducible tumor measurements that are indicative of overall disease response is imperative for the proper management of cancer patients, both those on study protocols and clinical protocols. Various methods to do this exist:
- Bi-dimensional tumor measurements.
- Uni-dimensional tumor measurements.
  - Used in the RECIST criteria (Response Evaluation Criteria in Solid Tumors), which was created to provide consistent measurement criteria across institutions.
- Volumetric tumor measurements—The most accurate method. Not currently widely available but likely to become so.

MRI

Due to the excellent soft tissue contrast obtainable with MRI, it is a useful imaging modality to evaluate structures in the abdomen and pelvis.

How are images acquired?
See chapter 1, Radiology Essentials, "MRI," p. 10. One of the limitations specific to MRI of the abdomen and pelvis is motion artifact. Sources of motion artifact include:
- Patient movement due to the long acquisition time.
- Normal respiratory and cardiac motion.
- Normal bowel motility.
- Ascites.

How to deal with breathing
The abdominal organs move with diaphragmatic excursion, and the abdominal wall moves with breathing.
Several techniques exist to counter this:
- Breath holding—can only be used for short sequences or rapidly acquired sequences. Requires patient cooperation.

- Respiratory triggering—images are acquired at end expiration, technique is based on patient's breathing pattern, and only works with regular respiratory rates.
- Respiratory gating—prospective or retrospective synchronization of image acquisition with a phase in the breathing cycle; can be done based on position of the diaphragm.

Protocols and technical considerations

Obtaining complimentary pulse sequences during an MRI of the abdomen and pelvis allows for discrimination of fat, fluid, blood products, and pathological processes.

> **Pulse sequences typically used in abdominal/pelvic imaging:**
> 1. Standard T1 and T2 weighted:
>   a. Characterize tissue type.
>   b. Anatomical identification.
> 2. Heavily T2 weighted sequences, sensitive for fluid:
>   a. MRCP.
>   b. MR Urography.
> 3. Fat saturation:
>   a. T2 increases conspicuity of edema/inflammation.
>   b. Characterization of macroscopic fat containing lesions.
> 4. In and out of phase imaging:
>   a. Identification of microscopic fat.
> 5. Balanced steady state free precession imaging:
>   a. Rapid acquisition (good for bowel).
>   b. May be referred to as FIESTA or true FISP.
> 6. Fat saturated T1 weighted:
>   a. Most commonly used pre- and post- contrast.

Fat suppression techniques

Fat suppression is frequently used in the abdomen. There are different methods to suppress the signal elicited from fat on MRI:

Fat saturation:

Fat saturation bands can be applied to a sequence to decrease the signal intensity of fat. Used to detect macroscopic fat (e.g., a fat containing ovarian tumor).

Opposed-phase imaging:

Protons in fat and water precess at different rates. These properties can be manipulated such that the signal from fat and water can be additive or cancel each other. This technique is used for:
- Evaluation of microscopic fat within organs (fatty liver).
- Evaluation of microscopic fat containing lesions (lipid rich adrenal adenoma) (see Figure 3.52, p. 177).
  - Lesions containing microscopic fat will lose signal and become darker on opposed phase images compared with in phase images.

Contrast enhancement
See chapter 1, Radiology Essentials, "What about Contrast?" p. 17.

MR enterography
Performed with same technique as CT enterography (see p. 138).
Spasmolytics to reduce peristalsis and artifacts that result from bowel motion are particularly important in MRE, due to the long acquisition time.

MRCP
MRCP (MR cholangiopancreatography) generates high resolution 2D and 3D images of the pancreatic and biliary ductal systems. MRCP is noninvasive and avoids the discomfort, morbidity, and potential complications of ERCP.

Indications
- Diagnosis of acquired and congenital abnormalities of the biliary and pancreatic ducts, including stone disease.
- Post-operative: Evaluation of suspected injury to the biliary tree, either leak or stricture.

Technique and protocol
- Very heavily T2 weighted coronal and axial images display the ducts as high signal intensity.
- Little background tissue seen.

MRA
See chapter 1, Radiology Essentials, "MRA," p. 13.
Indications include:
- Renal artery and mesenteric artery stenosis.
- Pelvic and peripheral vascular occlusive disease.
- Evaluation of IVC and pelvic vein patency.
- Evaluation of renal and hepatic transplant vasculature.

What do normal structures look on MRI?
Fat: T1 bright, T2 bright.
Simple fluid: T1 dark, T2 bright—gallbladder, bladder, bile ducts, pancreatic duct, renal collecting system, ascites.
Proteinaceous fluid: T1 bright, T2 bright.
Hemorrhagic fluid: T1 bright, T2 variable.
Solid organs: T1 and T2 intermediate.
- May be affected by fat content and protein content of organ (e.g., pancreas), edema, and pathologic processes.

Blood vessels: Dark flow voids on T2 images, bright on T1 post gadolinium.

Patterns of disease on MRI

Inflammation
- Increased T2 signal indicates edema and/or inflammation.
- Fat suppression techniques are used to distinguish the high T2 signal of inflammation from the normally high signal of fat.

CHAPTER 3 Abdomen/Pelvis Imaging

Fluid collections and abscess
- Localized region of fluid signal intensity—"fluid collection," non-specific.
- Rim enhancement of a contained fluid collection—abscess.
- Surrounding edema, fluid, and inflammatory changes may be present.
  - T2 weighted fat suppression sequences are essential to show this.
- Air causes a signal void at MRI; air within bowel or an abscess will appear black on the image.

Hemorrhage
- Complex MRI appearance, depending on age of the blood.
- Often T1 hyperintense.
  - Hemorrhagic renal or ovarian cyst.
  - Ovarian endometrioma.
- Often T2 hypointense.

Common conditions evaluated with CT and MRI

Trauma
CT is a fast and accurate way to diagnose traumatic injuries to the abdomen and pelvis. Injury frequency: liver>spleen>renal>bowel>pancreas.
- Allows for the diagnosis of acute ongoing bleeding.
- Intravenous contrast is essential to evaluate for solid organ injuries;
  - It increases the contrast between the enhancing organ and the non-enhancing, injured segment.

Traumatic injuries: definitions and findings

Hemoperitoneum:
- Blood within the peritoneal cavity, higher in attenuation than free fluid, typically 30–60 HU, depending on the time frame since injury.
- May see a hematocrit level, with higher attenuation dependently due to concentration of hemoglobin and blood products (see Figure 3.24).
- Indicative of injury to liver, spleen, bowel, or mesentery.
- Injuries to the pancreas, adrenal glands, and kidneys cause retroperitoneal bleeding.

Subcapsular hematoma:
- Crescentic or lenticular shaped, well circumscribed, low to intermediate density just below the capsule of the organ.

Laceration:
- Linear or stellate shaped area of low density in an otherwise enhancing solid organ. Represents disruption of parenchyma.
- If it extends to the organ surface, it is usually accompanied by adjacent blood clot and hemoperitoneum (liver, spleen) (see Figure 3.33).

Contusion:
- Less well defined focal area of low attenuation in solid organ, represents a region of non-enhancement and edema (see Figure 3.34).

Fracture:
- Complete disruption of an organ. Usually a complex injury extending from one surface of the organ to the other.

Active extravasation
- High attenuation blush of iodinated contrast located outside a vessel. Represents site of active bleeding (see Figure 3.32).

> Alert the clinical service if active extravasation seen; depending on the clinical status of the patient, angiogram and embolization may be indicated.

Sentinel clot sign:
- In cases of multi-organ injury, it can be difficult to determine the site of the most active bleeding.
  - Hemoperitoneum at the site of active bleeding has a higher attenuation than that more distant from the site of bleeding (see Figure 3.31).

Liver and spleen
Commonly injured by both blunt and penetrating trauma. Lacerations are the most common injuries (see Figure 3.33).

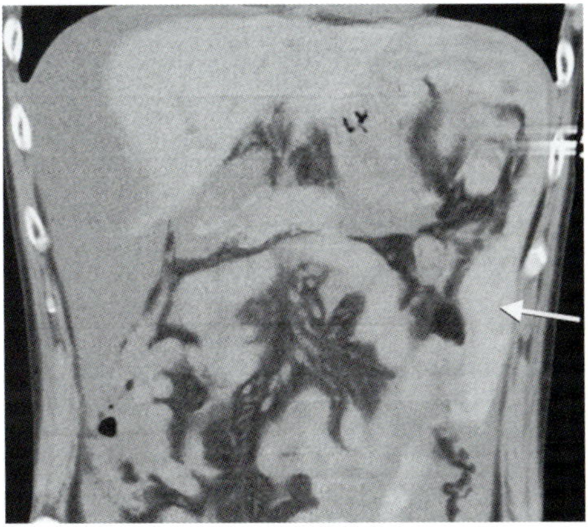

Figure 3.31 Hemoperitoneum with sentinel clot sign. Coronal unenhanced CT of the abdomen in a patient who sustained blunt injury to the spleen during a colonoscopy. There is diffuse hemoperitoneum, and the blood adjacent to the spleen and in the left paracolic gutter is higher in attenuation than that more distant from the spleen, consistent with sentinel clot sign (arrow).

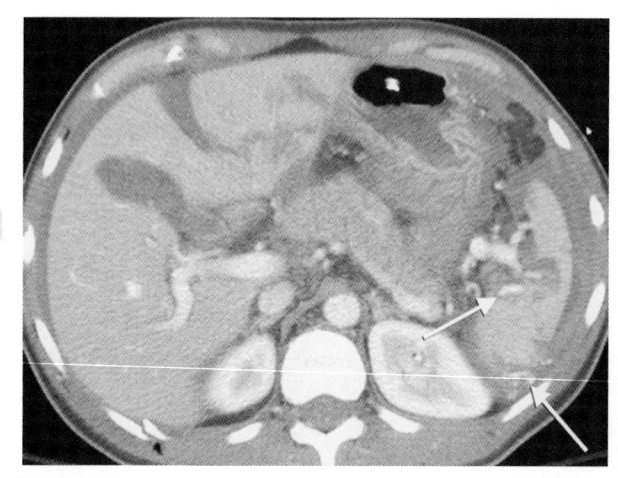

Figure 3.32 Active contrast extravasation. Axial contrast enhanced CT in a patient sustaining blunt trauma reveals splenic contusions and lacerations, with active extravasation of contrast near the lower pole laceration and near the hilum (arrows).

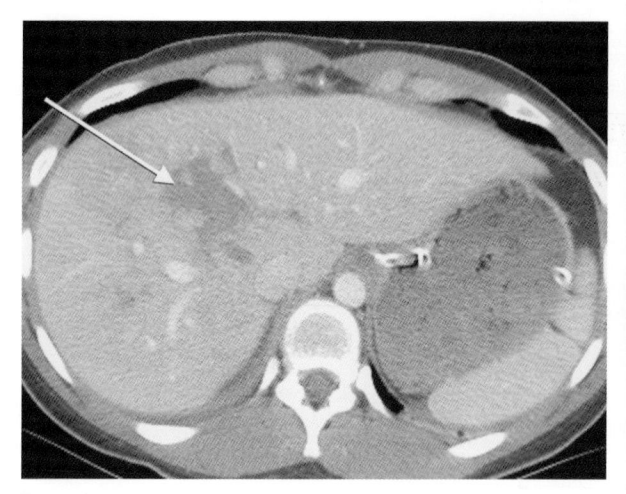

Figure 3.33 Complex liver laceration. Axial contrast enhanced CT in a patient s/p motor vehicle accident. There is a stellate shaped region of low attenuation in the central liver, near the porta hepatis, consistent with a grade III laceration (arrow).

Grading of hepatic and splenic injuries

The American Association for the Surgery of Trauma (AAST) has developed separate grading systems for classifying hepatic and splenic injuries. These serve as a means of accurately describing and communicating findings:
- Grades I through VI.
- Higher grades indicate more severe injuries.

Based on:
- Depth of laceration.
- Surface area of subcapsular hematoma.
- Presence of active bleeding.
- Amount of organ involved.
- Involvement of venous structures.

Pancreas

Trauma to the pancreas causes serious injuries that may be missed initially.
- Usually injured by blunt traumatic compression of the body of the pancreas against the spine (seatbelt, steering wheel, handle bars).
- More common in children, and nearly always associated with other injuries.
- Spectrum of injuries includes contusion, laceration, and transection (see Figure 3.34).
- It is important to look for duct disruption, which carries a higher mortality and requires surgical intervention.

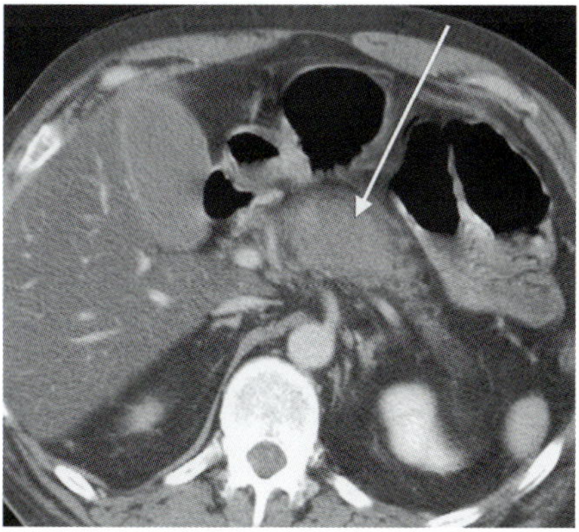

Figure 3.34 Pancreatic contusion. Axial contrast enhanced CT of the abdomen demonstrates focal enlargement and abnormal attenuation of the body of the pancreas, consistent with contusion (arrow).

Kidneys

Spectrum of injuries includes laceration, contusion, pedicle avulsion, collecting system disruption (see Figure 3.35).
- Pedicle avulsion results in a non-perfused, non-enhancing kidney on CT.
- Renal collecting system injuries result in leak of urine into the renal sinus and perinephric space.
- Delayed CT images should be obtained in patients with hematuria or renal injuries on CT to evaluate for extravasation of contrast enhanced urine.

> **Grading of kidney injury**
>
> The American Association for the Surgery of Trauma (AAST) has developed a grading system for classifying renal trauma. The severity of the grade correlates with the need for operative renal repair or nephrectomy.
> - Grades I to V.
> - Higher grades correspond to more severe injuries.
>
> <u>Based on:</u>
> - Depth and extent of laceration.
> - Extent and expansion of peri-renal hematoma.
> - Vascular injury.

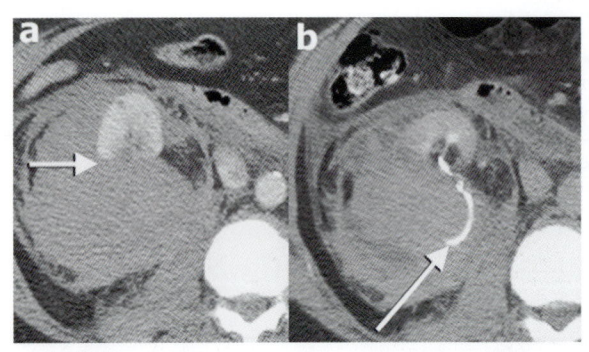

Figure 3.35 Renal fracture (a, b). Axial contrast enhanced CT reveals fracture through the lower pole of the right kidney with extensive peri-nephric hemorrhage (arrow). Five-minute delayed image (b) show extravasation of contrast opacified urine into the peri-nephric hematoma (arrow), consistent with a renal collecting system injury, a grade IV injury.

Bladder

Bladder injuries can occur with both blunt and penetrating trauma. Historically, diagnosis was made with fluoroscopic cystogram; however, CT cystography has become the imaging test of choice, with an accuracy approaching 100%.

Indications for CT cystography:
- Gross hematuria.
- Known pelvic fractures.
- Severe pelvic trauma.

Technique:
Varies from institution to institution. Commonly, CT of the pelvis is performed with two acquisitions:
1. Pre-contrast
2. Post-contrast: bladder is filled with dilute water soluble contrast via a Foley catheter by gravity drip, minimum of 250–300 cc must be instilled.

Key findings:
- Intraperitoneal bladder rupture:
  - Free fluid in pelvic cul-de-sac.
  - Contrast extravasation outlines loops of bowel.
  - Requires surgical repair.
- Extraperitoneal bladder rupture:
  - Fluid and stranding in the extraperitoneal space.
  - Contrast extravasation is streaky and irregular, often in the prevesical space (see Figure 3.36).

Bowel and mesentery
Look for focal areas of bowel wall thickening and enhancement in conjunction with free fluid +/− stranding and fluid at the mesenteric root.

> Bowel perforation can be diagnosed definitively based on the presence of free intraperitoneal air or extravasated oral contrast. However, these injuries are often difficult to diagnose on CT, and may be occult.

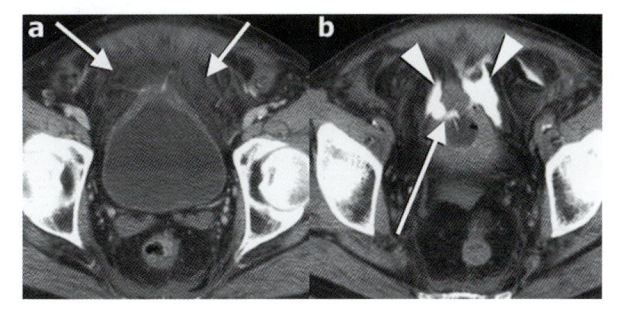

Figure 3.36 Traumatic extraperitoneal bladder rupture. Unehanced (a) and post bladder contrast (b) CT images show bladder wall thickening and extraperitoneal fluid and stranding (arrows, a). There is extravasation of contrast from the bladder (arrow, b) and into the extraperitoneal space (arrowheads).

CHAPTER 3 **Abdomen/Pelvis Imaging**

<u>Hypoperfusion shock bowel complex</u>
A specific constellation of findings resulting from profound hypotension and hypoperfusion (see Figure 3.37):

<u>Key findings:</u>
- Dilated small bowel with hyper-enhancing wall.
- Flattened IVC, small caliber aorta.
- Peri-pancreatic fluid.
- Hypoperfusion of the liver and spleen.

Appendicitis
The normal appendix originates from the base of the cecum near the ileocecal valve and measures less than 6 mm in transverse diameter.

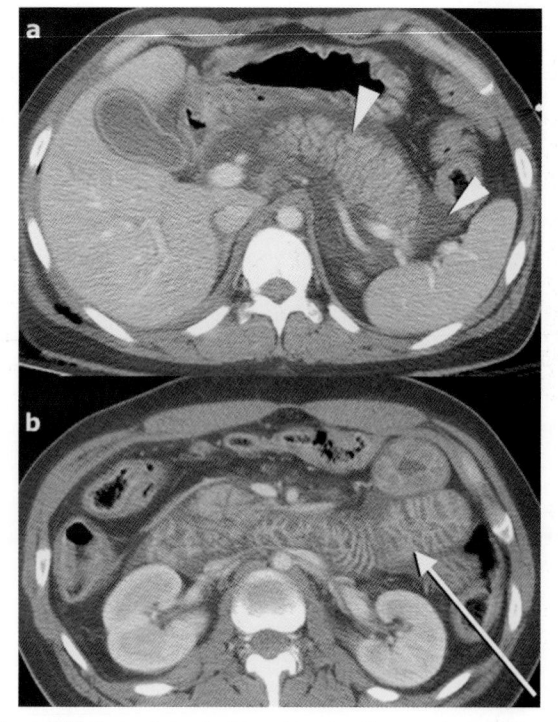

Figure 3.37 Hypoperfusion shock bowel complex. Contrast enhanced CT demonstrates enlarged pancreas with extensive peri-pancreatic fluid (arrowheads) (a), abnormal small bowel enhancement (arrow), flattened IVC, and small caliber aorta (b).

Acute appendicitis (see Figure 3.38)
Common findings on MRI and CT include:
- Dilated appendix > 6 mm in transverse dimension.
- Appendiceal wall thickening > 2 mm.
- +/− free fluid.
- Appendicoliths
  - Calcifications within lumen on CT.
  - Signal voids in lumen on MRI.
- Peri-appendiceal inflammatory changes in RLQ.
  - Fat stranding on CT.
  - Increased signal on T2 fat suppression sequences on MRI.

Perforated appendicitis
- Foci of air or a focal fluid collection adjacent to the appendix.
- Does not generally result in diffuse free air throughout the peritoneal cavity.

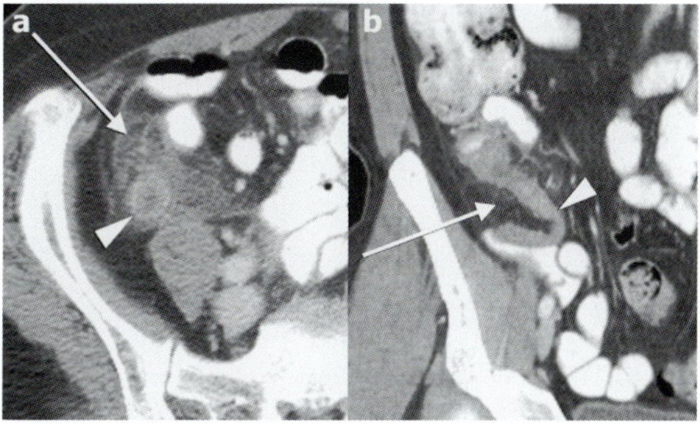

Figure 3.38 Acute appendicitis. Axial (a) and coronal (b) contrast enhanced CT images in two different patients show an obstructed, dilated, thick walled appendix (arrowheads). The accompanying inflammatory changes are severe in (a) and mild in (b) (arrows).

> **What if you can't find the appendix?**
> - It is not uncommon that the appendix cannot be identified.
> - Look for inflammatory changes in the RLQ.
> - In the absence of these, the likelihood of appendicitis is very low, although not zero.

Diverticulitis
Colonic diverticula are common, and the prevalence increases with age. 95% of diverticula are in the sigmoid colon.
- Hypertrophy of the longitudinal and circular muscles of affected segments results in colon wall thickening.

CT findings

<u>Uncomplicated diverticulitis:</u>
- Colon wall thickening of variable length and severity.
- Peri-colonic fat stranding.

<u>Contained perforations (see Figure 3.25):</u>
Are walled off/contained by the mesentery adjacent to the inflamed colon.
- Appearance varies, including:
  - Focal fluid collection with or without an enhancing wall, with or without air fluid levels.
  - +/− oral contrast extravasation into the collection.
- Managed non-operatively with antibiotics +/− percutaneous abscess drainage, depending on size and accessibility.

<u>Free perforation into the peritoneal cavity:</u>
- Diverticulitis plus pneumoperitoneum.
- Generally managed operatively.

Crohn disease

A chronic inflammatory disease that may involve the small bowel, colon, or both. Although traditionally diagnosed on SBFT, CT enterography (CTE) and MR enterography (MRE) have largely replaced SBFT, as they have the advantage of demonstrating the following:
- Abnormal bowel wall enhancement.
- Associated mesenteric inflammation.
- Associated vasodilatation.
- Potential complications: fistulas, abscess.

CTE versus MRE?

<u>Advantages of CTE:</u>
- Short acquisition time-useful in patients who cannot hold still.
- Better spatial resolution than MRI may aid in evaluation of fistulas.

<u>Advantages of MRE:</u>
- Lack of ionizing radiation—especially beneficial in:
  - Young patients.
  - Patients who may require multiple serial imaging examinations.

MR & CT enterography—key findings of Crohn disease
- Stratified mural enhancement (submucosal edema is low signal/low attenuation and sandwiched between the enhanced wall and mucosa).
- Comb sign (enlarged vessels of vasa recta).
- Transmural inflammation.
- Mural thickening.
- Mesenteric lymphadenopathy.
- Strictures, fistulae, and abscesses.
- Creeping (hypertrophied) mesenteric fat.

See Figure 3.39.

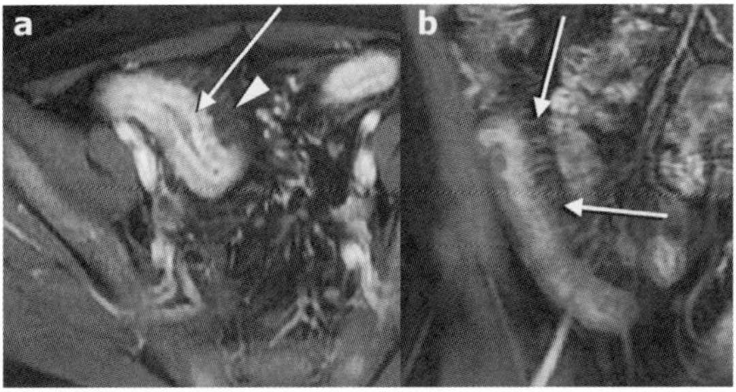

Figure 3.39 Crohn disease. Contrast enhanced fat saturated T1-weighted axial images from an MRE. The distal ileum shows mural thickening, intense mucosal and serosal enhancement (arrow, a), and adjacent fat stranding (arrowhead). Distended vasa recta adjacent to the involved bowel is called the "comb sign" (arrows, b).

Pancreatitis

Acute pancreatitis can be occult on CT. More severe cases have characteristic CT findings, although these findings do not correlate with the clinical severity of the disease.

CT findings
- Pancreatic enlargement and low attenuation due to edema.
- Inflammatory changes in the lesser sac and throughout the anterior pararenal space; "peri-pancreatic fat stranding"
- Extension into the small bowel mesentery and transverse mesocolon may also occur, and free intra-peritoneal fluid may develop.

Complications
- Pancreatic necrosis: focal non-enhancement of the parenchyma.
- Vascular: splenic vein thrombosis and arterial pseudoaneurysms.
- Pancreatic pseudocysts (see Figure 3.40).
  - Low density collections with a non-enhancing wall.
  - Contain necrotic tissue, secretions, and blood, and become walled off with a fibrous capsule.
  - Can occur within the pancreas or dissect and occur essentially anywhere in the extra-pancreatic abdomen.
  - Have even been reported in the mediastinum and retroperitoneal portions of the pelvis.
- Pancreatic phlegmon
  - A term used to describe an inflammatory mass that is not a walled off fluid collection; they cannot be drained.
  - Composed of inflammatory cells, fluid, exudates, and fat.
  - They may progress to suppuration, or may resolve spontaneously.
  - On CT, they are higher in attenuation than fluid.

Aortic aneurysms and dissection

CT angiography (CTA) is performed to evaluate the abdominal aorta and its branch vessels.

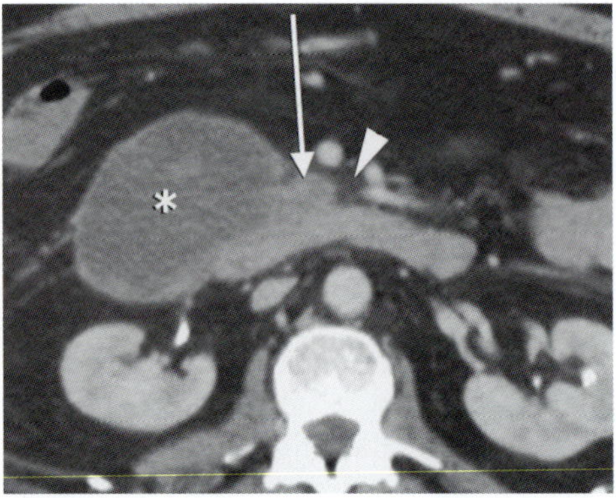

Figure 3.40 Pancreatic pseudocyst. Contrast enhanced axial CT at the level of the pancreatic head (arrow) shows residual peri-pancreatic inflammation (arrowhead) from pancreatitis. A large fluid collection adjacent to the pancreatic head (*) represents a pseudocyst.

Abdominal aortic aneurysm (AAA)
Definition:
- Maximal transverse diameter of the aorta > 2× normal.
- Most people use a threshold of 3 cm, however; in very small patients with small aortas, aneurysms may be present at smaller sizes.
- Generally followed by serial ultrasounds with CT used for pre-operative mapping and post-operative follow-up.

<u>Treatment threshold:</u> 5 cm diameter in males and 4.5 cm in females.

Recommended AAA follow-up:

Both sexes	>3 cm <4 cm	Annual US
Male	>4 cm <5 cm	q6 month US
Female	>4 cm <4.5 cm	q6 month US
Male	>5 cm	Vascular surgery consult and CTA
Female	>4.5–5 cm	Vascular surgery consult and CTA

Pre-operative evaluation of AAA: What to look for
- Location of AAA—suprarenal, juxtarenal, infrarenal.
- Branch vessel patency and origins—do they originate from the aneurysm?
- Maximal transverse diameter of the aorta.
  - Measure outer wall to outer wall (not the lumen).
  - Must measure this perpendicular to the long axis of the aorta.

- If endovascular repair is planned, several other factors must be assessed:
  - Aneurysm neck—is it long enough?
  - Size of the iliac arteries—are they large enough for the delivery sheath?

Post endovascular repair of AAA: looking for endoleaks

Endoleaks are a known complication of endovascular aneurysm repair.
- Defined as arterial flow within the aneurysm sac external to the endograft.
- On CT, a blush of contrast is seen within the sac either on the arterial phase or delayed images (see Figure 3.41).

> **Endoleak classification**
> A classification scheme has been developed to describe the different types of endoleaks that can occur.
> Type II is the most common type identified at CT, and represents inflow and outflow from patent branch vessels, most commonly the IMA and lumbar arteries.

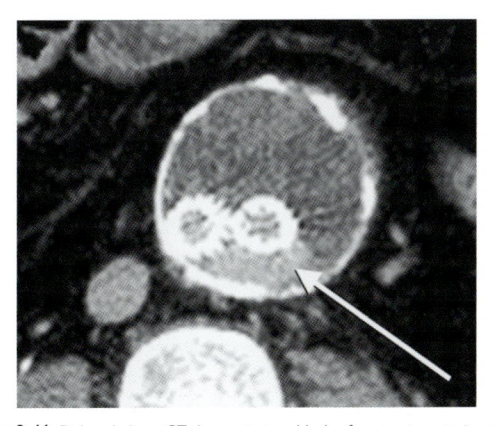

Figure 3.41 Delayed phase CT demonstrate a blush of contrast posterior to the stent graft (arrow), consistent with an endoleak.

Abdominal aortic dissection (AD)

Isolated abdominal aortic dissections are rare, accounting for only approximately 2% of all aortic dissections. More commonly, they extend from the thoracic aorta into the abdominal aorta.
- May be spontaneous, post-traumatic, or iatrogenic, most commonly related to catheter based interventions.
- Clinical presentation—abdominal pain, back pain, or limb ischemia.

CT findings (see Figure 3.42):
See chapter 2, Chest Imaging, "Dissection," p. 104 for general imaging findings in aortic dissection.
- Evaluate for end-organ ischemia.
  - Assess adequacy and symmetry of renal, splenic, and hepatic perfusion.
  - Look for signs of bowel ischemia (wall thickening, pneumatosis, portal venous gas).

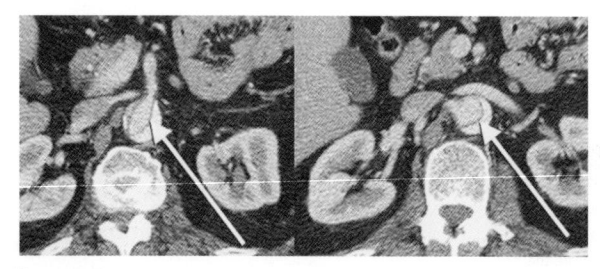

Figure 3.42 Axial contrast enhanced CTA demonstrates the intimal flap of aortic dissection (arrows). In this case, the true lumen is lower in attenuation than the false, indicating slower flow. The superior mesenteric and right renal arteries are perfused via the true lumen. The nephrograms are symmetric.

What about MRA?
MRA can demonstrate the same features of an aneurysm or dissection as CTA, and has the benefit of providing better soft tissue contrast than CT in patients who cannot receive iodinated contrast or gadolinium (see Figure 3.43).

Cirrhosis

Imaging findings
- Small liver with nodular surface and a heterogeneous enhancement pattern. Caudate lobe hypertrophy may occur.
- Main portal vein can occlude, and small serpiginous collaterals develop to supply the intrahepatic portal vein branches (called "cavernous transformation" of the portal vein).
- Signs of portal hypertension:
  - Splenomegaly and ascites.
  - Varices: esophageal, recanalization of the umbilical vein, spontaneous spleno-renal shunt.
- These patients have an increased risk of hepatocellular carcinoma (HCC) (see "Hepatocellular Carcinoma" p. 170).

Liver masses

Hypovascular masses
- Most conspicuous during peak hepatic parenchymal enhancement (during the portal venous phase).
- Do not require multi-phase imaging.

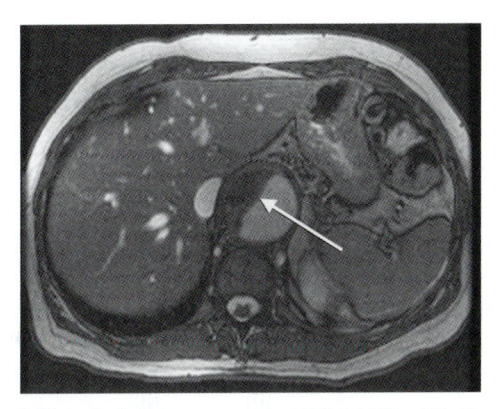

Figure 3.43 Aortic dissection on non-contrast MRI. Axial T2-weighted image demonstrates an aortic dissection flap (arrow) bisecting the true and false lumens. Note the differing signal intensities of the lumens, indicative of differential flow velocities. The dissection flap would not be visible on a non-contrast CT.

Hypervascular masses
- Most conspicuous during the late arterial phase of contrast enhancement. Tumors are brighter than the liver parenchyma during this phase.
- On the portal venous phase, these tumors may be brighter, darker, or the same intensity/attenuation as normal liver parenchyma.
- Dual phase (arterial and venous) imaging required for diagnosis.

The type of tumor suspected, any history of previous malignancy, and pertinent clinical history such as cirrhosis will guide prescription of the appropriate protocol.

Enhancement pattern of common hepatic masses
Hypovascular:
- Cyst.
- Metastasis from GI tract adenocarcinoma.
- Metastasis from breast, lung, pancreas cancer.

Hypervascular:
- Focal nodular hyperplasia and adenomas.
- Hepatocellular carcinoma.
- Metastasis from neuroendocrine tumors (islet cell, carcinoid, pheochromocytoma), GIST, renal cell carcinoma.

MRI versus CT
MRI is often used to characterize liver lesions that are indeterminate at US or CT scans. Certain conditions have characteristic MRI features that allow for a definitive diagnosis.

MRI: When do I use hepatobiliary gadolinium based agents?
- To distinguish focal nodular hyperplasia (FNH) from metastasis, hemangiomas, etc.
- To evaluate the biliary tree for mass, stricture, leak—usually done in conjunction with MRCP (see p. 153).

Benign hepatic tumors
Hemangioma
The most common benign hepatic tumor, with an estimated prevalence of 7–20%. May be multiple. There are different types of hemangiomas; only the "classic" will be described here.

Imaging findings:
- Lobular mass, high signal intensity on T2 MRI, occult on non-contrast CT.
- Progressive enhancement on successive phases of imaging, with nodular collections of contrast extending from the periphery of the lesion to the center.
- On delayed images, the lesion retains contrast and is isodense or hyperdense on CT (isointense/hyperintense on MR) (see Figure 3.44).

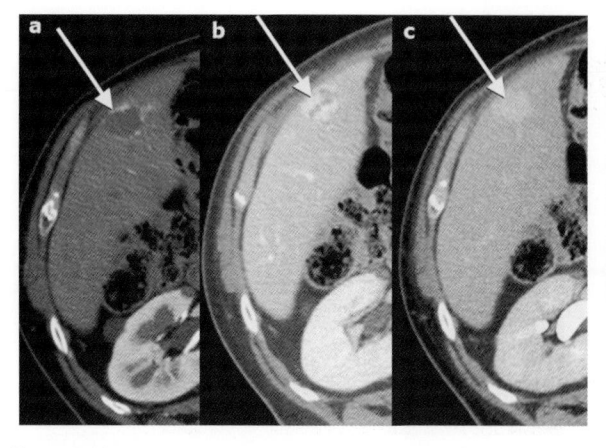

Figure 3.44 Hepatic hemangioma. Axial contrast enhanced CT images in the arterial phase (a), PV phase (b), and 5-minute delay (c). The lesion demonstrates progressive nodular enhancement, from the periphery to the center. On delayed images there is retention of contrast similar in density to that in the hepatic veins. This pattern of enhancement is very specific for hemangioma.

Focal nodular hyperplasia (FNH)
The second most common benign hepatic neoplasm, occurring primarily in young females. A benign vascular tumor of the liver containing hepatocytes, bile ducts, blood vessels, and Kupffer cells. Most accurately diagnosed with MRI using hepatobiliary IV contrast agents (see chapter 1, Radiology Essentials, "What about contrast?" p. 17).

Imaging findings:
- Brisk, uniform arterial phase enhancement +/− hypoenhancing central scar.
- Portal venous phase images: isodense/isointense to liver.
- Delayed (hepatocyte phase) images: retain contrast. Iso/hyperdense or iso/hyperintense to normal liver (see Figure 3.45).
- Progressive enhancement of the scar may occur.

Adenoma
A benign tumor of hepatocytes, lacking bile ducts and portal triad structures. Adenomas are more common in women, and they are associated with oral contraceptives.

CT and MRI findings:
- Brisk, uniform arterial phase enhancement.
- Portal venous and delayed images-occult, similar to liver.
- May be heterogenous on non-contrast CT or T1 MRI; they are prone to hemorrhage.

Adenoma can be difficult to distinguish from a well differentiated hepatocellular carcinoma (HCC).

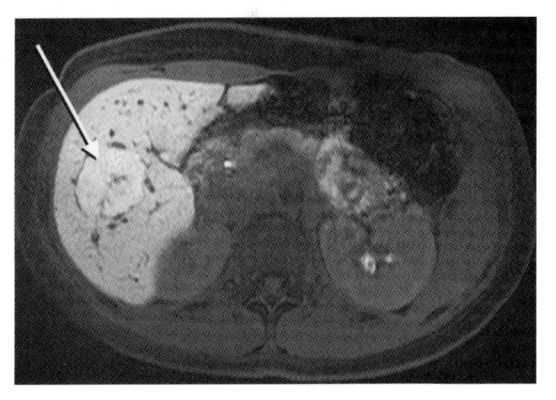

Figure 3.45 FNH. Axial contrast enhanced fat saturated T1-weighted image acquired 20 minutes following injection of a hepatobiliary contrast agent shows densely enhancing right liver lobe mass (arrow) with a central scar consistent with FNH. Other hypervascular lesions would be low signal intensity on these images. Note the expected excretion of contrast agent into the common bile duct.

Malignant hepatic tumor: Hepatocellular carcinoma
The most common primary tumor of the liver. Is associated with hepatitis B and C, and cirrhosis of any cause.

Classic CT and MRI findings:
- Brisk enhancement in the late arterial phase, brighter than adjacent parenchyma.
- "Wash out" in the portal venous phase such that they are low attenuation/intensity compared to normal enhancing liver.
  - May see pseudocapsular enhancement.
- Can be a focal mass or diffuse and infiltrative.
- Prone to invade the hepatic or portal veins—look for enhancing tumor thrombus in the veins.
  See Figures 3.46 and 3.47.

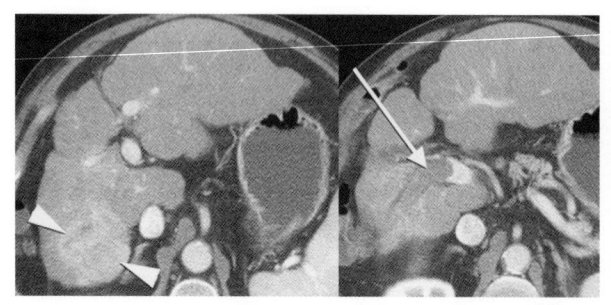

Figure 3.46 Hepatocellular carcinoma with portal vein invasion. Late arterial phase CT images demonstrate a hypervascular mass in the posterior right hepatic lobe (arrowheads). The low attenuation filling defect in the right portal vein represents tumor thrombus, from direct extension of tumor into the vein (arrow).

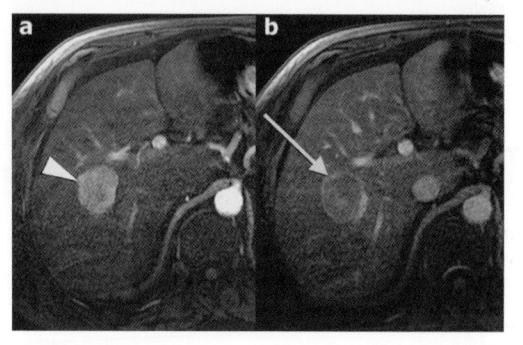

Figure 3.47 Hepatocellular carcinoma on MRI. T1 fat saturated contrast enhanced MRI in the (a) late arterial phase and (b) portal venous phase show avid enhancement of the tumor in the right hepatic lobe in the arterial phase (arrowhead), and rapid washout of contrast in the PVP. Note the peripheral enhancement of the pseudocapsule (arrow).

Imaging characteristics of other common liver lesions:

Simple cyst
- Circumscribed low T1 signal, very high T2 signal (MRI), or low density (CT).
- No enhancement.

Metastases (see Figure 3.26, p. 141)
- Variably low T1 signal, mildly increased T2 signal.
- Differential enhancement pattern will reflect vascularity of lesion
  - Some are hypervascular and some hypovascular
- Low signal intensity on 20-minute images obtained with hepatobiliary contrast agents.

Pancreatic masses

Enhancement pattern of common pancreatic masses

Hypovascular:
- Cyst.
- Adenocarcinoma.
- Cystic neoplasm—mucinous and serous.
- Most metastasis.

Hypervascular:
- Islet cell tumors (neuroendocrine).

CT versus MRI

Benefits of MRI over CT include:
- MRCP can be performed concurrently to evaluate the biliary and pancreatic ducts (see "MRCP" in "Protocols and Technical Considerations" p. 153).

Techniques and protocols—special considerations

Dual-phase imaging post contrast is essential to evaluate the pancreas.
- Late arterial phase: pancreatic parenchyma enhances maximally.
  - Assess degree and homogeneity of pancreatic enhancement.
  - Evaluate arterial encasement and narrowing.
- PV phase.
  - Assess patency and encasement of SMV, splenic and portal veins
  - Optimal time to evaluate for metastasis to liver.

Pancreatic adenocarcinoma

- Hypovascular solid mass. Can be subtle and infiltrative.
- Most conspicuous on the late arterial (pancreatic parenchymal) phase.
  - Low attenuation/intensity compared with brightly enhancing gland.
- Duct peripheral to the mass may be dilated, and gland may be atrophic.
- Lesions in the pancreatic head often cause both pancreatic and common common-bile bile-duct dilatation (known as the double double-duct sign) (see Figure 3.48).

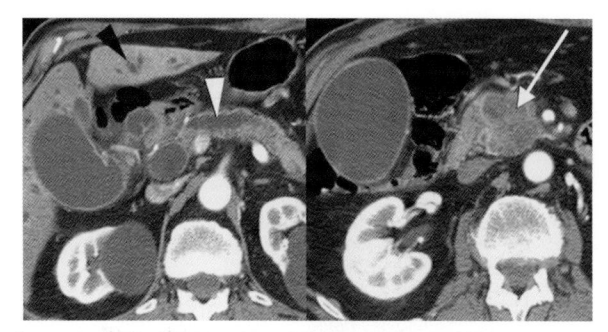

Figure 3.48 Pancreatic adenocarcinoma. Axial contrast enhanced CT (late arterial phase) in a patient with painless jaundice reveals a heterogeneously low density mass in the pancreatic head (arrow). The pancreatic duct peripheral to the mass (white arrowhead) and the intra-hepatic bile ducts (black arrowhead) are dilated, and the gallbladder is markedly distended.

- Vascular invasion/encasement (affects surgical respectability):
  - Narrowing or encasement of SMA or celiac axis.
  - Narrowing, occlusion, or encasement of the peri-pancreatic veins (splenic, superior mesenteric, portal).

Islet cell tumors
Hypervascular masses that enhance more avidly than the gland, and are best seen on early arterial phase images. These tumors include insulinoma, gastrinoma, and glucagonoma.

Choledocholithiasis and pancreatico-biliary ductal abnormalities

Choledocholithiasis
- On MRI, stones appear as a signal void (black) (see Figure 3.49).
- MRCP is more sensitive than CT and US for detection of choledocholithiasis (and more sensitive than CT for cholelithiasis).
- MRCP often obtained pre-operatively to exclude choledocholithiasis prior to cholecystectomy.

Bile duct strictures
- Diagnosed with MRCP.
- MRCP better than ERCP for depicting intrahepatic bile duct strictures, particularly in patients with CBD or CHD strictures.

Congenital abnormalities
- Pancreas divisum: Accessory pancreatic duct remains patent, draining the body and tail of the pancreas into the duodenum via the minor papilla, which is often stenotic.
- Annular pancreas: Pancreatic tissue lateral to descending duodenum.
- Accessory or aberrant cystic duct, biliary ducts.

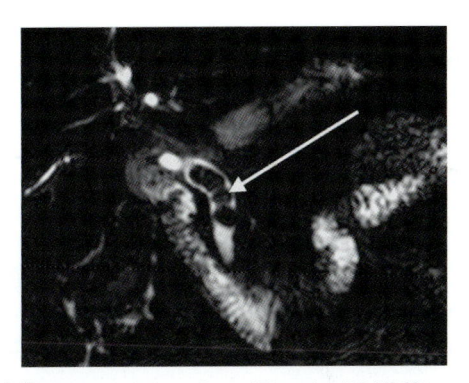

Figure 3.49 Choledocholisthiasis. Coronal T2-weighted 3D MRCP image demonstrates fluid in the biliary tree and small bowel as high-signal intensity. Three low signal foci are present within the common bile duct (arrow), consistent with choledocholisthiasis.

Urolithiasis and hydronephrosis
Urolithiasis
- Imaging test of choice is non-contrast CT.
  - The use of IV contrast does not improve diagnosis, and in fact excreted contrast in the collecting system may obscure the calculi.
- Low dose techniques are utilized to reduce the radiation dose in the young patient population commonly evaluated for this condition.

CT findings:
- Calculi are high attenuation on CT; similar to bone.
  - Look for dense foci within the renal collecting system and along the expected course of each ureter.
- Calculi may be obstructing or non-obstructing.
  - Look for associated signs of obstruction (Hydronephrosis). See Figure 3.50.

Pitfalls:
- Small calculi may only be visible on the thin section images.
- Phleboliths in pelvis may be confused with calculi.

Hydronephrosis
Dilated renal collecting system and/or ureter due to obstruction. Dilatation occurs to the level of obstruction.

> **Not all that is dilated is obstructed!**
> A dilated collecting system should only be called "hydronephrosis" if it is dilated due to obstruction. Collecting system may be dilated from other causes, including congenital, prior obstruction and chronic reflux. In these cases, the term *hydronephrosis* is not accurate.

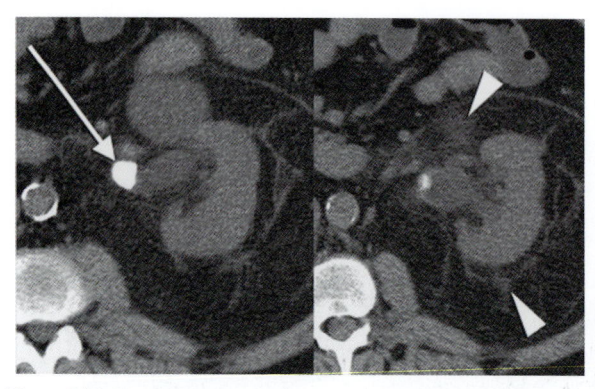

Figure 3.50 Obstructing calculus. Two non-contrast CT images demonstrate a large calculus in the left renal pelvis (arrow), with dilated renal collecting system and peri-nephric stranding (arrowheads) indicating acute obstruction.

CT findings:
- Dilated renal collecting system +/− ureter depending on the site of obstruction.
- Renal enlargement with peri-nephric and/or peri-ureteric stranding.
- On non-contrast study, can be difficult to distinguish dilated and obstructed versus dilated but not obstructed collecting system.
- Tc-99m MAG3 lasix study may be indicated. (see chapter 9, "Renal Imaging" p. 430.)
- If IV contrast has been administered, look for asymmetric nephrograms
  - The parenchyma of the obstructed kidney enhances more slowly and less avidly than the contralateral normal kidney (see Figure 3.51).

Pitfalls:
- Para-pelvic cysts can produce similar appearance.
  - Look to see if the fluid filled structures communicate (representing collecting system) or are separate (cysts).

Hydronephrosis: common causes
- Stones.
- Tumor-transitional cell carcinoma, prostate carcinoma invading the bladder base.
- Blood clot.
- Sloughed papilla.
- Iatrogenic/post surgical or stenting.
- Congenital ureteropelvic junction obstruction.
- Extrinsic ureteral compression from pelvic masses or adenopathy.

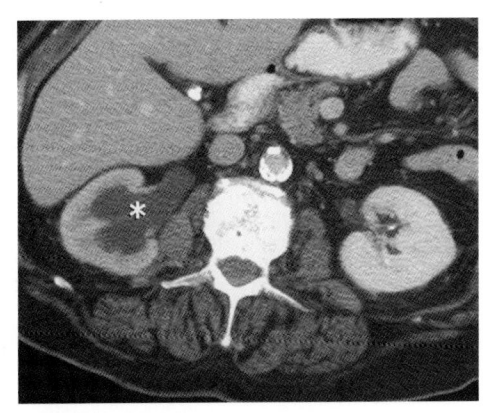

Figure 3.51 Right hydronephrosis. Contrast enhanced CT shows dilated right renal collecting system (star) and delayed enhancement of the right kidney ('delayed nephrogram') compared to the left due to renal obstruction.

Renal masses and hematuria

MRI versus CT
MRI is indicated in the following situations:
- To characterize renal masses that are indeterminate on CT: greater soft tissue contrast at MRI often permits the characterization of small renal masses.
- In the follow-up of equivocal renal lesions to avoid repetitive ionizing radiation.
- CT is preferred for hematuria, since calculi are a common cause and MRI is less sensitive for urolithiasis than CT.

Renal cysts
The most common renal mass, simple cysts arise from the cortex. They increase in size and number with age.

<u>Simple cysts: CT and MRI findings:</u>
- Well defined, round, non-enhancing.
- Uniformly fluid attenuation (<20 HU) on CT.
- Uniformly T2 hyperintense, T1 hypointense on MRI.
- Lack a discernable wall.
- Lack internal septations, calcifications, or nodularity.

<u>Complex cysts: CT and MRI findings:</u>
- Well defined, round or lobular, non-enhancing.
- Contain internal septations, calcifications, or mural nodules.
- If prior hemorrhage or high protein content:
  - High attenuation on CT.
  - T1 hyperintense on MRI.

> **Complex renal cysts may be cystic renal cell carcinoma**
> - Cysts are graded according to their imaging features using the Bosniak criteria (see box).
> - Risk of malignancy increases with increasing grade, and management is based on the grade:
>   - Category I and II lesions require no further workup or imaging.
>   - Category IIF lesions require follow up to prove their benignity by demonstrating stability.
>   - Category III and IV lesions are treated surgically.

> **Bosniak classification of renal cysts**
> I: Meets criteria for simple cyst.
> II: Cyst with few hairline-thin septa, fine calcification, or a short segment of thicker calcification.
> Uniform high attenuation lesions <3 cm with sharp margins.
> IIF: Does not clearly meet criteria for category II or III.
> Totally intra-renal high attenuation lesions >3 cm.
> III: Thickened irregular wall, measureable enhancement in wall or septa.
> IV Distinct, enhancing soft tissue component. These masses are clearly malignant.

Renal Cell Carcinoma (RCC)
<u>CT and MRI findings:</u>
- Round or lobular solid mass.
- Enhancement pattern varies:
  - Small lesions are often only mildly heterogeneous.
  - Large lesions may be markedly heterogeneous.
- Tumor extension into the renal vein, IVC, adrenal gland, and extension beyond the renal (Gerota's) fascia.
- Regional lymphadenopathy in the retroperitoneum.

Angiomyolipoma (AML)
A hamartoma, these lesions contain variable amount of fat, vascular elements, and soft tissue elements. These have a propensity to bleed.
- Heterogeneous mass—parts may enhance avidly.
- Diagnosed by presence of intralesional, macroscopic fat:
  - Very low density on CT-confirm with HU measurement.
  - Look at fat saturation images on MRI for loss of signal in lesion.

Adrenal masses
Small, uniform attenuation adrenal masses are encountered incidentally in ~ 1% of CTs. In the absence of a history of extra-adrenal malignancy, the vast majority of these masses are benign, non-functioning adenomas.

CT versus MRI
Both can be used to characterize adrenal lesions. Other than avoiding radiation with MRI, no specific benefits of MRI over CT exist.

Adrenal adenomas (see Figure 3.52)

Hormone producing adenomas are usually discovered clinically; however, *non-functioning* adenomas are typically incidental imaging findings. They can be confidently diagnosed on CT/MRI based on their intracytoplasmic lipid content and contrast washout characteristics (helping to distinguishing them from non-lipid rich lesions such as pheochromocytoma and metastasis).

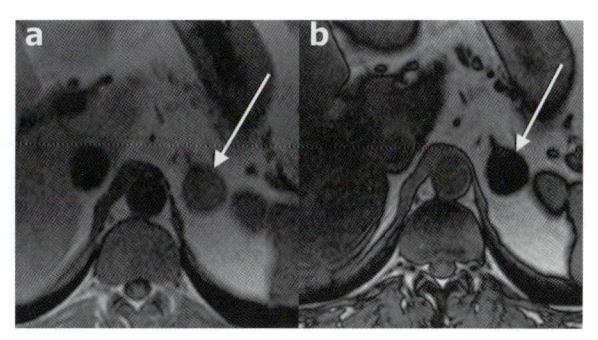

Figure 3.52 Adrenal adenoma. Axial T1-weighted (a) in phase and (b) out of phase MR images demonstrate a small left adrenal mass (arrow) with significant loss of signal on out of phase images due to the presence of intracytoplasmic lipid, diagnostic of adrenal adenoma.
Image courtesy of William Weadock, MD, University of Michigan

Imaging findings:
- Microscopic lipid content produces:
  - Low attenuation on unenhanced CT (< 10 HU).
  - Loss of signal on T1 out of phase MRI images (compared to inphase). See Figure 3.52.
- Not all adenomas contain sufficient lipid to be diagnostic.
- Adenomas enhance rapidly and washout quickly.
- The washout of contrast on delayed images gives an indication of the likelihood of adenoma:

Adrenal mass characterization on CT: Calculating washout

U=unenhanced E=enhanced D=delay (15 min)
Unenhanced images:
A HU measurement of <10 is 98% specific for adenoma.
Relative washout: [E-D/E]
Value >40% is 96% sensitive, 100% specific for adenoma.
Enhancement washout: [E-D/E-U]
Value >60% is 88% sensitive, 96% specific for adenoma.

Primary adrenocortical carcinoma
- Large at diagnosis, heterogeneous enhancement.
- Heterogeneous signal/attenuation depending on degree of hemorrhage and necrosis.
- Often contain calcification.

Adrenal metastases
- Variable size and density/intensity.
- Measure > 12 HU on non-contrast CT.
- No loss of signal on out of phase MRI.

Workup of incidentally discovered adrenal masses

<u>Imaging features diagnostic of benign etiology</u>
- HU < 10 on CT, or diagnostic features of myelolipoma.
  - No further workup..

<u>If imaging features non-diagnostic</u>
>4 cm size—consider PET, biopsy or resection.
<4 cm size—workup depends on history of cancer:
- If none and imaging features are benign, 12-month follow-up CT or MRI.
- If none and imaging features are suspicious, or if history of cancer:
  - Unenhanced CT or MRI, if needed, adrenal washout CT to attempt to characterize.
  - If unable to characterize, consider biopsy.

Common conditions best evaluated with MRI

Certain conditions are better evaluated with MRI than CT, either due to a need to avoid ionizing radiation (as in pregnancy), or because it provides excellent soft tissue contrast of specific structures that cannot be achieved with CT. MRI is superior to CT for imaging the female pelvis.

Acute abdomen in the pregnant and young patient

MRI produces high quality imaging of the abdomen and pelvis without ionizing radiation and, therefore, has unique applications in the pregnant patient or young patient. Rapidly acquired "turbo/fast" sequences help to minimize the artifacts caused by fetal motion, as well as other sources of motion.

Common uses in pregnancy (usually after initial evaluation with ultrasound):
- Abdominal pain.
- To exclude appendicitis.
- To exclude ovarian torsion.

Safety of MRI in pregnancy
The effects of the energy created at MRI upon the fetus are unknown, but to date no short- or long term fetal effects have been documented. Gadolinium based contrast agents are not routinely administered in pregnancy because their effects on the fetus are unknown.

Uterus
Leiomyomas
Most common uterine tumor. MRI usually performed following pelvic ultrasonography.

Benefits of MRI over ultrasonography:
- Tumor vascularity can be assessed; predictive of response to certain treatments (e.g., embolization).
- Location can be more accurately sub-typed (subserosal, submucosal, pedunculated, myometrial).
- Distinction of pedunculated fibroids from ovarian masses.

MR findings:
- Well defined uterine masses.
- Generally low to isointense on T1, hypointense T2.
- Appearance may vary secondary to hemorrhage, degeneration, edema, necrosis, and Ca++.
- Variable enhancement—some hypervascular, some isoenhancing to myometrium, some undergo cystic degeneration and don't enhance.

Adenomyosis
Ectopic endometrial tissue located within the myometrium, with associated smooth muscle hyperplasia. Clinical presentation overlaps that of leiomyomas; pelvic pain and dysfunctional uterine bleeding.

MR findings:
- Scattered foci of bright T2 signal (cysts, hemorrhage) within the junctional zone (the low signal intensity inner myometrium that borders the endometrium). May be focal or diffuse.
- Thickened, low T2 signal junctional zone (>12 mm).
- Isointense to myometrium on T1.

Meullerian duct anomalies
- MRI is the preferred method for evaluating these congenital anomalies.
- High quality, high resolution coronal and axial images of the endometrial cavity are obtained.

Ovary
MRI is excellent at characterizing benign ovarian lesions, such as cysts, hemorrhagic cysts, and dermoids. Malignant cystic lesions cannot be differentiated with certainty from complex benign cystic lesions.

MR technique and protocol
- Fat saturation techniques are mandatory to evaluate intra-lesional high T1 signal, which can be produced by fat or hemorrhage.
- IV contrast is utilized to assess for septal or mural enhancement.

MRI findings of common ovarian lesions

Cyst:
- Uniform low T1 signal, high T2 signal, non-enhancing.
- No discernable wall.

Hemorrhagic cyst:
- Heterogeneously bright on T1, no loss of signal with fat saturation.
- Variable on T2.
- No enhancement.

Dermoid (see Figure 3.53):
- Signal will depend on volume of fat and presence of Ca++.
- Loss of signal on T1 fat saturation images.
- Often has solid and cystic components.

Endometrioma: Ectopic endometrial glands/stroma forming cystic collection of blood products.
- Recurrent hemorrhage causes heterogeneity on MRI, with variable, high T1 signal, high T2 signal.
- May be better visualized on T1 fat saturated sequences.
- Wall enhances, central contents do not.

Ovarian carcinoma:
- Multicystic lesion.
- Septal thickening and enhancement.
- Mural nodularity, thickening, and enhancement.

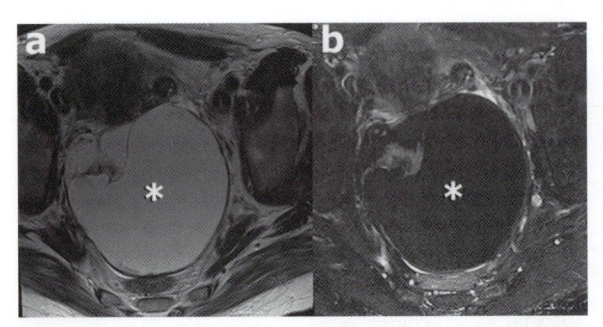

Figure 3.53 Large ovarian dermoid. (a) Axial T2 weighted and (b) T2 weighted fat saturation images through the pelvis demonstrate a large, predominantly high T2 signal pelvic mass (star) that loses signal with fat saturation.

Don't miss diagnoses

These critical diagnoses should not be missed on imaging as they require urgent treatment. The modality of choice for evaluation and the critical imaging findings to make the diagnosis are listed:

Aortic dissection (CTA)
- Spiraling true and false lumens; flap separates them.
- Differential luminal opacification or intramural hematoma.
- Branch vessel occlusion, organ hypoperfusion.

Ruptured abdominal aortic aneurysm (CT or CTA)
- Abdominal aortic aneurysm.
- Perianeurysmal/retroperitoneal hematoma.
- Aortic contrast extravasation outside of aortic lumen.
  - Indicates active bleeding during period of scan **URGENT** (see Figure 3.54).

Mesenteric ischemia/bowel infarction (radiography or CT)
- Pneumatosis intestinalis.
- Mesenteric and/or portal venous gas.
- Mesenteric arterial occlusion (CT).

Colonic volvulus (radiography)
- Single loop of markedly dilated bowel.

Toxic megacolon (radiography)
- Marked dilatation of the transverse colon.
- +/− wall thickening, thumbprinting.

Perforation and free air (upright CXR, decubitus abdominal radiograph and CT)
- Extraluminal air within peritoneal cavity and/or retroperitoneum.
- Enteric contrast extravasation.
- Abscess or air/fluid collection (contained perforation).

Emphysematous cholecystitis (CT and radiography)
Air in gallbladder lumen or wall.

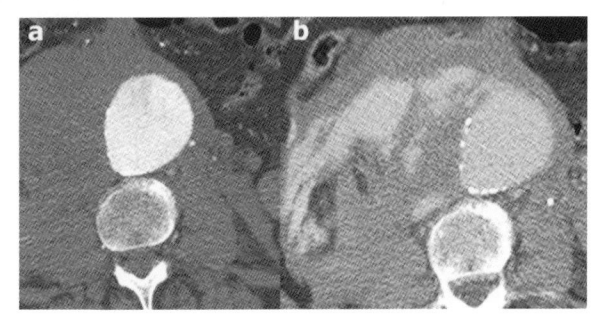

Figure 3.54 Ruptured AAA. (a) Arterial phase and (b) delayed images demonstrate extensive retroperitoneal hematoma obscuring the IVC and psoas muscles. The delayed image shows active contrast extravasation into the right retroperitoneal space from the AAA.

Emphysematous pyelonephritis (CT)
Air in collecting system or renal parenchyma.

References

Berland LL, Silverman SG, Gore RM, et al, Managing incidental findings on abdominal CT: White Paper of the ACR Incidental Findings Committee, *JACR* 2010; 7(10): 754–773.

Bosniak MA. The current radiological approach to renal cysts. *Radiology* 1986;158:1–10.

Dunnick, NR, Korobkin M, Imaging of adrenal incidentalomas: Current status, *AJR* 2002;179:559–568.

Horton KM, Corl FM, Fishman EK, CT evaluation of the colon: Inflammatory disease, *Radiographics* 2000; 20(2):399–418.

Leyendecker JR, Brown JJ, *Practical Guide to Abdominal & Pelvic MRI.* Philadelphia, PA: Lippincott Williams & Wilkins, 2004.

Moeller TB, Reif E, *Pocket Atlas of Sectional Anatomy. Computed Tomography and Magnetic Resonance Imaging. Volume II: Thorax, Heart, Abdomen, Pelvis*, New York: Thieme, 2007.

Moore EE, Cogbill TH, Jurkovich MD, et al. Organ injury scaling: Spleen and liver (1994 revision). *J Trauma* 1995;38(3):323–324.

Moore EE, Shackford SR, Pachter HL, et al. Organ injury scaling: Spleen, liver, and kidney. *J Trauma* 1989;29(12):1664–1666.

Normal CT anatomy: www.dartmouth.edu/~anatomy

Ryan S, McNicholas M, Eustace S, *Anatomy for Diagnostic Imaging*, 3rd ed. Edinbugh, Saunders, 2010.

Vaccaro JP, Brody JM, CT cystography in the evaluation of major bladder trauma, *Radiographics* 2000 (20);1371–1381.

Chapter 4

Musculoskeletal Imaging

Donna Magid, MD, Avneesh Chhabra, MD, and Albert J. Song, MD

Normal anatomy *184*
Radiography *184*
   Requesting musculoskeletal radiographs *184*
   How are images acquired? *184*
   How do I read an extremity/joint radiograph? *185*
   Describing the findings on MSK radiographs *187*
   Interpreting the findings *189*
   Pitfalls and problems *191*
Cross sectional imaging *191*
   CT *191*
   MRI *195*
   Ultrasound *197*
Patterns of disease *199*
   Descriptors of radiologic findings *199*
   Fractures *201*
   Internal derangements *204*
   Inflammation *206*
   Arthritis *207*
   Joint effusions *209*
   Other soft tissue abnormalities *209*
   Masses and neoplasms *212*
   Abnormalities of bone marrow *214*
Common conditions *215*
   Pelvis and hip *215*
   Knee *221*
   Ankle *225*
   Shoulder *227*
   Elbow *230*
   Wrist and hand *233*
Joint replacements (arthroplasty) and orthopedic hardware *234*
Procedures *236*
References *238*

Normal anatomy

Illustration and discussion of normal musculoskeletal anatomy is beyond the scope of this text. Suggested reference for radiologic anatomy covered by body region: www.dartmouth.edu/~anatomy

Radiography

Requesting musculoskeletal radiographs

Requisition must include the following clinical information
- Type of injury.
- Specific site of symptoms (e.g., pain, swelling, etc.).
- What you suspect clinically.

Selecting the site to be imaged
Focus and center exam on site of concern. For example:
- To evaluate the knee and ankle, order separate "knee" and "ankle" studies; do not order "tibia-fibula."
  - Long bone radiographs only provide limited exam of joint above/below.
- For finger (or toe) trauma, specify which finger (toe); do not order "hand" or "foot" (see Figure 4.1).

> Appropriate image acquisition depends on precise information in the patient history! Always include EXACTLY where the problem is— e.g., site of pain/tenderness.

How are images acquired?

(See Chapter 1, Radiology Essentials, "Radiography" p. 3 for additional information).

If radiographs are not ordered or performed correctly, the examination may not detect or define abnormalities.

Factors that maximize sensitivity of radiography
- Having the area of concern in the center of the study and making the center of the x-ray beam perpendicular to this site.
- Taking smallest film possible of relevant area.
- Obtaining the appropriate angled views for the area of concern.

Views

At least two and often three or four views are performed for initial assessment of all MSK pathology.
- Frontal (AP, PA).
- Lateral (90 degrees to frontal).
  - A "cross-table lateral" is a lateral radiograph that is taken with the patient supine, i.e., the x-ray beam is horizontal.
- Obliques—these are site specific (e.g., scaphoid view, radial head view).

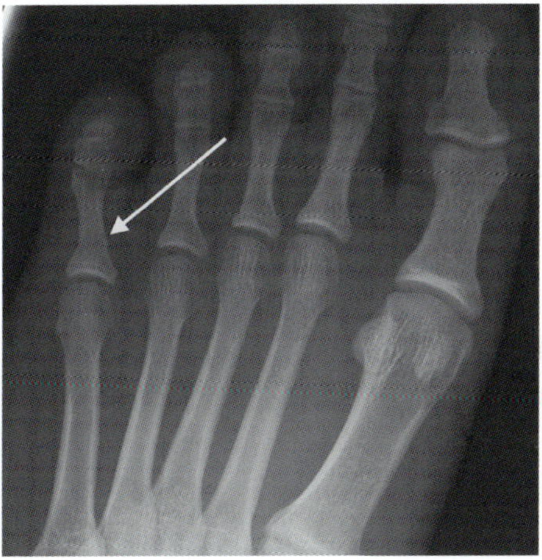

Figure 4.1 Coned and centered view of the small toe demonstrates a subtle, non-displaced metaphyseal fracture of the proximal phalanx small toe (arrow). This was not visible on the 3 view foot radiographs.

Additional views for problem solving
- Additional obliquities—to exclude subtle fracture.
- Contra-lateral extremity for comparison—is it a normal variant?
- Weight bearing or traction views—used most commonly for foot, knee, hip, and acromioclavicular radiographs.
  - May show ligamentous disruption or altered mechanics not appreciated on non-weight bearing views.

How do I read an extremity/joint radiograph?
MSK radiograph interpretation requirements
- High resolution monitors (not laptop!).
- Consistent, meticulous search patterns.
- (Mental) checklists specific both to the anatomic area imaged and to the potential diagnostic/clinical concern.
- Habitual double-checks of "miss" areas.
- Get in the habit of describing what you are seeing *before* you start thinking about the diagnoses.

Search strategies
For all studies you MUST look at the following:

Bones
- Trace the outer contours of the cortex and articular surfaces for discontinuities or step-offs.
- Follow the fine trabecular lines of the medullary spaces to see if they are continuous or disrupted.

CHAPTER 4 **Musculoskeletal imaging**

Joint spaces
- Assess symmetry of cartilaginous spaces.
- Look for narrowing or widening.

Soft tissues
Assess soft tissue/fat/fascial/muscle planes for:
- Displacement or effacement, e.g., by an effusion (see Figure 4.2).
- Density changes, e.g., calcifications, gas or edema in tissues.
- Contour change, e.g., diffuse swelling, tendon enlargement (e.g., Achilles).

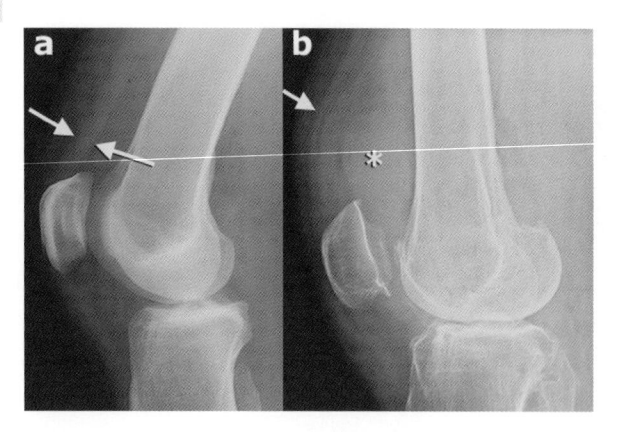

Figure 4.2 (a) Normal lateral knee. Well defined quadriceps tendon (arrows), parallels anterior distal femoral cortex. (b) Joint effusion. Lateral view of the knee shows anterior displacement of the quadriceps tendon (arrow) due to mass effect from a large knee joint effusion (*).

General strategies
- Look for symmetry when possible.
  - May be particularly helpful in children, especially in assessing epiphyses.
  - If necessary (indeterminate findings) obtain a contra-lateral view.
- Review common "miss areas": e.g., anterior process of calcaneus, scaphoid, sacral arches, etc.
- Compare to older studies or reports to assess for chronicity or change.
- When you identify an abnormality, confirm on more than one view.

Unfamiliar or possibly abnormal findings?
- Correlate with history and exam and if possible, old films.
- Consult a "Normal Variant" book (see references) (see Figure 4.3).
  - E.g., normal variant posterior sesamoid bone (called fabella) is seen in up to 30% of knee radiographs.

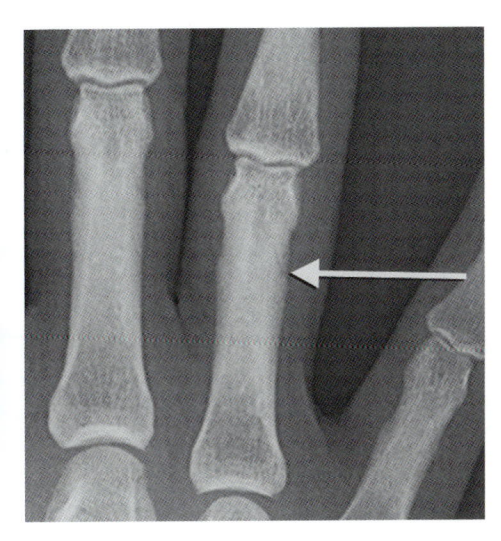

Figure 4.3 Normal variant. The subtle oblique linear radiolucency in the medial cortex of the proximal phalanx of the ring finger (arrow) was NOT point tender and is a normal nutrient foramen.

Describing the findings on MSK radiographs

Semantics

Digits
Thumb (first ray or digit), index (second), long (third), ring (fourth), small (fifth).

Hand/wrist/forearm
- Anterior—use: *palmar, ventral,* or *volar.*
- Posterior—use *dorsal.*
- Medial—use *ulnar.*
- Lateral—use *radial.*

Foot
- Sole—use *plantar.*
- Top—use *dorsal.*

Vague non-medical terms, i.e. *"near," "behind," "next to,"* or *"in front of"* are imprecise and can lead to significant miscommunication or misunderstanding.

CHAPTER 4 **Musculoskeletal imaging**

Terminology
Position descriptors
- All positional descriptors are related to the normal anatomic position:
  - Supine, arms and legs extended straight.
  - Hands supinated, feet plantigrade (at right angles to ankles).
- For describing fracture fragments. See p. 201, "Describing Fractures."

Density
Describes the degree of radioopacity of a lesion.

<u>Sclerotic:</u>
- Hyperattenuating, high density.
- New or reactive bone, osseous proliferation, matrix mineralization.
- Blastic: subset of sclerotic lesions, implies neoplasm.

<u>Lucent:</u>
- Hypoattenuating, low density.
- Lytic: subset of lucent, implying destroyed or resorbed bone as seen with aggressive processes (infection, neoplasm).

Shape
- Linear, round, stellate, ovoid.

Location within long bones (see Figure 4.4)
- Longitudinal location.
  - Epiphyseal, metaphyseal, diaphyseal.
- Axial location.
  - Medullary (central or eccentric), cortical, periosteal.
- Intra-articular.

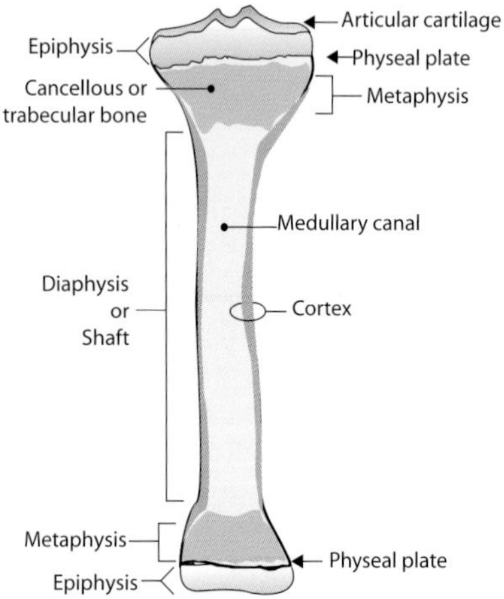

Figure 4.4 Diagram of the zones of a long bone.

Interpreting the findings
Acute or chronic injury?
Chronic findings
- Tend to be smooth, well defined, rounded, corticated.
  - More like river rocks than broken glass.
- Stable from older exams.
- Adjacent fascial planes or soft tissues normal.

Acute findings
- Fractures are sharply defined with disrupted trabeculae or cortex.
- Infection or masses may be ill-defined.
- New or changed compared to older exams.
- May have associated soft tissue changes.
- Swelling, effusion, loss of fat planes.

What to do with "negative" films and high clinical suspicion in trauma?

> Soft tissue injuries (e.g., ligaments, menisci) are almost always occult or associated with non-specific findings on radiographs.

Many fractures are initially extremely subtle or occult. Some fractures (scaphoid, proximal femur, femoral neck, cervical spine) are notorious for being occult on initial radiographs (see Figures 4.5 and 4.6).

If the radiograph is normal and there is high clinical suspicion, consider:

<u>Additional radiographs:</u> (See "Additional Views for Problem Solving," p. 185)

<u>Delayed radiographs:</u>
- Obtain 10–14 d after limb immobilization (cast, splint). These may reveal:
  - Increasing lucency or sclerosis at fracture site.
  - Developing periosteal reaction.

<u>Fluoroscopy:</u>
- "Real time" dynamic imaging may demonstrate injuries not captured with static images (e.g., subluxation, joint instabilities).

<u>CT:</u>
- Useful for complex joints such as subtalar or hip joint.
- Osteopenic patient

<u>MRI:</u>
- Sometimes indicated in osteopenic patient (e.g., proximal femoral fracture looking for marrow edema) (see Figure 4.5).

<u>3-phase bone scans:</u>
A sensitive (though less specific) modality for patients who can't tolerate MRI.

> Negative radiographs do *not* exclude fractures if there is high clinical suspicion. Treat the patient, not the radiograph.

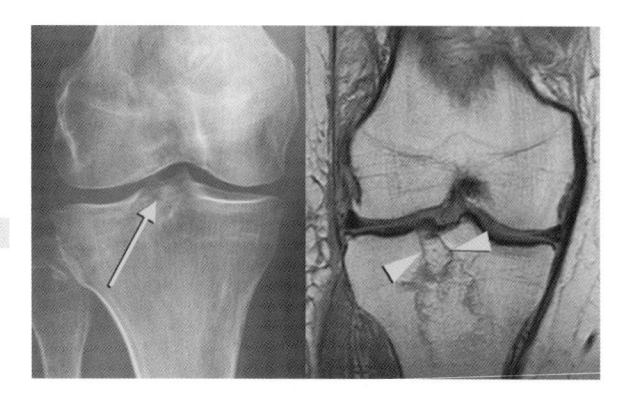

Figure 4.5 Tibial plateau fracture. AP film on day of injury has very subtle subchondral trabecular irregularity and possible radiolucent fracture line (arrow). Joint effusion was seen on the lateral view. Coronal T1-weighted MRI more clearly depicts the multiple tibial fracture lines.

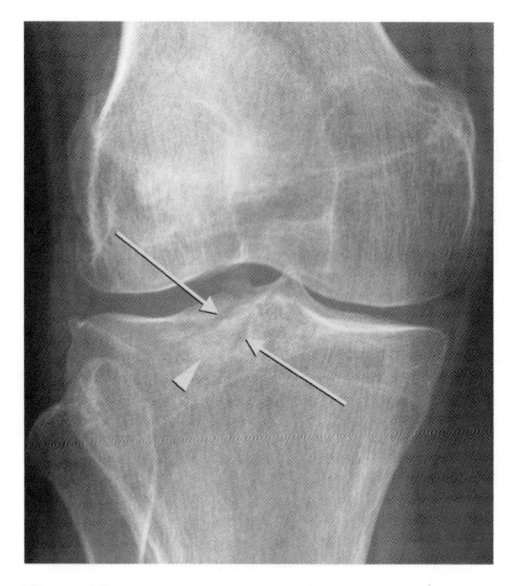

Figure 4.6 Six-week follow-up. AP film now shows both osteoclastic activity with increased lucency of the fracture lines (arrows), and osteoblastic healing as increasing subchondral bone density (arrowhead).

Pitfalls and problems
Radiographs (2D technique) may not visualize non-displaced or complex fractures
- Cross sectional or provocative (e.g., traction) imaging may be required.

Technique dependent
- Radiographs must be obtained in the correct position/rotation
- Inadequate technique may obscure findings
  - Repeat the radiographs if images are substandard

Radiographs are limited in patients with osteopenia
- Nondisplaced fractures can be missed.
- CT/MRI/bone scan may be required.

Pediatric patients
- Bones of children are malleable, fractures may be occult.
- Physeal injuries can be subtle. (see Salter-Harris fractures, p. 315).
- If initial study is negative or equivocal, obtain follow-up radiographs in 10–14 days; may demonstrate healing fracture.

Limited evaluation of soft tissue structures—ligaments, tendons, etc.
- MRI is required.

Cross-sectional imaging

Although radiography is important for the initial screening and diagnosis of musculoskeletal (MSK) pathologies, cross-sectional imaging has revolutionized the care of patients.

Radiographs should always be performed prior to CT/MRI to assist in interpretation of the cross-sectional findings:
- Some lesions can look worrisome for neoplasm based on the MRI findings, yet the plain film may have specifically benign characteristics and prevent a false diagnosis (e.g., myositis ossificans).
- The radiograph can identify unknown orthopedic hardware/devices that may cause artifact on CT or MRI images.

CT

How are images acquired?
General concepts
- High-resolution techniques and thin-slice acquisition are necessary.
- ALARA (as low as reasonably achievable) principle:
  - Focus imaging to the target area so that radiation dose can be minimized.
- No specific patient preparation is necessary other than for CT arthrograms when contrast is injected into the joint.

Reformatting
- Multiplanar reformats are standard. Allows scan to be acquired with extremity in any orientation.
- 3D reformats (see Figure 4.7):
  - Display joint alignment and fracture fragment alignment.
  - Aid in pre-operative planning. Increase diagnostic accuracy.

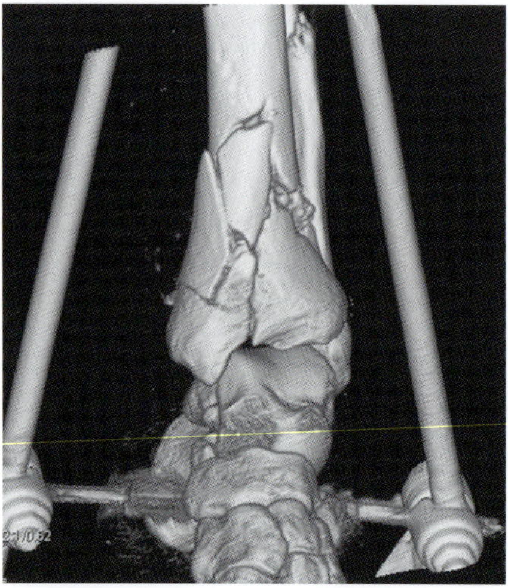

Figure 4.7 Comminuted distal tibial fracture. 3D CT image demonstrates comminuted intra-articular distal tibial metaphyseal and epiphyseal fracture and distal fibular diaphyseal fracture after closed reduction and external fixation.

When to use IV contrast
Rarely indicated.
- Useful for suspected infection, inflammation, or tumors. However, MRI is more sensitive for all of these entities, and CT should be reserved for cases in which MRI is contraindicated.

When should I do a musculoskeletal CT?

Trauma
- Pre-operative evaluation of complex fractures.
  - E.g., pelvic fractures, intra-articular fractures (see Figure 4.8).
- Persistent significant clinical findings with negative radiographs.
- Spine injury.
- To assess for tendon entrapment at the fracture site.
- Suspected vascular injuries associated with fracture/dislocation (CTA).

Infection (osteomyelitis)
- Identify cortical destruction and look for sequestrum (dead piece of bone separated from the surrounding bone within the nidus of infection).
- Intraosseous (Brodie) or soft tissue abscess.
- Secondary findings:
  - Overlying ulcer, sinus tract, or fistula.
  - Foreign body.
- MRI is more sensitive than CT for both bone and soft-tissue infection.

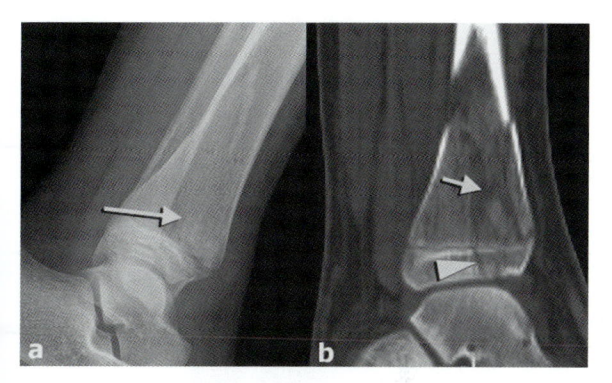

Figure 4.8 Distal tibial fracture in 11-year-old girl with acute ankle injury. (a) Lateral view of ankle shows an oblique fracture through the distal tibial metaphysis (large arrow) with widening of the anterior physeal plate. (b) Sagittal CT reformat demonstrates that the fracture is comminuted, with extension through the metaphysis (small arrow) and epiphysis (arrowhead), a Salter-Harris IV fracture.

Bone tumors
CT is superior to MRI for the evaluation of:
- Periosteal and cortical lesions (see Figure 4.9). These are difficult to see on MRI.
- Internal calcified matrix of lesions (see "Internal Characteristics of Lesions" in "Patterns of Disease," p. 200).
- Integrity of cortex.
  - Endosteal scalloping increases the risk of pathologic fracture.
  - Cortical break through, pathologic fracture.

Prosthesis imaging
CT is used as an adjunct to conventional radiographs to assess for hardware complications, although hardware causes "beam-hardening artifacts" (produces streaking across images).
- See "Joint Replacements and Orthopedic Hardware," p. 234.

CT Arthrography
See "Arthrography Technique," p. 238.

Pitfalls and problems
Soft tissue evaluation
- Soft tissue structures (e.g., tendons, ligaments, and muscle) are similar in density, and can be difficult to resolve on CT.
- Soft tissue lesions and abnormalities (e.g., inflammation and edema) are often isodense or of similar attenuation to muscle, obscuring the lesion.
- MRI has superior soft tissue resolution.

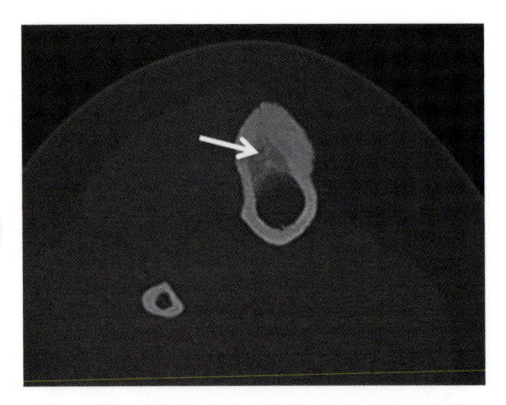

Figure 4.9 Osteoid osteoma. 19-year-old girl with leg pain at night relieved with aspirin. Axial CT image shows a classic lucent nidus (arrow) of an intra-cortical osteoid osteoma with surrounding exuberant cortical thickening and periosteal reaction in the tibia.

Bone marrow pathology
The marrow is sub-optimally assessed with CT.
- Marrow infiltration and replacement disorders, such as leukemia, lymphoma, and metastasis may be missed.
- Red marrow conversion can simulate a marrow replacing process.

Stress injuries
Stress response/transient osteoporosis/trabecular and subchondral fractures may all be occult on CT (MRI is superior to demonstrate the associated marrow edema).

How do I read a musculoskeletal CT?
General strategies

Soft tissue and bones
Although can be assessed on any reformatted series, axial images are typically used.
- Look at bones on the bone algorithm series (enhances edges).

Alignment and longitudinal extent of the pathology
Coronal and sagittal images best display this.

3D images
Evaluate alignment of joints and fracture fragments.
- Often used by orthopedic surgeons for pre-operative planning.

Search strategies: What are you looking for?

Bones
- Cortical interruption, expansion, destruction, or lucency.
- Cortical thinning, thickening, endosteal scalloping, or external erosion (see Figure 4.15, p. 203).

- Medullary trabecular interruption, impaction, or destruction.
- Periosteum—new bone formation, periosteal reaction.

Joints
- Alignment: subluxation or dislocation.
- Widening or narrowing of joint space.
- Effusions.
- Intra-articular fragments, loose bodies.

Soft tissues
- Thickening, masses/lesions, effacement of fat/SQ tissues.
- Muscles: swelling, intramuscular masses/lesions, fat atrophy.
- Fascial planes: displacement or effacement, inflammation/edema, intermuscular masses/lesions.

Neurovascular bundle
- Displacement or encasement of arteries and veins.
- Nerves: thickening, subluxation/dislocation, interruption.

MRI

MRI is a significant advance in MSK imaging for the diagnosis and treatment of many bone, joint, and soft tissue pathologies. MRI provides better soft tissue contrast than CT, and allows excellent evaluation of small ligaments, cartilage, and tendons, which cannot be evaluated on CT.

How are images acquired?
Protocols and technical factors
Each exam uses a combination of pulse sequences, often with fat suppression (fs) to increase the conspicuity of edema on T2 images, or enhancement on post-contrast T1 images.

T1: Good for anatomic evaluation.
PD (proton density): Good for evaluation of knee menisci and articular cartilage.
T2 fat sat / STIR: Fat is hypointense (dark) on both of these sequences.
- Good for evaluation of ligaments, tendons, soft tissue or bone marrow edema or lesions.

3Tesla imaging (high field scanners):
- Better imaging of the labro-ligamentous and articular cartilage anatomy.
- Faster image acquisition, shortening scan times with less motion artifacts

When to use IV contrast
Gadolinium enhanced, fat-suppressed scans should be obtained in suspected infections, inflammatory processes, or tumors.

When should I do a musculoskeletal MRI?
Trauma
- Muscle, tendon, ligament, meniscal, chondral and labral injuries (see Figure 4.29, p. 224).
- Peripheral nerve entrapment and injuries.

- Clinically suspected vascular injuries associated with MSK trauma- use MRA.
- Spine: suspected spinal cord compression.

Infection
Preferred modality for the assessment of soft tissue and bone infection including:
- Joint and osseous involvement, osseous sequestrum.
- Sinus tracts, fistuli, and abscesses as well as devitalized soft tissues.
- Foreign bodies.

Tumors
Preferred modality for assessing:
- Tumor extent.
- Tumor composition.
- See "Masses/Neoplasm," p. 212.

Internal derangement
Preferred modality to assess injury or damage to structural components of a joint including: cartilage, ligaments, tendons, and fibrocartilagenous structures (e.g., labrum, mensicus).
- Knowing the origin, insertion, and normal morphology of these structures is crucial.

Arthritis
Can be used as an adjunct to conventional radiographs for early diagnosis of inflammatory or infectious arthritis.
- Assess for articular cartilage abnormality.
- Diagnose synovitis and joint effusions.
- Diagnose extra-articular manifestations such as tenosynovitis.
- Identify specific diagnostic features of uncommon diseases:
  - E.g., T2 hypointensity seen with hemosiderin deposition in pigmented villonodular synovitis and hemophilia (see Figure 4.10).

Marrow abnormalities
Excellent soft tissue contrast of MRI and the ability to suppress the signal from fat makes MRI suitable for detecting marrow abnormalities and pathology. MRI is more sensitive than radiographs and CT, and more specific than nuclear scans for these pathologies.
- See "Abnormalities of Bone Marrow," p. 214.

Pitfalls and problems

Cortical bone
Cortical bone has low signal intensity on all sequences.
- Small cortical and periosteal lesions may not be identified.
- MR image slices are usually thicker than CT.
- Subtle cortical abnormalities are much better characterized on CT.

Intralesional mineralization/matrix
- Difficult to identify compared to radiographs and CT.
- Soft tissue calcifications, intra-articular bodies are better identified on radiographs and CT.

Patient tolerance
- May not tolerate MRI scans (longer imaging time and claustrophobia).
- Motion artifacts may degrade imaging.

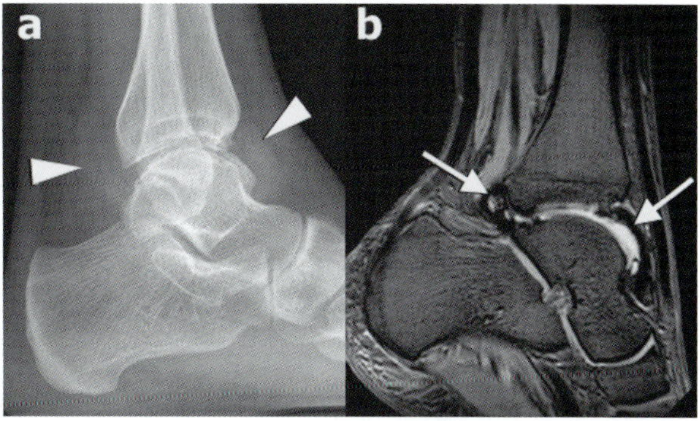

Figure 4.10 Early degenerative joint disease in 18-year-old with hemophilia. (a) Lateral radiograph of the ankle shows a large joint effusion (arrowheads) and early degenerative joint disease characterized by osteophyte formation and eccentric joint space narrowing. (b) Sagittal gradient echo MR image demonstrates a hypointense and thickened joint capsule (arrows) due to hemosiderin deposition from chronic intra-articular hemorrhage.

"Magic angle" phenomenon
Artifactual increased signal in tendons and ligaments when oriented 55 degrees to the main magnet.
- Common in the rotator cuff of the shoulder and tendons of the ankle.
- Must be aware of this entity when interpreting MSK MRI exams.

Ultrasound

US has high spatial resolution for superficial structures, particularly of the hand, wrist, and ankle. US guidance is also commonly used for musculoskeletal procedures such as aspiration/injections, nerve blocks, and tenotomies.

How are images acquired?
- Use high-frequency linear probes: 9–18 MHz:
  - These provide high-resolution images for superficial structures but don't allow penetration to deeper tissues.
  - Lower frequency sector probes may be used for deeper structures, but with lower resolution.
  - Use transducers with a small footprint ("hockey stick" probes) to assess small structures, (e.g., interphalangeal joints).
- Obtain images in the long and short axes.
- Dynamic imaging can be used to diagnose snapping/friction syndromes and impingement.

When should I do a musculoskeletal ultrasound?

Trauma—acute and repetitive injury
- Tendons:
  - Tendinosis, calcific tendinopathy, tenosynovitis.
  - Rupture, subluxation/dislocation, snapping/friction syndromes.

- Impingement syndromes—using dynamic imaging.
- Muscles—strains/tears, rupture, atrophy.
- Evaluation of soft tissue hematoma.
- Foreign body localization (see Figure 4.11).

Neuropathies
- Peripheral nerve entrapment/impingement syndromes.
- (e.g., carpal tunnel syndrome).
- Nerve thickening, subluxation/dislocation.

Infection
- Assessment of soft tissue extent including sinus tract, abscess, and foreign body.

Masses/cysts/tumors
- Differentiation of solid versus cystic mass.
- Evaluate for vascular malformations (marked Doppler flow).

Arthritis
- Ultrasound use is increasing as an adjunct to conventional radiographs.
- Early detection of inflammatory/infectious arthritis, synovitis/tenosynovitis and joint effusions, erosions.

Pitfalls and problems
- The vast majority of osseous pathology cannot be evaluated with ultrasound.
- MR is more specific for the evaluation of vast majority of bone and soft tissue masses. These often appear nonspecific on US.
- Tendon tears can be difficult to differentiate from tendinosis.
- Deeper structures (menisci, glenoid labrum) are poorly resolved or incompletely visualized, and are better evaluated with MRI or CT arthrogram.
- Operator dependent and time consuming as compared to CT and MRI.

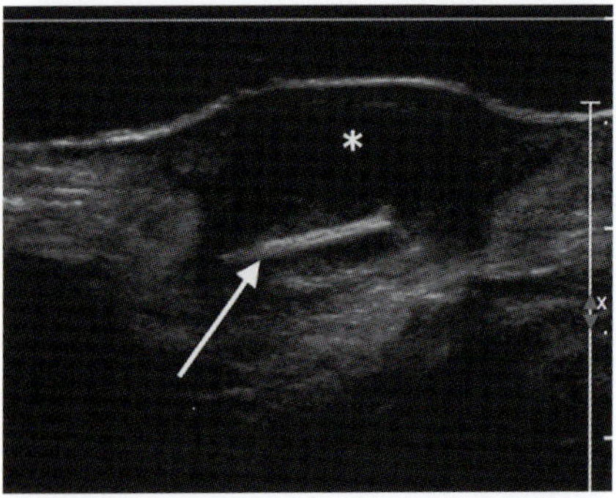

Figure 4.11 Foreign body. US of the thumb shows a splinter as a linear echogenic structure in the subcutaneous soft tissues (arrow) surrounded by fluid (star). Wood is not dense, therefore, this foreign body was not detected on radiographs.

> **What is anisotropy?**
> - Artifact resulting in loss of echoes. Occurs when the incident US beam is not 90 degrees to the tendon fibers. Can mimic pathology.
> - When evaluating tendon or ligament abnormalities, probe angle must be adjusted to differentiate true pathology from artifact.

Patterns of disease

When evaluating an image, the decision process is:
1. Is this abnormal?
2. Is this pattern worrisome for an aggressive process?
3. Is this pattern characteristic for a specific process?

Descriptors of radiologic findings

The radiological findings in MSK lesions have specific descriptors that convey the aggressiveness of a process, and may lead to a specific diagnosis.

Periosteal reaction

The peritosteum is the connective tissue membrane forming the external layer of cortical long bone. When stimulated by trauma, infection, tumor, etc., the cells generate bone matrix that gradually ossifies and creates distinctive patterns (see Figure 4.12).

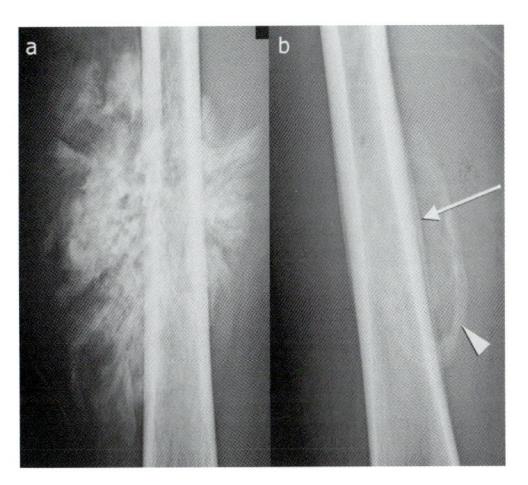

Figure 4.12 (a) Aggressive periosteal reaction. Clouds of periosteal new bone, some nearly perpendicular to cortex, attest to aggression and speed of growth of this high-grade malignancy (osteogenic sarcoma). (b) Non-aggressive periosteal reaction. Second patient, four weeks out from horse kick. A fine, layered periosteal reaction parallels the cortex (arrow) and the oval soft tissue hematoma shows early peripheral calcification or ossification (arrowhead).

- The morphology of the reaction is used to date fracture healing and assess aggressiveness of neoplastic or inflammatory lesions.
  - Slow growth/reaction produces a single, thick, well-defined layer.
  - More active growth/reaction produces layers like onion skin.
  - Rapid/aggressive reaction produces a perpendicular and spiculated pattern (see Figure 4.12).

Lesion margins ("zone of transition")

These are terms used to describe the margins or borders a lesion makes with adjacent bone.
- Sharp: You could draw a fine pencil line around the lesion.
- Ill-defined: Lesion too fuzzy or indistinct to draw a fine line around.
- Marginal sclerosis: Reaction creating a definite radiodense periphery.
- Punched out: Sharply punched out of surrounding bone, like a cookie cutter; no sclerosis.
- Permeative or moth eaten: Multiple ill-defined lesions.

Internal characteristics of lesions

The following terms are used to describe the ossification/calcification of lesions/findings:
- Dystrophic—non-specific calcification.
- Amorphous—featureless, like milk.
- Matrix mineralization—tumor is making calcified tissue, either bone or cartilage. Occurs with benign and malignant processes (see Figure 4.13).
  - <u>Cartilage-forming or chondral</u>: arcs, whorls, and smoke rings. A calcified matrix implies cartilaginous origin lesion such as enchondroma, osteochondroma (see Figure 4.21, p. 213)

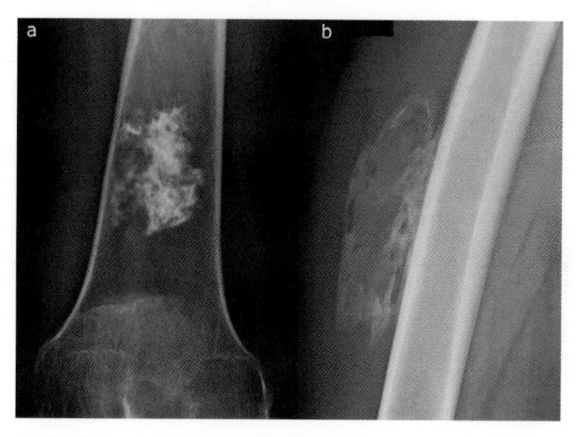

Figure 4.13 (a) Enchondroma. Calcified matrix characterized by well-defined rings and arcs of calcifications clustered in the medullary canal. (b) Post-traumatic myositis ossificans. Ossified matrix characterized by trabeculation and sharp definition progressing from perimeter toward center.

PATTERNS OF DISEASE

- Bone-forming or osseous: looks trabeculated, corticated or amorphous. An osseous matrix generates a different differential diagnosis, such as bone island, heterotopic ossification or neoplasm.

Fractures

Fractures occur due to a failure of osseous structural integrity. The nature of the causative force (twisting, bending, compressive, repetitive, etc.) creates different fracture patterns and indicates where to look for associated injuries. For example:
- Axial loading/jumping injuries with compression of calcaneus, high association of lumbar vertebral compression fractures.
- Twisting injuries producing ankle fractures, likely involvement of specific ligaments, tendons.
- Repetitive actions in certain sports produce characteristic overuse injuries or stress fractures.

Describing fractures

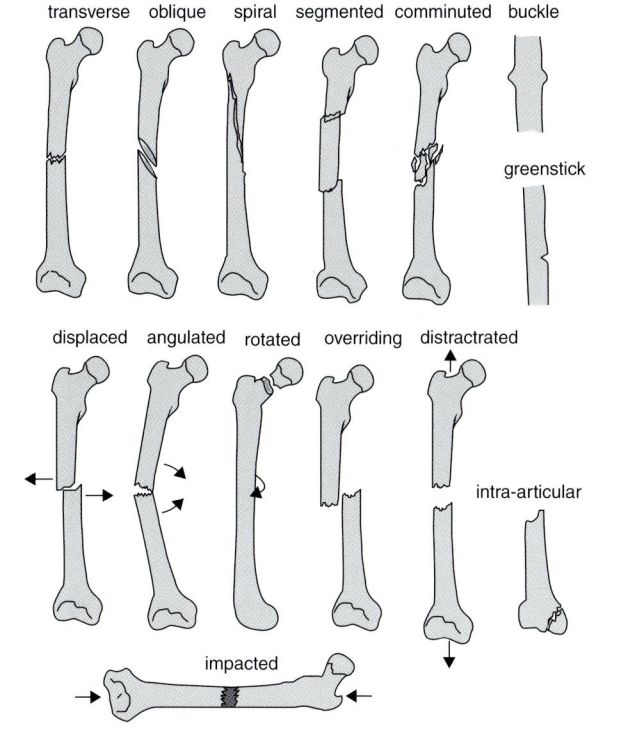

Figure 4.14 Fractures

Displacement:
Position of DISTAL fragment in axial plane (ant/post, med/lat).
- E.g., "3mm lateral displacement of major distal fibular fragment" (see Figure 4.16)

Angulation:
The angulation created by the two bone fragments, deviating from the normal long axis of a bone or extremity.
- Report exact degree measurement.
- Can be referenced to where DISTAL fragment went relative to PROXIMAL or by direction of resultant apex of angulation between fracture fragments.

Rotation:
Relative clockwise or counterclockwise rotation of fragment around long axis.
- Described relative to more proximal point (e.g, a femoral diaphyseal fracture rotating laterally/externally would position the knee externally rotated relative to the hip).
- Even in children, rotation does not remodel; it must be reduced.

Override:
The degree to which the distal portion overlaps the proximal portion.

Distraction:
The degree to which the two portions are separated (see Figure 4.34, p. 232).

Comminuted: A fracture with three or more fragments.
Intra-articular: Extending through an articular surface (see Figure 4.16).
Impacted: Shortening of the bone due to compression.

Simple or closed:
Overlying soft tissue/skin is intact. No contamination from environment.

Compound or open:
Communicates with environment.
- Bones may disrupt skin ("inside out").
- Skin/soft tissue punctured or ruptured from externally ("outside in").
- Greatly ↑ risk of infection, osteomyelitis, and/or septic arthritis.
- Urgent need for rapid debridement.

"Greenstick" fracture:
Incomplete, single-cortex, or bowing fracture deformity typical of children's more elastic bone tissue.

Fractures involving the physis:
For pediatric fractures and the Salter-Harris classification see p. 315.

Stress or fatigue fracture:
Abnormal repetitive forces on a normal bone.
- E.g., new military recruits on 20-mile march.

Insufficiency fracture:
Normal repetitive stress on abnormal bone.
- E.g., osteopenia or prior radiation therapy weakening bone.

Pathologic fracture:
Fracture through a pre-existing bony abnormality (cyst, tumor, infection, drill hole, or hardware) (see Figure 4.15).

If there is ≥ 50% cortical destruction on radiographs there is a high risk of impending fracture especially in a weight-bearing bone (lower extremity). Clinicians need to be made aware of this as often prophylactic intramedullary rods or other preventative procedure may be performed.

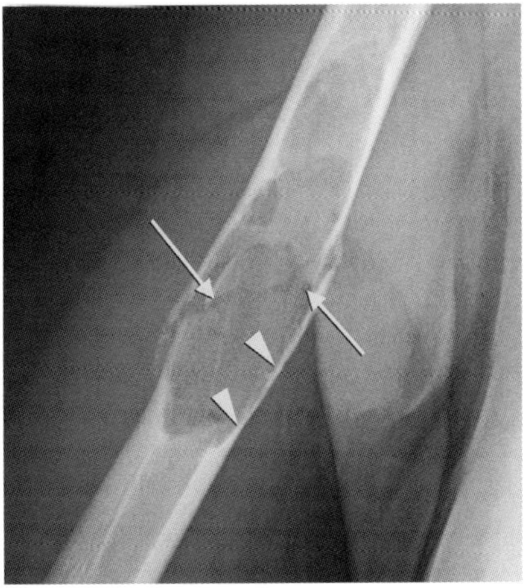

Figure 4.15 Pathologic fracture proximal humerus; renal cell carcinoma metastasis. A radiolucent fracture line (arrows) extends through a minimally expansile lytic medullary diaphyseal lesion, which has caused endosteal cortical thinning (arrowheads) and fine cortical deformity. Note the subtle lateral angulation of distal portion.

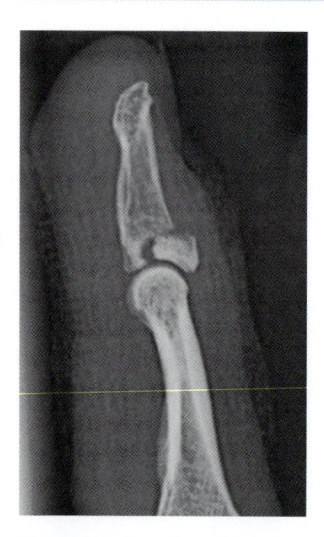

Figure 4.16 Coned lateral finger demonstrates a fracture of the dorsal base of distal phalynx with intra-articular extension and 2 mm dorsal displacement, which creates a 2 mm gap in the articular surface.

Fracture reduction

Reduction refers to manipulation that positions the fracture fragments into more anatomic alignment.

Closed reduction

Without surgery; often with cast, brace, boot, or splint.

Open reduction

Surgical, often with hardware.

Internal fixation

Surgically or percutaneously placed hardware (pins, plates, screws, etc.).

Internal derangements

This term implies an abnormality of the tendons, ligaments, cartilage, or other supporting structures of a joint. Injuries to joints are initially evaluated with radiographs followed by MRI if radiographs are negative or non-specific.

Radiography

Most internal derangements are occult on radiographs. Findings that may be seen include:
- Associated avulsion fractures (origin or insertion of tendon/ligament can avulse and pull off a sliver of bone).
- Associated effusions.
- Swelling of some tendons is visible due to the adjacent more radiolucent fat on lateral views (e.g., Achilles tendon).

MRI

MRI is superior for the evaluation of soft tissue injuries of joints. Knowing normal anatomy and the mechanism of injury will help you identify the abnormality.

Tendons

<u>Tendinosis/tendinopathy:</u>
- Thickened, with increased or heterogeneous signal.

<u>Calcific tendinopathy:</u>
- Globular hypointense signal abnormality, with or without edema.

<u>Tears/ruptures:</u>
Defects in the substance of tendons are usually filled with fluid and, therefore, hyperintense on fluid sensitive sequences. (*Beware of the magic angle phenomenon, p. 196 "MRI Pitfalls and Problems.") Classification of tendon tears:
- *Partial thickness.*
  - Defect can involve either the articular or bursal surface. Does not involve the full thickness of the tendon.
- *Full thickness, incomplete.*
  - A through and through tear of one portion of the tendon, not involving the complete width of the tendon.
- *Full thickness, complete.*
  - Complete rupture of the tendon—both thickness and width (see Figure 4.32).
- *Retraction.*
  - Degree of proximal displacement of the myotendinous junction due to a complete full-thickness tear.

Ligaments

<u>Grade I:</u> Strain. Increased signal and thickening on all sequences.
<u>Grade II:</u> Partial tears. Interruption of fibers, not involving the entire thickness of the ligament. Increased signal.
<u>Grade III:</u> Complete rupture (see Figure 4.29).

Cartilage

Cartilage is intermediate signal on T2- and PD-weighted sequences with homogeneous signal or can have a trilaminar appearance (thin superficial hypointense rim, subjacent high signal layer, and deep low signal lamina).

<u>Degeneration:</u> Contour or signal abnormalities (alteration of trilaminar appearance, heterogeneous).

<u>Fissuring or defects:</u> Usually filled with fluid. Appears as linear high signal on fluid sensitive sequences.

<u>Subchondral bone abnormalities:</u> Cyst formation, edema, trabecular fractures.

<u>Loose bodies:</u> From dislodging and seeding of cartilage debris. Appear as filling defects in joint fluid.

MR arthrogram (see p. 238 "Arthrography")
Fluoroscopically guided intra-articular injection of gadolinium provides increased soft tissue contrast and better visualization of tears and defects.

US
Ultrasound evaluation of internal derangement of joints is increasing in frequency as probe technology improves. Accuracy of this technology is very operator dependent.

Tendons and ligaments
<u>Normal appearance:</u> Fibrillar appearance on long axis imaging.
- Fine, linear echoes: small dots when tendon imaged in axial plane, linear when imaged longitudinally.

<u>Tendinosis and ligament strain:</u>
- Thickening, heterogenous echotexture with loss of normal fibrillar appearance.

<u>Tears/ruptures:</u>
- Hypoechoic or anechoic defects.

Subluxation/dislocation
Subluxation
- Partial loss of contact of two articular surfaces.
- Implies compromise of stabilizers (ligaments, tendons).

Dislocation
- Complete loss of contact of apposed articular surfaces.

Inflammation
Inflammation refers to the tissue response to irritants, either exogenous biologic agents as in infection, or to harmful stimuli such as toxins, immune reactions, or trauma (e.g., physical, chemical, thermal).
- Clinically, patients present with focal redness, swelling, heat, pain, and reduced mobility/function, +/– joint effusion.

Common inflammatory conditions include:
- Infection (osteomyelitis, septic arthritis).
- Inflammatory arthropathies (e.g., rheumatoid arthritis, gout).
- Other autoimmune disorders (e.g., lupus).
- Friction or trauma.

Radiologic findings
Decreased bone radiodensity
- Focal osteoporosis, erosions, lytic areas, cortical loss.

Soft tissue abnormalities
- Displacement of fascial planes, ligament/tendon swelling.

Subluxations
- Chronic inflammation affects the integrity of stabilizing ligaments or tendons.

Joint effusions

Arthritis
There are two main categories of arthritis:
Degenerative joint disease, E.g., osteoarthritis (OA).
Inflammatory arthropathies, E.g., rheumatoid arthritis (RA).

Radiographic evaluation and descriptors
Often arthropathies are evaluated with a four view radiographic evaluation of both hands (AP, oblique, ball-catchers, and lateral). Joint specific radiographs can be performed when evaluating localized joint pain.

The following factors must be assessed and described:

Joint space
- Narrowing: eccentric (OA) or symmetric (inflammatory).
- Widening (septic).
- Intact (e.g., gout).

Reactive bone formation
- Osteophytes (OA).
- Periosteal bone formation (buttressing in OA or "whiskering" in psoriatic arthritis).
- Subchondral bone formation (sclerosis in OA).
- Overhanging edge (erosions with bone formation in gout).

Soft tissues
- Periarticular swelling.
  - Fusiform (RA).
  - Dactylitis (sausage digit in psoriatic arthritis).
  - Eccentric or "lumpy-bumpy" (gout).

Erosions
- Marginal (inflammatory).
- Central (erosive or inflammatory OA).

Distribution
- Unilateral, bilateral asymmetric or symmetric.

Mineralization
- Generalized osteopenia or juxta-articular osteopenia (RA).

Alignment
- Ulnar subluxation and deviation (RA).
- Swan neck or boutonniere deformity (RA).

Degenerative joint disease (DJD)
Referred to as osteoarthritis (OA) when involving synovial joints, it is the most common type of arthritis. This "wear and tear" arthritis, most common in hands, and weight bearing joints such as knees, hips, posterior elements spine, or other chronically over-used joints.

Risk factors include:
- Age.
- Obesity.

- Prior trauma.
- Abnormal mechanical forces, e.g., chronic joint malalignment.
- Other focal insult, e.g., prior infection, hemarthrosis, inflammation.

> **Radiographic findings of osteoarthritis**
> - Cartilage loss causing asymmetrically or eccentrically narrowed joint spaces.
> - Subchondral sclerosis.
> - Subchondral cysts.
> - Osteophyte formation at margins of joints.
> - +/− Joint effusions.
> - Asymmetric joint involvement.

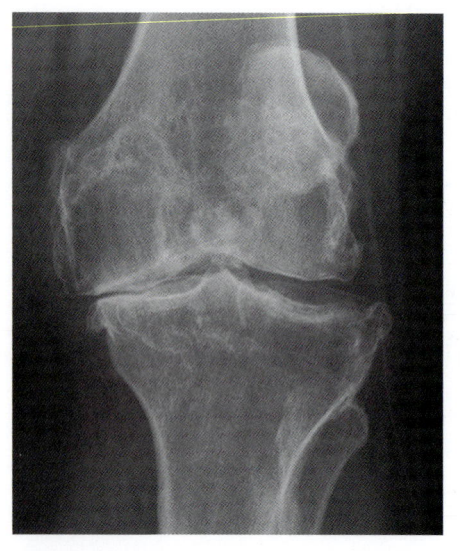

Figure 4.17 Classic osteoarthritis. AP knee radiograph shows marked medial compartment narrowing (representing loss of meniscus and cartilage), medial osteophytes, subchondral sclerosis, and articular surface changes.

Inflammatory arthritis
Types of inflammatory arthropathies
- Seropositive (Rh positive) – Rheumatoid arthritis.
- Sereonegative (Rh negative) spondyloarthropathies:
  - Psoriatic, reactive arthritis, ankylosing spondylitis, enteropathic arthropathies.

- Crystal induced arthropathies:
  - Gout.
  - Pseudogout—calcium pyrophosphate dihydrite (CPPD) disease.
- Infectious—septic arthritis.

> **Radiographic findings of inflammatory arthropathies**
> - Symmetric joint space narrowing.
> - Symmetric joint involvement.
> - Erosions.
> - Peri-articular demineralization.
> - Soft tissue swelling.
> - Subluxations.
> - Proliferative bone:
>   - Spikes of bone in periarticular region.
>   - Occurs in sero-negative arthropathies.
>   - Does NOT occur in rheumatoid arthritis.

See Figure 4.23, p. 216.
- MRI is sometimes indicated in the evaluation of these diseases. Arthritis tends to be understated on radiographs, and MRI allows for earlier detection

Joint effusions

Increased fluid, blood, or pus within a synovial joint. If large, may distend the capsule. Etiologies include:
- Chronic irritation/trauma (e.g., OA).
- Acute trauma (often hemarthrosis).
- Inflammation.
- Rheumatoid arthritis—often in MCP joints.
- Crystal arthropathy e.g., gout.
- Infectious.

Radiographic findings

Depends on the joint.
- Fluid creates increased density in the soft tissues.
- Easiest to identify when it displaces adjacent lucent fat, such as in the knee and elbow. (Radiography is less reliable in other joints.)
- The lateral view is usually the most helpful.

> A fat-fluid level in a joint effusion (usually seen on a cross-table lateral radiograph, also on CT or MRI) indicates an intra-articular fracture (see Figure 4.28, p. 222).

Other soft tissue abnormalities

Fat
Changes (e.g., displacement) of the fat in the subcutaneous tissues and intermuscular fascial planes can provide important clues to the localization of pathology on all modalities.

- Blurring of fat—muscle/tendon interfaces may represent trauma, inflammation, or infiltration (e.g., neoplasm).
- Subcutaneous edema, subcutaneous "honeycombing" or "stranding."
- Displacement of pericapsular fat may indicate joint effusions (see Figure 4.33, p. 232).

Foreign bodies
Foreign matter is often relatively superficial.

Radiography
<u>Radiodense</u> and visible on X-rays: Leaded glass, metals, gravel.
<u>Radiolucent</u> and occult on X-rays: Wood, plastic, small glass fragments.
- Local edema or fascial plane obliteration may be only visual clue on radiographs.

Ultrasonography
- Useful for both radiodense and radiolucent foreign bodies.
- Usually seen as echogenic areas with posterior acoustic shadowing.
- (see Figure 4.11, p. 198).

Air
Air in soft tissue MUST be explained:
- Recent penetrating trauma?
- Surgery or other procedure?
- Otherwise suspect infection—necrotizing faciitis is a medical emergency caused by several bacteria including staphylococcus aureus, clostridium perfringens ("gas gangrene"), bacteroides fragilis.

Calcium/bone

Calcium within tendons
Calcific tendonitis in shoulder is often milky, homogeneous, rounded, and in the path of the rotator cuff (see Figure 4.18, p. 211).

Calcium/bone within masses
Pattern of progression aids in determining the diagnosis:
- Progressing from the center of a mass toward the periphery: suspicious for neoplasm.
- Starting at the perimeter of a mass and progressing inward: more likely to be posttraumatic myositis (see Figure 4.13, p. 200).

Heterotopic bone
May form adjacent to joints or bones or in muscle following surgery or trauma (see Figure 4.19, p. 211).
- Exact etiology unknown.
- Can occur in large joints following closed head or spinal cord injury, repetitive trauma, and/or immobilization.
- Some patients are exuberant bone formers and may need further surgery/treatment to maintain range of motion.

PATTERNS OF DISEASE

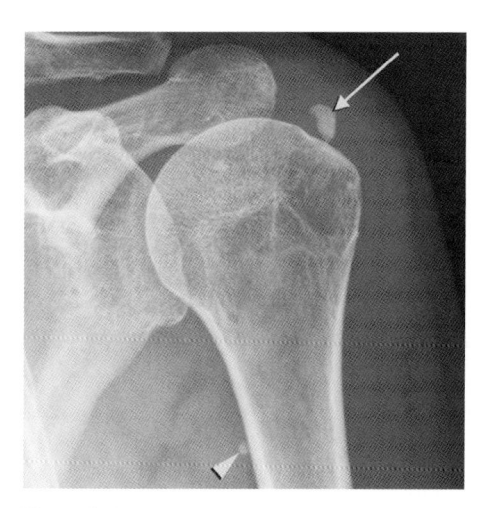

Figure 4.18 Calcific tendonopathy. Dense oval calcification in expected location of the rotator cuff tendons, between inferior acromion and supero-lateral humeral head (arrow). Smaller 2 mm round radiodensity medial to proximal diaphysis in biceps tendon (arrowhead).

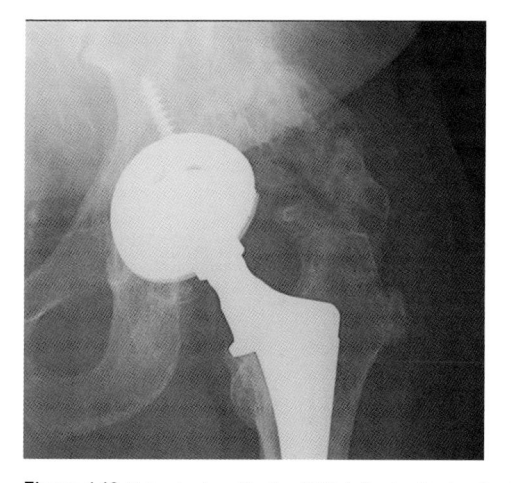

Figure 4.19 Heterotopic ossification. Well-defined and trabeculated mature bone extends from greater trochanter toward lateral acetabulum, nearly bridging this space. Patient is s/p hip arthroplasty.

Masses and neoplasms

The word *mass* describes a space-occupying lesion (could be neoplasm, fluid, fibrosis, inflammation). *Neoplasm* more specifically refers to new tissue growth (benign or malignant). The differential diagnosis is wide and beyond the scope of this book. Some general guidelines are included here.

Approach to interpretation
Decision 1: Is there a mass?
Look carefully for the following:
- Disruption or distortion of the fine trabecular pattern of bone.
- Increase or decrease in the cortical thickness.
- Areas of sclerosis or lucency.
- Change from previous studies.

Old studies are vital to improve your detection of lesions.

Decision 2: Do I need to worry or not worry?
Before you can decide if you need to worry about a lesion, you need to assess the following:
- Origin: where is the "center" of the mass (soft tissue/cortical/medullary space/periosteal)?
- Longevity: new, newly discovered, or previously documented?
- Characterize margins*
- Characterize internal matrix*
- Is there a periosteal reaction?* If so, what type?
- Are the adjacent soft tissues abnormal—are fascial planes blurred or displaced?

*See p. 200 for details.

Aggressive features of MSK masses
- Periosteal reaction: spiculated or radial.
- Margins: ill defined, wide zone of transition.
- Longevity: new.
- Soft tissues: displacement of fascial planes, edema.
- Transgression of compartments (e.g., epiphyseal extension of a metaphyseal mass) (see Figure 4.20).
- Cortical scalloping or break through.
- Necrosis.

Benign features of MSK masses
- Periosteal reaction: fine, linear, wavy.
- Margins: well defined, narrow zone of transition.
- Longevity: old, chronic.
- Soft tissues: normal.

Lytic lesions in adults over 45 are "metastasis or myeloma until proven otherwise."

PATTERNS OF DISEASE

What is the role of CT in MSK masses?

Evaluation of bone structure, matrix mineralization, and soft tissue calcifications is better with CT than MRI. CT is used to:

- Assess the internal matrix: Is it a chondroid or osseous lesion? (see Figure 4.21).

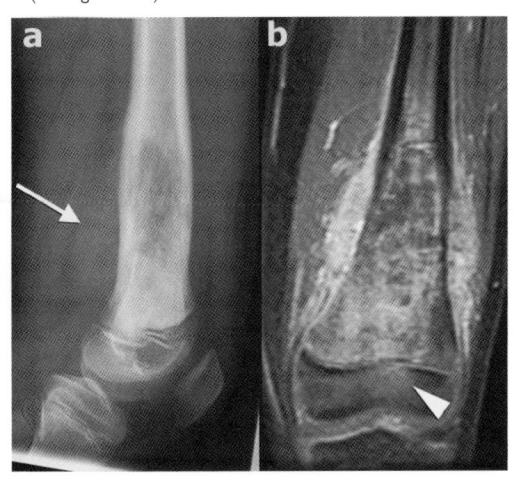

Figure 4.20 Osteosarcoma. (a) Lateral radiograph shows lucency of the distal femur, with posterior aggressive periosteal reaction and soft tissue mass (arrow). (b) Contrast enhanced MRI shows tumor enhancement in the medullary space, extending into the soft tissues and through the growth plate (arrowhead). Note the cortical thinning.

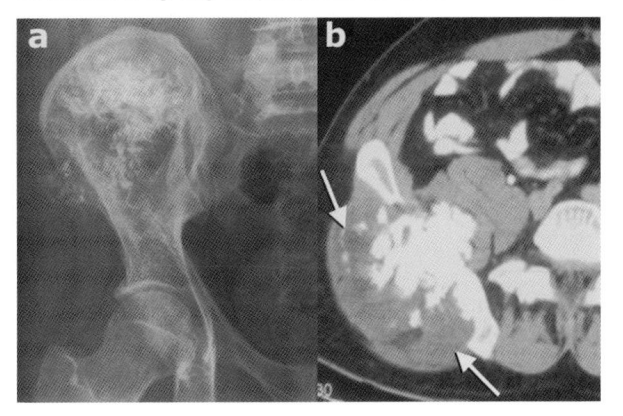

Figure 4.21 Chondrosarcoma. (a) Large calcified chondroid matrix mass overlies most of right iliac wing. (b) CT demonstrates the large calcified mass centered over the iliac bone. Peripheral soft tissue portion extends postero-laterally (arrows).

- Assess the risk of impending or pathologic fracture.
- Follow progression or regression of osseous disease.
- Perform image guided biopsy.

What is the role of MRI in MSK masses

MRI is far superior to CT for the characterization and assessing the extent of musculoskeletal masses.

Tumor composition/characterization
- Blood-fluid levels (e.g., aneurysmal bone cyst).
- Vascular components (e.g., hemangioma, vascular malformations).
- Cartilaginous lesions:
  - Lobular and hyperintense on T2W sequence with peripheral septal enhancement on post contrast images.
- Cystic versus solid: cystic (peripheral enhancement), solid (internal nodular enhancement).

Anatomic assessment
- Localization to a compartment (e.g., intramuscular, SQ).
- Association with specific soft tissue structure (e.g., schwannomas with nerves, giant cell tumor of the tendon sheath with tendons).
- Neurovascular involvement.

Marrow evaluation
- Replacement with tumor, reconversion.

Abnormalities of bone marrow

Marrow conversion

Red marrow (hematopoetically active, isointense to muscle on T1) converts to yellow marrow (fatty marrow, hyperintense on T1) in a predictable pattern starting in early childhood:
- First in the appendicular skeleton, from distal to proximal.
- The axial skeleton (spine, pelvis, sternum, ribs, and skull) is the last to convert.
- Red marrow reconversion (hematopoietic hyperplasia) occurs in smokers, obesity, marathon runners, and menstruating females.

Marrow infiltration by malignancy or infection
- Foci of signal abnormality, iso to hypointense to muscle on T1 images (see Figure 4.22).
- T2 images are non-specific; some of the increased T2 signal will be due to edema rather than the pathologic process itself.

Trauma
- Bone contusions: appear as bone marrow edema.
  - Pattern and distribution is specific to the mechanism of injury (e.g., kissing contusions of the lateral femoral condyle and posterolateral proximal tibia in ACL injuries).
- Fracture: linear hypointense fracture line or cortical step-off or interruption. Associated with bone marrow edema.
- Stress injuries: periosteal soft tissue and bone marrow edema occur in stress reaction, with or without a linear fracture line.

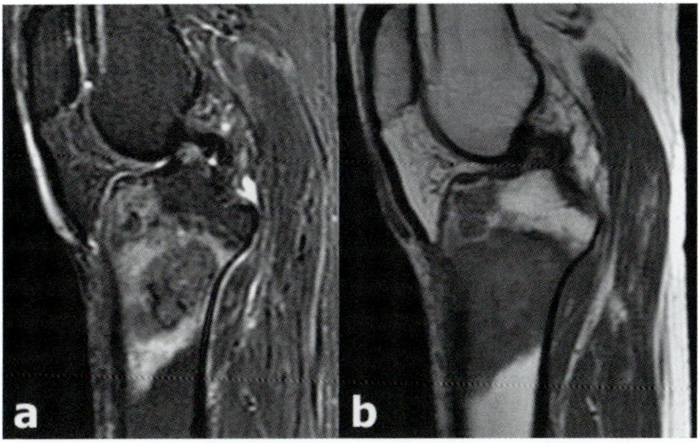

Figure 4.22 Osseous metastatic disease. 68-year-old female with diffuse metastatic melanoma. (a) Sagittal STIR image shows a heterogeneously hyperintense mass in the proximal tibial metaphysis and anterior epiphysis. (b) Corresponding sagittal T1 MR image of the knee shows replacement of the normal hyperintense bone marrow with hypointense soft tissue.

Common conditions

Rheumatoid arthritis

Rheumatoid arthritis (RA) is a chronic multisystem (most commonly MSK, but also pulmonary, pericardial, dermatologic) inflammatory disease. Characteristically, RA is bilateral, symmetric, most commonly affecting the hands, feet, cervical spine, and occasionally larger joints.

Radiographic findings of RA (see Figure 4.23)
- Fusiform periarticular soft-tissue swelling.
- Symmetric joint space narrowing from cartilage destruction.
- Periarticular (marginal) erosions.
- Diffuse osteoporosis.
- Muscle atrophy or wasting.
- Joint effusions.
- Ulnar subluxation and deviation from ligamentous inflammation, laxity, rupture.

PELVIS AND HIP

Fractures

Pelvic fractures are very common in trauma, particularly motor vehicle accidents.

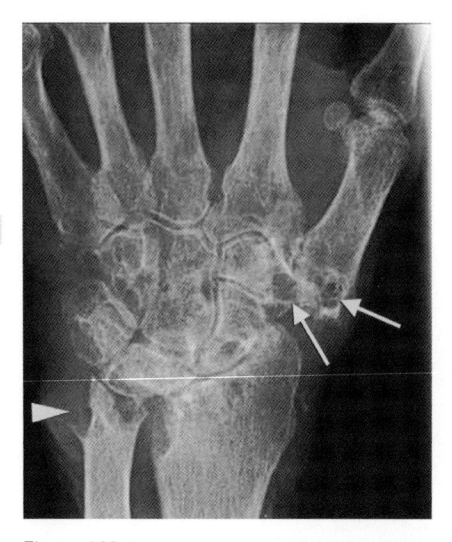

Figure 4.23 Severe rheumatoid arthritis of the wrist and hand. AP image shows periarticular demineralization, marginal erosions (arrows), and involvement of the ulnar styloid process (arrowhead). Note the symmetric narrowing of the radiocarpal joint.

Pelvic ring fractures
Occuring with severe acute trauma, pelvic ring fractures are the third leading cause of shock and death following blunt trauma, with high early mortality due to:
- Close proximity to major organ systems.
- Intensely rich osseous vascularization.
- Severity of force required to disrupt this biomechanically strong structure.

Rapid and accurate initial clinical and radiographic assessment are key to reducing morbidity and mortality in all pelvic injuries.

Radiography
<u>Views</u> AP pelvis and pelvic inlet/outlet views.
- Assesses for pelvic ring integrity without moving patient.
- Tube tilted caudally (inlet view).
- Tube tilted cephalad (outlet view).

<u>Indications</u>
- To assess pelvic ring integrity in lieu of CT (which has mostly replaced these views in the acute setting).
- To provide baseline for further follow-up, pre-op, post-op.

How to look for pelvic fractures
- Look at pelvic ring integrity

- In the pelvis there are specific lines that need to be followed for continuity and symmetry (see Figure 4.24).
- Evaluate symmetry of SI joint width and normal width of symphysis pubis
- Medial pelvic wall soft tissues—look at fascial planes, muscles, and bladder.
  - Displacement (e.g., of the bladder) may indicate hematoma.

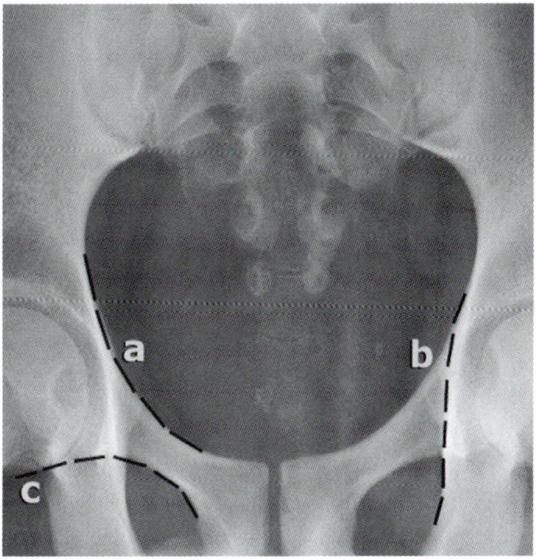

Figure 4.24 Normal lines of pelvic ring. (a) iliopectineal line, (b) ilioischial line, (c) Shenton's line.

Femoral neck fractures

Over 350,000 proximal femur fractures occur in the US each year, increasing as the population ages. Patients at higher risk are older, thin postmenopausal females.
- Fracture risk begins to double every 5 years over 50 years of age.
- Fracture can occur following even seemingly minor trauma or no trauma at all with relatively minor symptoms and signs.
- Remember that "hip" pain can come from the low back, the pelvis, femur or knee.

> **Correct your vocabulary!**
> "Hip" refers to the entire joint, that is, the acetabulum, proximal femoral head and neck. *Hip fractures* usually mean "proximal femoral fractures," which are common and a source of great morbidity and mortality in elderly.

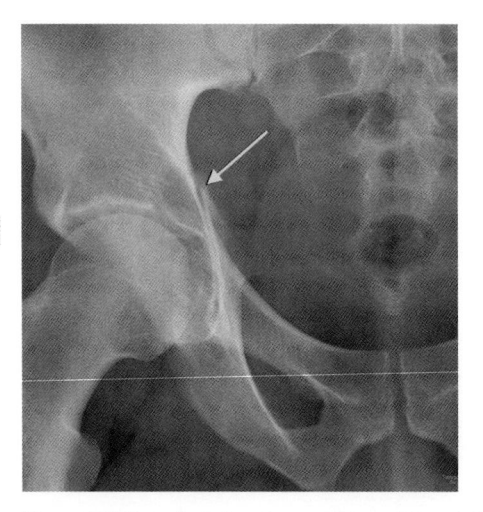

Figure 4.25 Minimally displaced fracture of the medial acetabular wall. Coned AP pelvis of a patient after fall from horse. Note the discontinuity and step-off of the pelvic inlet (iliopectineal line) (arrow).

Radiography

Views: AP and lateral hip.
- Coned AP hip—centers film on area of concern.
- Lateral hip/proximal femur:
  - "Frog leg" view (hip flexed and externally rotated).
  - Cross-table lateral when patient cannot move.

Indications:
- If initial pelvic AP is inadequate.
- If there is a high clinical suspicion of hip fracture.

How to look for proximal femoral fractures
- Check adequacy of proximal femoral neck visualization:
  - Can you see the lesser trochanter? This confirms internal rotation of the hip, which is needed to accurately evaluate the femoral neck. (Hip pain typically leads to external rotation).
- Step off of the femoral neck cortex.
- Subtle interruptions in the trabecular pattern of femoral neck.
- Is the femoral head in the acetabulum or is it dislocated?

Never interpret an inadequately viewed femoral neck as "negative." This leads to unacceptable medical and legal risk. Do alterative imaging. Proximal femoral fracture is one of the most expensive diseases to patient, society, and physicians.

When do I order a CT/MRI in pelvic or hip trauma?
- Poor visualization on radiography because of:
  - Obesity.
  - Marked osteopenia.
  - Superimposed structures e.g., marked air and feces.
- Obvious pelvic ring or acetabular deformity should trigger prompt CT, to characterize fractures and assess for associated soft tissue injuries.
- Osteopenic patients, or those with high clinical suspicion.
  - Consider MRI to evaluate for bone marrow edema.
  - A limited "quick" scan (coronal STIR or fat suppressed T2-weighted) can exclude an occult proximal femoral fracture.

> MRI is far more sensitive than CT for the evaluation of occult hip/pelvic injuries. However, CT is faster and more accessible on an emergent bases, and still is commonly performed, probably more often than MRI.

Osteoarthritis (OA)
Half of all patients with OA have hip involvement. The cartilage of "ball and socket" joint wears away, eventually producing abnormal biomechanics and motion.
Certain processes accelerate the development of OA, including:
- Femoral acetabular impingement (FAI)—abnormal bone contact or friction with extreme flexion or abduction of the hip.
- Hip dysplasia (see chapter 6, developmental dysplasia of the hip, p. 321).

Radiographic findings in the hip
- Eccentric loss of joint space, most commonly medial (centrally) or superiorly (see Figure 4.26).
- Osteophytes at the head-neck junction and acetabular rim.
- Medial femoral neck cortical buttressing (thickening).

Avascular necrosis (AVN)
Caused by femoral head devascularization. The femoral head blood supply is retrograde from intertrochanteric circumflex vessels.

Predisposing factors:
- Femoral neck fractures.
- Systemic etiologies—SLE, steroid use, collagen vascular diseases, alcohol abuse, pancreatitis, sickle cell dyscrasias, decompression.

Radiographic findings
Up to 55% will be bilateral although often asynchronous.

Earliest changes:
- May be occult.
- Geographic areas of sclerosis and lucency in superior femoral head.

Subsequent changes:
- Subchondral radiolucency (crescent sign) in superior femoral head—implies impending femoral head collapse.
- Femoral head collapse (see Figure 4.27).
- Secondary degenerative joint disease.

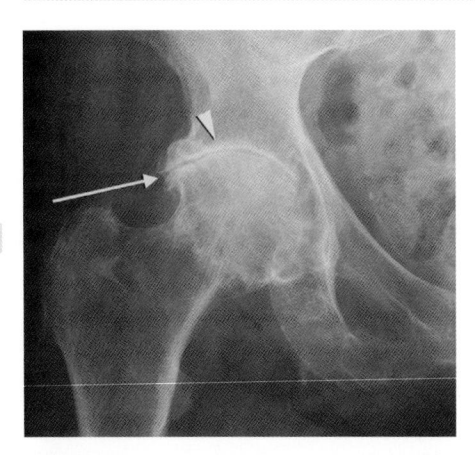

Figure 4.26 Osteoarthritis of right hip. AP view shows eccentric loss of joint space superiorly and medially, large acetabular and femoral osteophytes (arrow), and subchondral sclerosis (arrowhead).

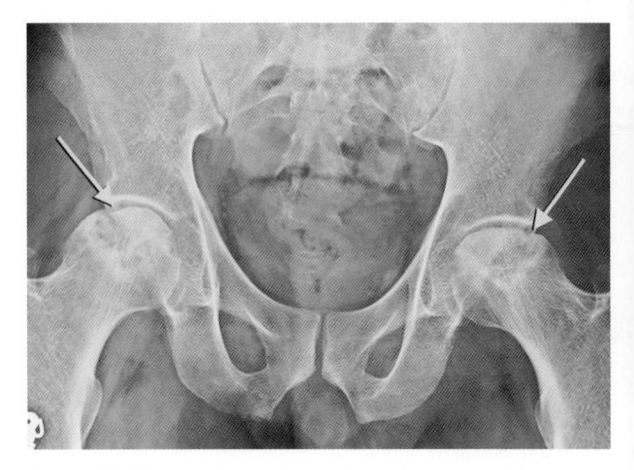

Figure 4.27 Bilateral AVN femoral heads. Geographic sclerotic and lucent changes are present in the superior portion of each femoral head. Note the disruption of the usual spherical femoral heads from early collapse (arrows).

MRI findings
Far more sensitive for early changes than radiography:
- Bone marrow edema (which is nonspecific).
- Double-line sign on fluid-sensitive sequences (T2, STIR).
  - Hyperintense inner zone represents granulation tissue.
  - Hypointense outer zone represents sclerosis.
  - Often serpiginous.

Internal derangement
MRI is commonly used to evaluate hip and groin pain, to assess for internal derangement.

Labral tears
- 3T MRI or MR arthrogram required for diagnosis.
- Linear or complex signal abnormalities or defects in the labrum.
- Perilabral cysts are associated with labral tears.

Cartilage
Thinning, fissuring, defects.

Synovitis and bursitis/bursal effusion
- Iliopsoas and greater trochanteric bursitis common.
- Fluid-signal intensity.

Tendon injury
Common tendons to be injured include gluteus medius and minimis, hamstring, iliopsoas, adductor compartment (see p. 205).

KNEE
Primarily a flexion/extension "hinge" joint. Includes the articulations between femur and tibia, femur and patella, and proximal tibia and fibula.

Radiography
Views
- AP.
- Lateral (femoral condyles should be superimposed).
  - Standing.
  - Cross table lateral (if unable to stand).

Supplementary views
- Patello-femoral ("sunrise") view:
  - To assess for patella injuries, mal-alignment, arthritis.
- Flexed AP ("schuuss view"):
  - To assess joint space and look for intra-articular bodies.
- Weight bearing "standing alignment view":
  - Images from pelvis to feet.
  - Identifies altered mechanical axis of the lower extremities, usually from varus/valgus angulation of the knees.

What to look for on knee radiographs
- Joint effusion.
- Definition of the quadriceps and patellar tendons.
  - Posterior margin should be well defined by the adjacent fat pads (see Figure 4.2).

- Position of the patella.
  - Subluxation is almost always lateral.
- Calcifications.
  - Calcified menisci: chondrocalcinosis.
  - Vascular: usually posterior to joint.
  - Intra-articular loose bodies (osteochondral fragments): usually round, sometimes lamellated. May change position between exams, and can enlarge over time.

Knee joint effusion
Best visualized in the suprapatella bursa (a misnomer—communicates with joint space unlike true bursa), located between the quadriceps tendon and anterior cortex of the distal femur.

Radiographic findings
- Focal oval opacity deep to the quadriceps tendon, between the patella and distal femur.
- Anterior bulge or displacement of tendon (see Figure 4.2, p. 186).
- Suprapatellar fat/fluid level.
  - Seen on cross table lateral view.
  - Indicates an intra-articular fracture (e.g., occult tibial plateau fracture). Caused by fat leakage from marrow layering with fluid/blood

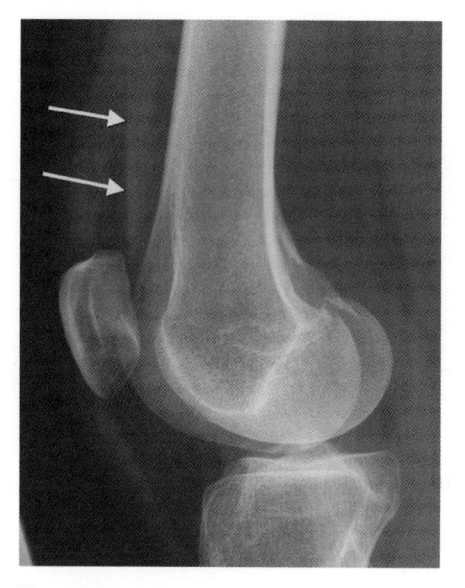

Figure 4.28 Lipohemarthrosis. Cross table lateral of knee in a patient with an occult tibial plateau fracture (identified on CT). Fat-fluid level (arrows) is a sign of an intra-articular fracture.

Fractures
Distal femoral fractures
- Usually supracondylar, associated with ACL tears.
- Osteochondral injuries (injury to cartilage and underlying bone).
  - Deep notch sign: valgus stress and rotation causes impaction of the lateral femoral condyle with the posterior tibial plateau, creating a compression of the femoral condyle. Associated with ACL injuries.

Tibial plateau fractures
- Lateral plateau is most common.
- Compression of the plateau: tends to occur in older patients.
- Split compression fractures (where the plateau separates from the proximal tibia): tend to occur in younger patients.
- Can be subtle, look for fat-fluid level in effusion (see Figure 4.28).

See Figures 4.5 and 4.6, p. 190.

Proximal fibular fractures
- Arcuate sign—an avulsion fracture of the fibular head, associated with postero-lateral corner injuries and ACL tears.
- Fibular head and neck fractures.
  - Usually associated with tibial plateau fractures.
  - Can be seen with Maisonneuve fractures of the ankle. See p. 223.

Osteoarthritis
Osteoarthritis is extremely common in the knee, especially in obese patients and as a consequence of prior traumatic injuries. It is the most common indication for a total knee arthroplasty.

Specific findings of knee OA
- Asymmetric involvement of compartments:
  - Medial and patellofemoral compartments are more frequently affected than lateral.
- Asymmetric joint space narrowing of the medial/lateral compartments causes valgus or varus angulation and altered weight bearing.
- Joint effusions are common.

See Figure 4.17, p. 208.

Internal derangement
Ligamentous, tendon and meniscal injuries of the knee require MRI for evaluation. Please refer to 'internal derangement', p. 205 for MRI findings of ligament and tendon injuries. Findings specific to the knee are discussed.

Ligaments
<u>Collateral ligaments (MCL and LCL):</u>
Medial and lateral stabilizing structures that resist valgus and varus stress, respectively.
- Medial (tibial) collateral ligament (MCL).
  - Much more commonly injured than the LCL, but rarely injured in isolation.
- Lateral collateral ligament complex (LCLC).
  - Comprised of the LCL, iliotibial band, biceps femoris tendon.
  - Rarely injured.

CHAPTER 4 **Musculoskeletal imaging**

Cruciate ligaments (ACL and PCL):
- Located in the intercondylar notch, intracapsular but extrasynovial.
- Stabilize the knee from anterior and posterior tibial translation.
- Anterior cruciate ligament (ACL) tears:
  - Injuries much more common than PCL.
  - Tears can be partial or complete.
  - *Radiography*: secondary signs—effusion, Segond and arcuate fractures (avulsion fractures of the lateral proximal tibia and fibular head, respectively).
  - *MRI*: Best seen on sagittal PD and T2 sequences. Thickening, increased T2 signal, partial or complete disruption (see Figure 4.29).
- Posterior cruciate ligament (PCL):
  - Thicker, involved in hyperextension injuries.
  - MRI: Best seen on sagittal PD and T2 sequences. Thickening, increased T2 signal, partial or complete disruption.

Menisci

C-shaped fibrocartilagenous structure located peripherally between the articular surfaces of the medial and lateral compartments of the knee.

MRI findings:
- They appear as dark triangles on coronal and sagittal cross sectional images.
- Menisci are hypointense on all MR pulse sequences.
- Tears appear as linear or complex foci of increased signal that extend to an articular surface, as blunting of their triangle shape, or as loss of volume (they simply look too small).

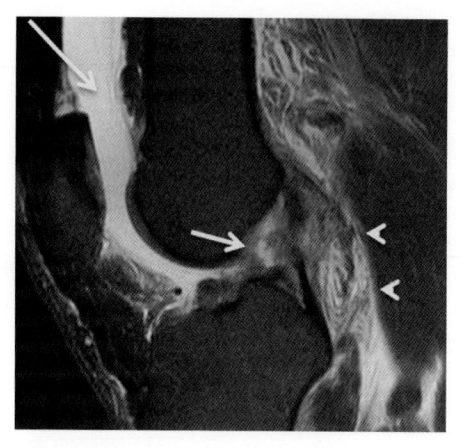

Figure 4.29 Ligamentous and soft tissue injury. Sagittal T2 fs MR image in a 45-year-old man with injury during soccer game. There is a complete anterior cruciate ligament tear (small arrow). A moderate joint effusion (large arrow) and posterior capsular rupture with fascial edema (arrow head) are also seen.

Tendons
Injuries are rare. Patellar tendon injuries most common.

When do I order a CT/MRI of the knee?
- Unexplained lipohemarthrosis: fracture can be diagnosed on either CT or MRI. MRI has the advantage of assessing for internal derangement concomitantly.
- High clinical suspicion for internal derangement or fracture with negative radiographs (or only showing joint effusion).
- Knee pain not explained by radiographs (MRI).

ANKLE
Ankle injuries are common and account for millions of ED visits annually. Serious injury may involve the bones and/or stabilizing ligaments. About 90% of presenting ankle complaints are radiographed, 15% require immobilization/follow-up.

Radiography
Views
Three views are commonly obtained:
- AP: Fibula partially obscures lateral talus.
- Oblique: Shallow internal oblique, foot internally rotated, mortise joint visualized well.
- Lateral.

What to look for on ankle radiographs
- Integrity of the trabecular pattern.
    - Subtle distortion of trabeculae may imply occult impaction fractures (e.g., of calcaneus).
- Integrity of talar dome and articular surfaces.
    - Articular surfaces should be smooth.
    - Look for subchondral lucencies (osteochondral fracture commonly causes persistent pain).
- Ankle mortise integrity
    - Assess on internal oblique view (profiles mortise).
    - Joint space normally 3–4 mm and uniform. Widens with unstable ankle injuries (see Figure 4.30).
- Joint effusion (lateral view)—"dumbbell" opacity immediate anterior/posterior to tibio-talar joint (see Figure 4.10, p. 197).
- Soft tissues
    - Achilles tendon: anterior margin should be sharply defined against the lucent fat on lateral view.
    - Look for symmetry of subcutaneous tissues over the medial and lateral malleoli with preservation of fascial planes (fat and muscle).

Even small (1 mm) asymmetries in medial/lateral ankle mortise width are significant and imply relative talar subluxation under tibia.
- Can be chronic or occur from an acute ligamentous injury

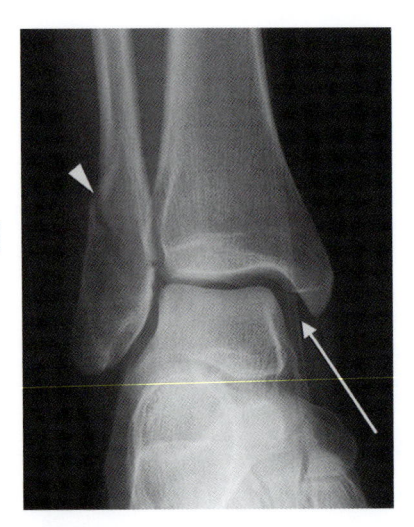

Figure 4.30 Disruption of ankle mortise. Internal oblique view of ankle demonstrates an oblique fracture through distal fibula (arrowhead). The ankle mortise is abnormally wide medially (arrow) indicating damaged deltoid (medial) ligament.

Fractures

Knowledge of ankle ligaments and their attachment and mechanism of injury is key to understanding and identifying fracture patterns.

<u>Classification:</u>

Weber type A
- Fracture of lateral malleolus below level of ankle joint.

Weber type B
- Most common (>60%).
- Fracture of lateral malleolus at level of ankle joint.

Weber type C
- Fracture of fibula above the level of the ankle joint.

Maisonneuve fracture
- Traumatic forces may transmit proximally along the syndesmosis and result in high (proximal) fibular fractures.

Images of the proximal lower leg should be obtained when there are isolated medial or posterior malleolus fractures or medial ankle soft-tissue injury in the absence of lateral malleolus fractures.

Common "miss" areas in the ankle
- Calcaneal (Achilles) tendon abnormalities:
  - Rupture, tendonitis, calcification.
- Anterior process calcaneus fractures.
- Subtalar joint abnormalities.
- Base of 5th metatarsal fractures.
- Tibio-fibular joint widening.

When do I order a CT or MRI to evaluate the ankle?

CT indicated for
- Patients with suspected complex/multiple ankle fractures, especially when subtalar joint and calcaneus fractures are involved.
- Suspected talar dome osteochondral injuries can be evaluated with MR or CT.

MR indicated for
- Soft tissue injury involving ligaments, muscles (gastrocnemius injury or tear), tendons (Achilles), plantar fascia.
- Early osteomyelitis.
- Suspected bone contusions or non-displaced fractures.

SHOULDER

A ball and socket joint, the shoulder joint is the most mobile joint. This mobility is obtained at the sacrifice of stability. The socket is shallow, and the glenoid labrum plays a minimal role in stabilizing the humeral head.

"Shoulder joint" includes: the gleno-humeral (GH), acromio-clavicular (AC) and sterno-clavicular (SC) joints.

Radiography

Views

For most purposes, three views suffice:
- Internal rotation AP view.
- External rotation AP view.
- Either an axillary view or scapular Y view—to assess for dislocation/subluxation.

What to look for on shoulder radiographs
- Size of subacromial space.
  - Narrowed in supraspinatous tears.
- Position of humeral head in the glenoid.
  - Best seen on axillary or scapular Y views.
- Width and alignment of AC joint, spurs.
- Perarticular calcifications (calcific tendonitis see Figure 4.18, p. 211).

Fractures

Humeral fractures

Proximal humeral fractures more common with advancing age.
- Anatomic neck—at the fused physeal plate just distal to the articular surface of the proximal humerus.
- Surgical neck—structurally weaker area just distal to the tuberosities, usually about 2 cm distal to the anatomic neck.

- Greater or lesser tuberosity.
- Are described as "two, three, or four part" fractures depending on the number of fragments.

Scapula fractures
- Rare, usually due to direct blunt trauma.
- Often poorly seen on radiographs and require CT.

Clavicular fractures
- Common, and distal fractures may present with shoulder pain.

Sternal fractures and sterno-clavicular dislocation are poorly seen on radiographs and should be evaluated with CT.

Dislocations/subluxations
Glenohumeral (GH) joint
<u>Antero-inferior:</u>
- 95–98% of GH dislocations are antero-inferior.
  - Represents weakest point of stabilizing structures.
- Associated fractures:
  - Superior-lateral humeral head (Hill-Sachs).
  - Inferior glenoid (Bankart).

<u>Posterior:</u>
- Only 3% of GH dislocations are posterior.
- Associated with seizures, electric shock.
- Associated fracture: anterior humeral head (reverse Hill-Sachs).

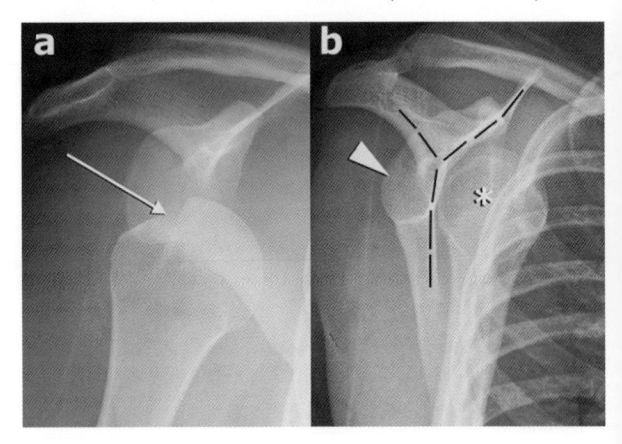

Figure 4.31 GH dislocation. (a) AP view. The humeral head is displaced inferiorly; note the "uncovered" glenoid. The head has impacted the inferior glenoid, creating a Hill Sachs deformity on the supero-lateral head (arrow). (b) Scapular Y view shows anterior displacement of the humeral head (*), with an uncovered glenoid fossa (arrowhead). Dashed lines indicate the "Y."

Pseudosubluxation:
- Drooping shoulder due to presence of joint effusion.
- Alignment will be normal on scapular Y and axillary views.

Acromioclavicular joint

Radiographic classification of injuries:
- Type I—Sprain of the acromioclavicular ligaments without tear, AC joint remains normally aligned (radiographically occult).
- Type II—Tear of the acromioclavicular ligaments, widening of the acromioclavicular space (usually <4 mm, but can be normal up to 7 mm).
- Type III—Tear of the acromio- and coracoclavicular ligaments resulting in widening of the ac joint space and coracoclavicular interval (>12 mm) and elevation of the distal clavicle (>5 mm).

If radiographs are negative and you have high suspicion for AC joint injury, consider obtaining bilateral AC joint radiograph with stress (weights).

Rotator cuff (RC) injuries

This cuff of muscles stabilizes the shoulder joint, holding the humeral head in the glenoid throughout the range of motion of the joint.
The rotator cuff is comprised of the following muscles:
- Supraspinatus.
- Infraspinatous.
- Teres minor.
- Subscapularis.

Mechanism of injury

Injuries may be acute or chronic:
- Acute: Associated with trauma/sports activities with overhead components (e.g., pitching, weight-lifting, tennis).
- Chronic: Injuries often also involve some degree of impingement of rotator tendons in the narrow subacromial space during range of motion.

Radiography

- Often occult.
- Subacromial interval may be narrowed with rotator cuff tears.
  - Normally >9 mm on AP view.
- Acromio-clavicular joint inferior osteophytes or hooked acromion may cause impingement, predisposing to tears.

MRI

Study of choice if ligamentous, RC injury or cartilage/labrum injury suspected. See "Internal Derangements," p. 205 for descriptors of tendon injuries on MRI.
- Supraspinatus tendon most commonly involved.
- Subscapularis tears may be associated with subluxation or dislocation of the long head of the biceps tendon from the biciptal groove.
- Teres minor rarely affected.
- For full thickness complete tears, evaluate degree of muscle atrophy and retraction.

MR arthrogram
- Intra-articular gadolinium injection distends the joint and fills defects in cartilage and tendons.
- Ideal for evaluating partial thickness articular surface RC and labral tears and capsule-ligamentous injuries.
- CT arthrogram can be performed if there are contraindications to MRI.

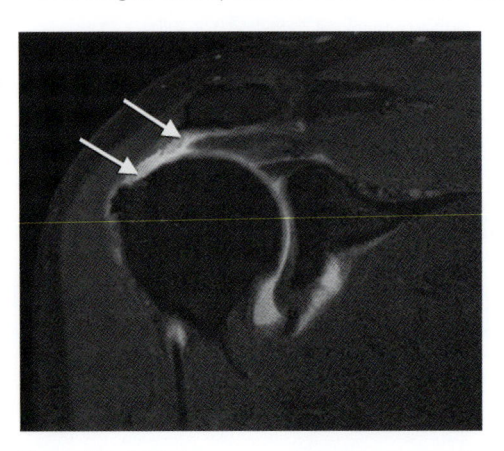

Figure 4.32 Full thickness rotator cuff tear: MR arthrogram. Coronal T1fs image shows a full thickness tear of the supraspinatus tendon. Hyperintense fluid in the joint (injected gadolinium) extends from the humeral head to the subacromial space, confirming full thickness tearing of the rotator cuff (arrows).

US
Used in some centers for RC assessment. See p. 197, "Ultrasound" section for general tendon assessment.
- May be helpful for assessing biceps tendon.
- Operator-dependent and at this time less reliable, but it is a developing modality (cheaper).

Labral injuries
The glenoid labrum is a fibrocartilagenous structure that plays a role in glenohumeral stability. In cross section, the labrum appears triangular in shape. Tears do not usually occur inferiorly. Best evaluated with MR arthrography.

When should I order a CT/MRI of the shoulder?
Suspected rotator cuff tear, tendinopathy, labral injuries (MRI).
Suspected labral tear (MR arthrography).

ELBOW
Primarily a hinge joint. Three articulations: humerus-ulna, humerus-radius, radio-ulnar.

Radiography
Views
- AP.
- Lateral.
- Addition of oblique radial head-capitellum view may demonstrate more subtle radial head fractures.

What to look for in the elbow
- Displacement of fat pads by joint effusion on lateral view.
- Alignment of radio-capitellar joint and ulno-trochlear joints.

Joint effusions
- Anteior fat pad elevation often looks like a sail, and is known as the "sail sign" (see Figure 4.33).
- Posterior fat pad typically not seen; if seen, indicative of joint effusion.
- If an effusion is present, have high suspicion for occult fracture.
  - Radial head in adults.
  - Distal humeral in children.

> **Do not ignore elbow effusions!**
> If no fracture evident, get follow-up in 10–14 days.

Fractures
Radial head
Translates and rotates along ulna groove to participate in supination/pronation of the forearm.
- Most common adult elbow fracture is radial head.
- Suspect radial head fracture when joint effusion seen in adult trauma (see Figure 4.33).

Olecranon
Most common proximal ulnar fracture in adult.
- Either from direct blow or fall on outstretched arm, allowing triceps to avulse the olecranon.
- Usually requires surgical fixation to overcome triceps contraction and restore the articular surface.

Distal humeral fractures
The anatomic classification is complex and includes level of fracture with respect to the condyle, presence/absence of intra-articular extension, and separation of the condyles.
- <u>Intercondylar</u>: fracture line that separates the capitellum and trochlea.
  - Most common distal humerus fracture in adult.
  - Associated with neurovascular damage due to proximity of neurovascular bundle to fracture fragments.
- <u>Supracondylar:</u> above condyles.
  - Most common in children see chapter 6, Pediatrics, "Salter-Harris Fractures," p. 315.

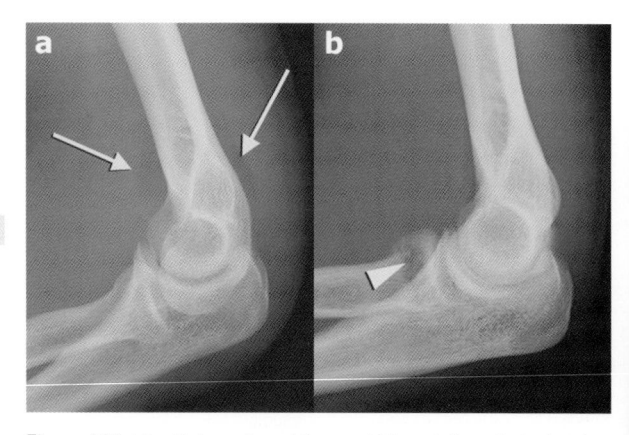

Figure 4.33 Joint effusion and occult fracture: (a) Lateral elbow obtained on the day of injury demonstrates fat pad elevation consistent with joint effusion (arrows) but no definite fracture is identified. (b) Follow-up lateral 16 days later confirms radiolucent radial head-neck junction fracture line (arrowhead).

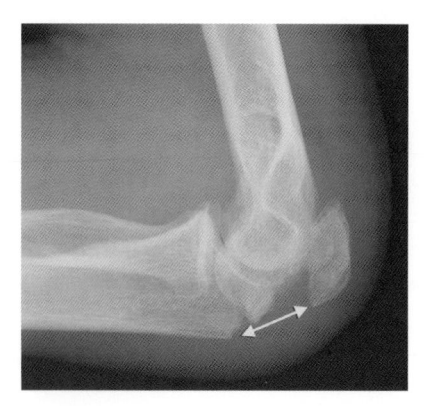

Figure 4.34 Olecranon fracture. Lateral view of elbow demonstrates proximal displacement (avulsion) of olecranon fragment due to contraction of the triceps. This creates a wide distraction of the fracture fragments.

Epicondylitis
More properly termed an "overuse tendinosis."
- Colloquially called:
  - "tennis elbow" (lateral, common extensor tendon)
  - "golfers elbow" (medial, common flexor tendon)

- Radiography:
  - Tiny osseous irregularities or enthesophytes about the lateral or medial epicondyles on radiographs (due to chronic tendon "tugging").
  - May be occult.

MRI: See p. 205 for MR findings of general tendon pathology.

When should I order a CT/MRI of the elbow?
- Suspected internal derangement (MRI).
- Complex fractures, or suspected fracture with negative radiograph (CT).
- Neuropathies (MRI).

WRIST AND HAND

The wrist consists of the distal radius and ulna, and the eight carpal bones.

Radiography

Views
- AP.
- Lateral.
- Oblique.
- Supplementary views:
  - In adult trauma, a "scaphoid" view should be added (PA view of the wrist in ulnar deviation with tube angled radially by 20–30 degrees.)
  - In arthritis, add "ball-catchers view" (hands are oblique by 45 degrees in a cupping position). Helps identify and characterize erosions.

Note, the wrist and hand should be imaged separately.

What to look for in the wrist

AP view:
- Assess the integrity of the carpal arcs (3 lines that define the carpal rows. Disruption suggests fracture or mal-alignment).
- Assess intercarpal joint spaces:
  - Should be symmetric, no greater than 2 mm.
  - Widening suggests fracture or ligament tear.
- Scaphoid fat pad (radial to the scaphoid).
  - Displaced with scaphoid fractures.

Lateral view
- Assess alignment. Should be able to draw a straight line through long axis of distal radius, lunate, capitate.
- Look for elevation of the pronator quadratus fat pad from hemorrhage or edema (volar surface of distal radius); displaced with distal radial fractures.

Fractures
Most common mechanism of injury is fall on an outstretched hand.

Distal radius fracture
Distal radial fractures are very common, especially in the older patient and patients with osteopenia. Often require internal fixation, especially if comminuted.

- Assess for intra-articular extension and impaction.
- Assess degree of angulation of the articular surface of the distal radius:
  - For normal functioning of the wrist, the distal radial articular surface needs to be angled slightly anterior volar.
  - 'Colles' fracture is a common distal radial fracture with dorsal angulation of the articular surface
- Secondary finding: displaced pronator quadratus fat pad.

Scaphoid fracture

Scaphoid fractures account for 85% of all carpal fractures; disproportionate morbidity and lawsuits due to non-union/avascular necrosis (AVN).
- When a scaphoid fracture is suspected (e.g., "snuffbox tenderness"), a scaphoid view must be obtained.
- Most common site of fracture is the scaphoid waist.
- These are at risk for AVN of the proximal pole.
  - Blood supply of scaphoid is intraosseous, from distal to proximal.
  - Associated with 30% of waist fractures, up to 100% of all fractures involving the proximal fifth.
  - Radiographs: sclerosis and/or collapse of the proximal fragment.
  - MR: loss of T1 marrow signal.

<u>What if initial radiographs are negative?</u>
- Immobilize and get follow-up study.
- Continue to immobilize patient as long as point-tender even if radiographs negative.

Arthritis

OA and RA are the most common arthritic diseases of the wrist, and occur frequently. See p. 207 for detailed findings of OA and RA; abnormalities specific to the wrist and hand are listed here.

Osteoarthritis
Commonly affects the first ray and distal interphalangeal joints.

Rheumatoid arthritis
- Early involvement of ulnar styloid process.
- Commonly affects MCP joints.
- Ulnar deviation and subluxations at MCP joints (see Figure 4.23).

When should I order a CT/MRI of the wrist or hand?
- Early detection of inflammatory arthropathies (MRI).
- To evaluate for AVN associated with scaphoid fractures (MRI or CT).

Joint replacements (arthroplasty) and orthopedic hardware

There is an enormous spectrum of internal and external fixators, implants, hardware, cement, and graft materials commonly used.

Fixation of implants to bone can be:

Active: Using screws and other mechanical devices.
Passive: Cemented or "grouted" via a chemical interaction.
Biofixated: By ingrowth of the patient's bone into a rough or fenestrated implant surface.

Combinations of fixations
Spinal fusions and reconstructions often employ both anterior and posterior fixation and disc space implants, grafts, or cages.

Terminology
Total arthroplasty
The articular surfaces on both sides of a joint are replaced.

Hemiarthroplasty
- Only one articular surface is replaced.
  - <u>Unipolar</u>— prosthesis consists of one single component.
  - <u>Bipolar</u>—Consists of two sliding components, allowing for greater longevity and range of motion.

ORIF
- Open reduction internal fixation (of fracture) with hardware.

Radiography of orthopedic hardware and fixation devices
What do you need to look for?
Immediate post-operative imaging
Images are usually obtained in the operating or recovery room, and then again before discharge. Assess for:
- Anatomic alignment.
- Adjacent fractures.
- Dislocation.
  - Arthroplasty components may dislocate, especially in the peri-operative period before healing, or if the components are less stable than usual (e.g., unusual tilt of a cup relative to the implant head) (see Figure 4.35).

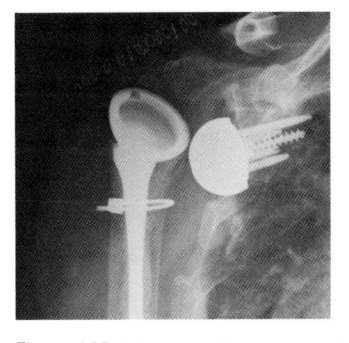

Figure 4.35 Arthroplasty dislocation immediately post-op. AP view of a reverse total shoulder arthroplasty. The humeral cup is laterally, superiorly dislocated from the prosthetic glenoid head.

Follow-up imaging
Old films improve detection of subtle changes in hardware or hardware-bone interfaces. Assess for:
- Hardware position stability.
  - Has subsidence or migration occurred?
  - Screws may "back" out, leaving screw head projecting into soft tissue. Compromises fixation, immobilization, and restoration of ROM.
- Hardware integrity.
  - Screws, plates, and other metal structures can fracture.
- Interface with adjacent bone.
  - Is bone well opposed to hardware?
  - Is there an abnormal lucency at bone/hardware/cement interface?

> Metal-bone, metal/cement, bone/cement interfaces should be tight, with < 1 mm radiolucency between implant (or cement) and bone. *Increasing lucency over time is worrisome, and may indicate:*
> - Infection.
> - Osteolysis-particle disease (see below).
> - Loosening.

Infection
Radiography
- Causes poorly marginated cystic lucencies or irregular widening of bone/metal or bone/cement interface.

If clinically suspected, further evaluation with:
- Joint aspiration/irrigation under fluoroscopy.
- Radio-labeled leukocyte scan (+/– Tc-99m sulfur colloid scan).
- Bone scan (loosening tends to have focal uptake, whereas infections demonstrate diffuse radionuclide uptake).

Osteolysis (particle "disease")
Wear of polyethylene causes tiny particles of foreign matter to shed. These particles cause a sterile inflammatory response. This induces peri-prosthetic bone resorption (see Figure 4.36).
- Inflammatory process, painful.
- Increased risk of peri-prosthetic fracture.

Procedures

Joints
- Aspiration (diagnostic).
- Injection (pain studies).
- Contrast injection (prior to cross sectional imaging).

Risks
- Pain, infection, bleeding, allergy to contrast, radiation exposure (minimal).
- Steroid flare—post injection pain may occur for up to 7 days after steroid injection due to irritation from steroid.

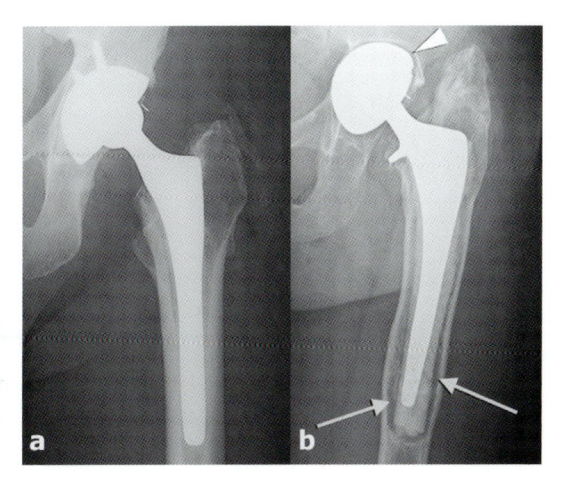

Figure 4.36 (a) AP hip shows normal in-growth of uncemented hip arthroplasty components and no lucency at metal/bone or bone/cement interfaces. (b) Second patient with pain. AP hip shows 2–4 mm lucency (arrows) at interfaces around the entire stem, and 2 mm lucency at superior cup/bone interface (arrowhead). Note the resultant thinning of the femoral cortex.

Technique—general
- Sterile technique utilized.
- Fluoroscopic or ultrasound guidance can be used:
  - Depends on site and indication.

Joint aspiration
Indications:
- Suspected infection: Signs, symptoms, history (e.g., prior arthroplasty, IV drug abuse, immunocompromised), or initial radiographs suggesting possible infection.
- Pre-arthroplasty: Patients about to undergo primary or, more commonly, revision arthroplasty may have baseline aspiration to ensure there is no subclinical infection present.

Joint injection-pain study
Indications:
- Confirm that the joint is actually the source pain.
  - If symptoms not relieved by injection, search for other causes.
- Provide temporary (hours/weeks, not predictable) relief from pain.
  - Although symptoms may be improved, unchanged, or more uncomfortable (steroid flare) post procedure.
- Improve range of motion.

Procedure:
- Inject steroid and anesthetic mixture.

Arthrography (contrast joint injection)
Indications
Intra-articular dilute contrast enhances visualization of cartilage (menisci, labrum), joint capsule, rotator cuff tears.
- Most commonly done pre-MRI (with gadolinium).
- In patients whose metal implants (orthopedic, pacemakers or defibrillators, vascular/aneurysm clips, etc.) preclude MR, can be performed using iodinated contrast pre CT.

Technique
- Dilute gadolinium or iodine injected.
- MR/CT must follow injection promptly; long delays compromise image quality as contrast is reabsorbed.

Biopsies and soft tissue aspirations and injections
Indications
- Diagnosis of bone lesions, soft tissue masses.
- Ganglion or cyst aspiration.
- Lesion injections/sclerotherapy.

Technique
CT, US, fluoroscopic or MR guidance can be used. (See chapter 10, Interventional Radiology, "Methods of Imaging Guidance," p. 450.)
- Must consider *number and choice* of compartments breeched.
- Chose route in conjunction with orthopedic oncologist to limit tumor "seeding" in needle track (subsequent en bloc excision of malignancy must include needle track).

References

Buckwalter KA, Farber JM. Application of multidetector CT in skeletal trauma. *Semin Musculoskelet Radiol.* 2004;8(2):147–156.

Dartmouth human anatomy website: http://www.dartmouth.edu/~anatomy.

Finnoff JT, Smith J, Nutz DJ, Grogg BE. A musculoskeletal ultrasound course for physical medicine and rehabilitation residents. *Am J Phys Med Rehabil.* 2010 Jan;89(1):56–69.

John Hopkins Radiology website: http://www.teamrads.com.

Keats TE, Anderson MW. *Atlas of Normal Roentgen Variants That May Simulate Disease.* 8th ed. Elsevier Mosby, Philadelphia, PA: 2006.

Ragsdale BD, Madewell JE, Sweet DE. Radiologic and pathologic analysis of solitary bone lesions. Part II: Periosteal reactions. *Radiol Clin N Am* 1981;19:749–783.

Resnick D, Kransdorf MJ, *Bone and Joint Imaging.* Philadelphia, PA: Elsevier Saunders. 2005. 78–136.

Chapter 5

Ultrasound

Stephanie P. Yen, MD

How are images acquired? *234*
  Types of ultrasound *236*
Tissue characteristics and patterns of disease *240*
Abdomen *243*
  What examination should I order and how is it performed? *243*
  Normal anatomy *244*
  Common conditions *247*
Pelvis *255*
  What examination should I order and how is it performed? *255*
  Normal anatomy *256*
  Common conditions *256*
  Prostate *262*
Reproduction *263*
  First trimester pregnancy *263*
  Common conditions *265*
  Second and third trimester pregnancy *268*
  Common conditions *272*
    Imaging guidance for procedures 276
Scrotal ultrasound *276*
  Anatomy on the testicular ultrasound *276*
  Common conditions *277*
Other small-parts ultrasound *278*
  Thyroid ultrasound *278*
  Find the foreign body *280*
Vascular ultrasound *280*
  Venous ultrasound *280*
  Arterial ultrasound *282*
Ultrasound guided procedures *283*
Other applications of ultrasound *284*
References *284*

How are images acquired?

Ultrasound uses high frequency sound waves to create images. No ionizing radiation is involved. It has both advantages and disadvantages as an imaging modality as listed on Table 5.1.

The sound wave
The ultrasound probe transmits high frequency sound waves into the body, which travel until they hit an interface of tissues of differing acoustic impedance. Some of the sound waves then get reflected back to the probe and others continue to travel further until they reach another boundary and get reflected. The reflected waves get picked up by the transducer probe and transmitted to the ultrasound machine. The machine then calculates the distance from the probe to the tissue boundary where the sound wave was reflected from the time of each echo's return and the data are used to generate a two-dimensional (2D) image.

The acoustic window
An appropriate window, called an "acoustic window," must be available to image the structure of interest; images cannot be obtained through air (e.g., lung or bowel) or bone.
- A conductive jelly is used to improve transmission between the transducer and the skin.
  - This must also be used inside sterile probe covers.
  - Sometimes a solid jelly "standoff pad" is used to improve the imaging of superficial structures (e.g., skin lesions, foreign bodies).
- Often we need to "move organs" into the acoustic window (e.g., by having the patient take a deep breath when imaging the liver)
- In pelvic ultrasound, the urine-filled bladder is used as the transabdominal acoustic window to image the pelvis.
- Patients may need to be turned on their sides to find the right window.

Table 5.1 Advantages and disadvantages of ultrasound

Advantages	Disadvantages
No ionizing radiation	Operator dependent
Non-invasive	Patient dependent (body habitus, mobility, etc.)
Widely available	
Portable	Limited depth penetration
Relatively inexpensive	Resolution variable with depth
Images acquired in any plane	Problems with penetrating air-filled structures
	Lacks penetration of calcified structures

Technology

Ultrasound transducers
Ultrasound transducers come in different sound frequencies and configurations and are chosen depending on the area of the body that is to be imaged and the resolution needed; for examples, see Figure 5.1. Probes may be placed inside sterile covers for use in the OR or intracavitary. There is a trade-off between depth of penetration and resolution:
- Higher frequencies produce better spatial resolution.
- Higher frequency waves do not penetrate as deeply into the body, and they can only be used for relatively superficial structures.
- Most probes produce a range of frequencies that can be selected by software settings.

Curved or sector probes
- Image larger areas, such as abdominal imaging for liver and kidneys.
- Produce wedge-shaped image with good depth.

Linear probes
- Image "small parts" (e.g., breast, thyroid, testis, joints, and vascular).
- Higher resolution images than with curved/sector probes.
- Produce a rectangular field with less depth than sector probes.

Intracavitary probes
- High resolution probes used for transvaginal (endovaginal) pelvic ultrasound and transrectal prostate ultrasound.
- Wedge-shaped fields with limited depth.
- Good resolution.

Specialist small probes
- Available for neonatal/pediatric and musculoskeletal applications.

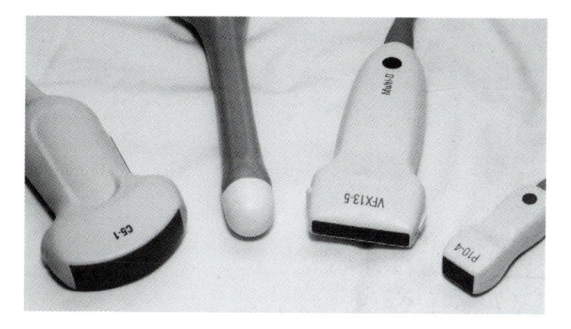

Figure 5.1 Common ultrasound probes. From left to right: curved, endovaginal, linear, and pediatric probes are shown.

Types of ultrasound

M mode ultrasound
- Graphical display of the echoes from a single, thin ultrasound beam (Y axis) recorded against time (X axis).
- Used for some cardiac echocardiography applications and measuring cardiac activity in embryos due to its low energy (see Figure 5.2).

2D ultrasound
- The standard "gray-scale" technique as already described.

3D ultrasound
- Sound waves are not reflected straight back to the transducer as in 2D scanning, but instead are sent at different angles.
- Requires special probes and software.
- Computer program then processes the returning echoes and creates a three-dimensional (3D) volume image that can be rendered ("resliced") in different planes or a surface rendering of the structure can be created.
- Most popular in obstetrical ultrasound (see Figure 5.3).

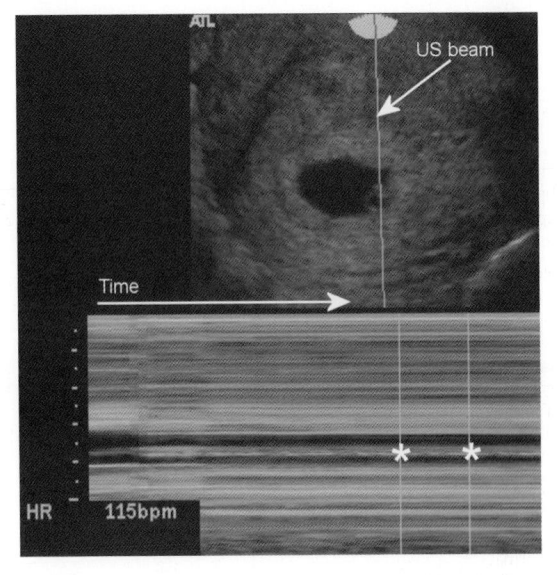

Figure 5.2 M-mode ultrasound of a 6-week embryo showing the recording of echoes along a single beam (arrow), with time. *-* marks where the tech has identified the start and end of a heart tube contraction to calculate the heart rate.

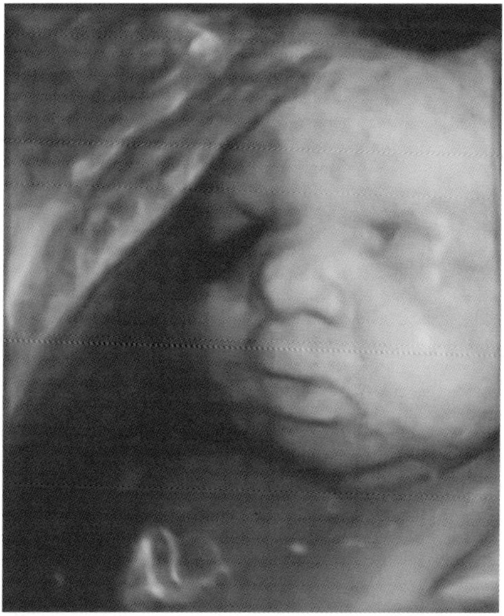

Figure 5.3 3D image of the fetal face. See Color Plate 2.

Doppler Ultrasound
Doppler ultrasound is used to evaluate blood flow, specifically its direction and velocity.

Color Doppler (see Figure 5.4):
- Measures velocity of the blood flow and assigns a color to the blood flow depending on its direction (e.g., flowing toward or away from the transducer).
- Most typically: red = toward transducer, blue = away from transducer, green = turbulent flow.
- Typical indications: to evaluate flow direction in the portal vein; to evaluate patency of transjugular intrahepatic portosystemic shunts (TIPS); to identify renal arteries and veins.

Power Doppler:
- More sensitive for detection of blood flow (e.g., slow flow and/or flow in small vessels), but does not give directional flow or velocity information.
- Typical indications: to look for flow within a mass or a suspected torsed ovary or testis.

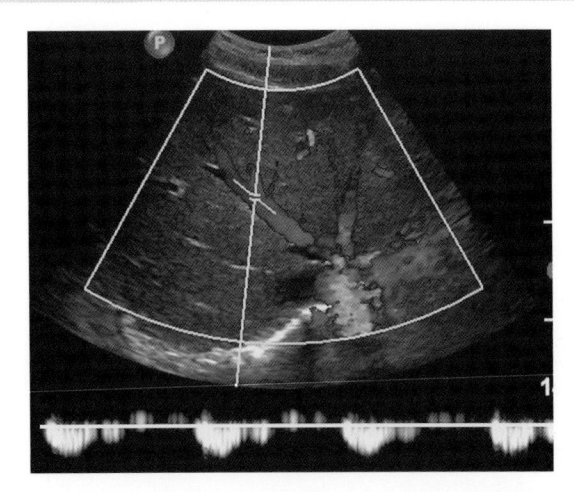

Figure 5.4 Normal color Doppler image and spectral waveform of the hepatic veins. The tracing below the baseline and the blue color shows flow away from transducer. Both cardiac and respiratory pulsatility should be seen. See Color Plate 3.

Pulsed wave Doppler (see Figure 5.4):
- Displays the blood flow as a graphed waveform, giving information about:
  - Direction of flow.
  - Flow velocity.
  - Flow characteristics such as resistive indices (RI) = a ratio of (peak systolic velocity—min diastolic velocity)/peak systolic velocity) and other systolic/diastolic ratios.
- Typical indications: Identifying vessel stenoses, transplant rejection, evaluation of the umbilical artery in obstetrical imaging, and screen for fetal anemia (which results in increased intracerebral bloodflow).

Image display

Images are generally displayed in gray scale. By convention, the skin surface/transducer surface is depicted at the top of the image. By convention, the probe is held so the left side of the image as viewed is the right or the cranial side of the patient, depending on the projection.

Terminology

"Echogenicity" describes the gray-scale appearance of a structure. Often, the echogenicity must be described in relation to another structure (see below).

Anechoic ("black")
- Fluid-filled structures without debris.

Hypoechoic ("gray")
- Solid masses or complex fluid.
- Organs such as liver, kidneys, spleen. Normal liver tends to be more echogenic than normal kidneys.

Echogenic/hyperechoic ("white or bright")
- Structures that contain fat, air, calcium, or bone.

"Shadowing" (see Figure 5.12)
- Darker areas behind a structure, which is caused by the soundwave transmission being blocked (e.g., by calcium or bone).

"Increased through transmission" or "posterior acoustic enhancement" (see Figures 5.16 and 5.20)
- Areas that are brighter (whiter) behind a structure due to increased sound wave transmission (e.g., usually by fluid in a cyst, gallbladder or the bladder).
- Note: uniform solid masses can sometimes have increased through transmission, e.g., hemangiomas, some malignant nodes.

> We cannot image air-filled structures such as the lungs on ultrasound because the sound waves do not penetrate air well; nearly all are reflected. Similarly, as ultrasound does not penetrate calcium, we cannot see behind or into calcified structures.

Real time imaging versus static images

Static images
- Refers to a single ultrasound image taken at one point in time.
- Images the radiologist reviews.

Real-time imaging
- Refers to multiple individual ultrasound images taken rapidly in succession to simulate motion; they may be recorded and viewed in cine mode.
- This is what is displayed on the ultrasound monitor when imaging the patient with the transducer in hand. With real-time ultrasound, you get information about both anatomy and motion, e.g., peristalsis, cardiac motion.

Measurements in ultrasound

Ultrasound can be used to make anatomic measurements, such as organ size and measurements of the fetus, as well as measurements of masses, stones, and other structural pathology. Angles such as acetabular roof angles in baby hips can be measured. Ultrasound can also measure blood-flow velocities. These measurements are done at the time of scanning and are recorded on the images.

Accuracy
- Ultrasound measurements overall tend to be less accurate than in CT and MRI due to operator variability and inherent differences of the ultrasound machines
- The higher the resolution probe and the smaller the field being imaged, the more accurate the measurement. Submillimeter accuracy can be obtained in some circumstances, e.g., nuchal translucency measurements (p. 272).

Tissue characteristics and patterns of disease

Fluid
Fluid appears anechoic or "black" on ultrasound, with increased posterior through transmission of sound (i.e., the image is "brighter" behind the fluid).
- Fluid is simple if free of echoes, septations, and debris.
- Fluid is complex if echoes, septations, or debris are present.

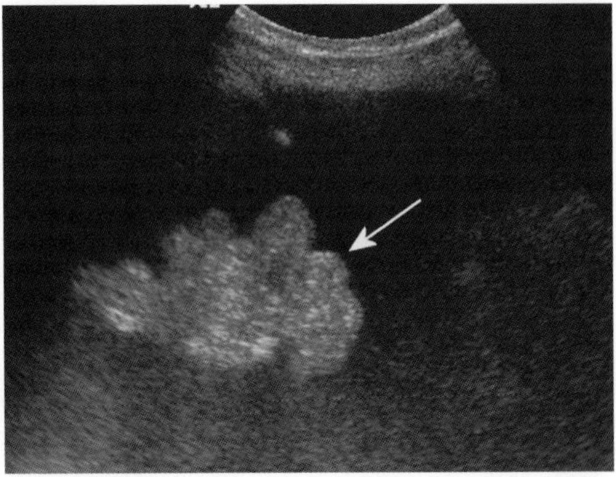

Figure 5.5 Simple intra-abdominal ascites (black). Note the floating bowel loops within the fluid (arrow).

Cysts

Cysts occur in multiple organs and are easily identified with ultrasound. Simple cysts have specific ultrasound criteria that are diagnostic. These include:
- Round or oval and anechoic.
- Smooth posterior border, with posterior acoustic enhancement.
- No discernable walls, septations, or mural nodules.
- No internal blood flow.

See Figure 11.13 for an example of a breast cyst and Figure 5.20 for an example of a renal cyst.

Calcium

Calcium is echogenic or "bright" on ultrasound.
  - Often will have posterior acoustic shadowing.
  - May not be evident if the calcification is quite small.
- Common calcified structures seen on ultrasound include bone, gallstones (see Figure 5.12), and renal stones (see Figure 5.19).

Air

Air is echogenic or "bright" on ultrasound.
- Posterior shadowing is usually "gray" rather than "black" as seen in calcified structures, often referred to as "dirty shadowing."
- Ultrasound waves cannot penetrate air; the incident beam is reflected and tissues deep to air cannot be imaged (e.g., if the stomach is gas filled, the pancreas will not be seen behind it).
- Examples of abnormal air: emphysematous cholecystitis; air in wounds, and so forth.

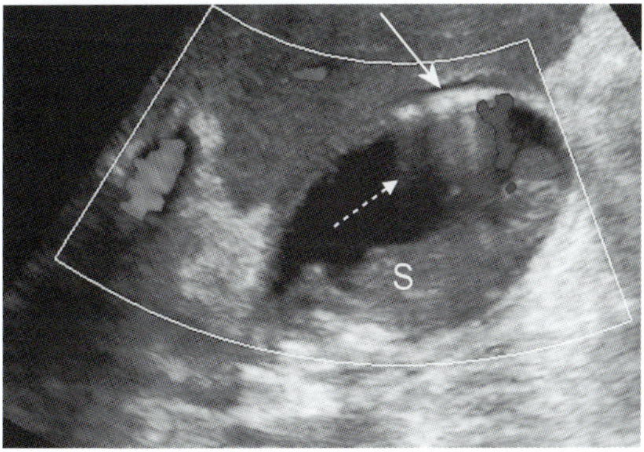

Figure 5.6 "Dirty shadowing" (dashed arrow) behind air in the wall of the gallbladder (arrow) in a patient with emphysematous cholecystitis. S = sludge.

Masses

Anechoic masses
- Are cystic, comprised of simple fluid (e.g., simple renal cyst).

Hypoechoic masses
- May be solid.
- May be complex cystic – appear "gray" on ultrasound (see testicular mass p. 285).

Hyperechoic (noncalcified) masses
- Echogenic or "bright" on ultrasound, but do not have the posterior acoustic shadowing as seen with calcified lesions. May be benign or malignant. For example:
  - Hemangioma of the liver is a benign, uniformly hyperechoic lesion with characteristic posterior acoustic enhancement.
  - Certain primary malignancies, such as renal-cell carcinoma, and some metastases can present as hyperechoic masses.
- In some cases, echogenicity reflects the presence of fat, as in an angiomyolipoma of the kidney (see Figure 5.7).

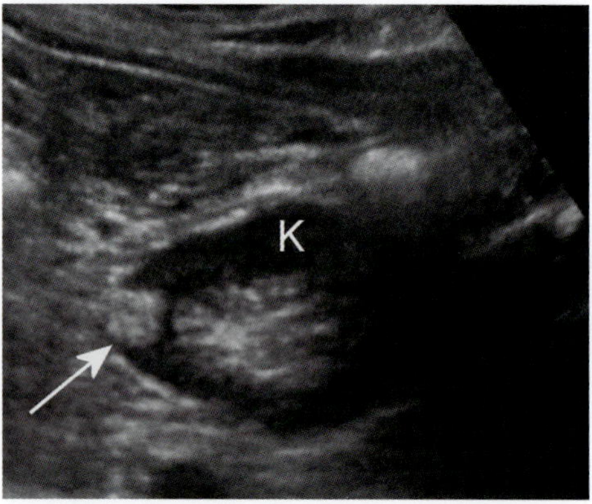

Figure 5.7 Transverse image of the left kidney (K) shows an angiomyolipoma (arrow). In contrast to the echogenic gallstones in Figure 5.12, there is no shadowing seen posterior to this echogenic mass.

Wall thickening

The wall thickness of hollow organs can be fairly accurately measured with ultrasound. Wall thickening is a common presentation of many disorders, including inflammation and infection. Structures that are commonly measured with ultrasound include the gallbladder, appendix and gastric pylorus. Ultrasound is infrequently used in the bowel:

- It is not the imaging modality of choice for evaluation of bowel edema/thickened folds or other bowel pathology, as air within the bowel loops obscures the image (CT is generally more useful).

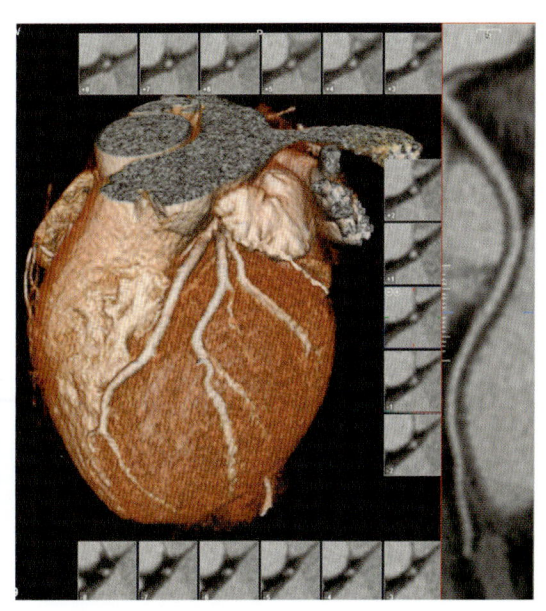

Color Plate 1 3D volumetric depiction of the heart in color, as well as reformatted images along the long axis and short axis of one coronary artery (see Figure 2.64).

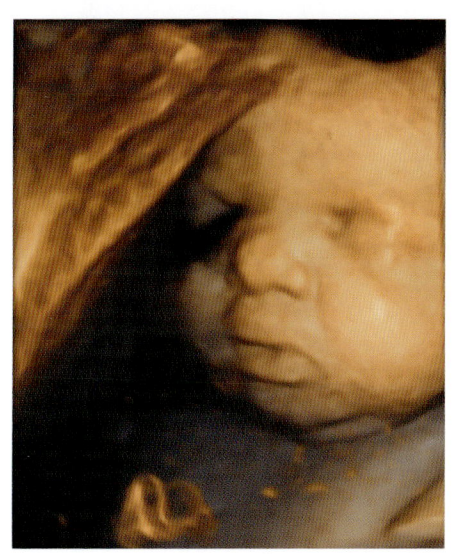

Color Plate 2 3D image of the fetal face (see Figure 5.3).

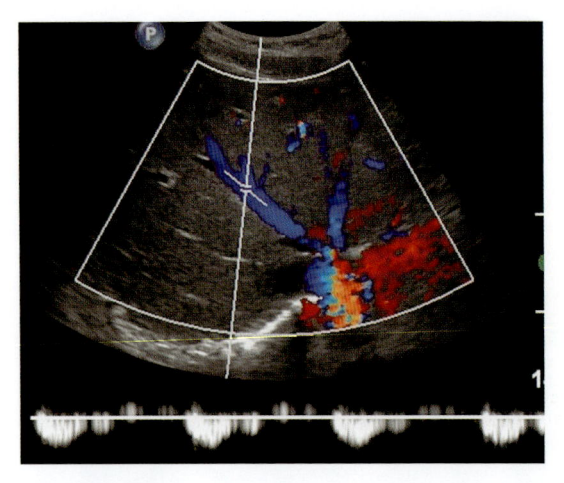

Color Plate 3 Normal color Doppler image and spectral waveform of the hepatic veins. The tracing below the baseline and the blue color shows flow away from transducer. Both cardiac and respiratory pulsativity should be seen (see Figure 5.4).

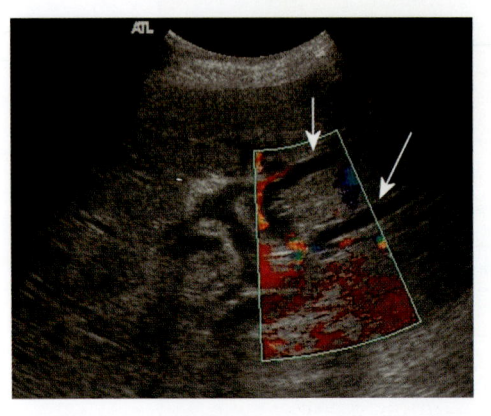

Color Plate 4 Intrahepatic biliary ductal dilatation. Dilated intrahepatic bile ducts (arrows). Note how the color Doppler distinguishes these from vessels (see Figure 5.17).

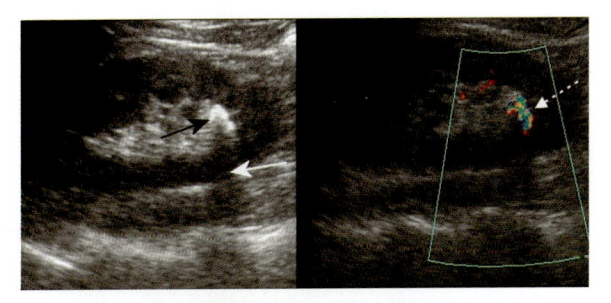

Color Plate 5 Renal calculus. Sagittal image of the kidney on grey scale (left) and color Doppler (right) shows a small echogenic stone in the lower pole (black arrow). Note the posterior shadowing (white solid arrow) and twinkle artifact (white dashed arrow) (see Figure 5.19).

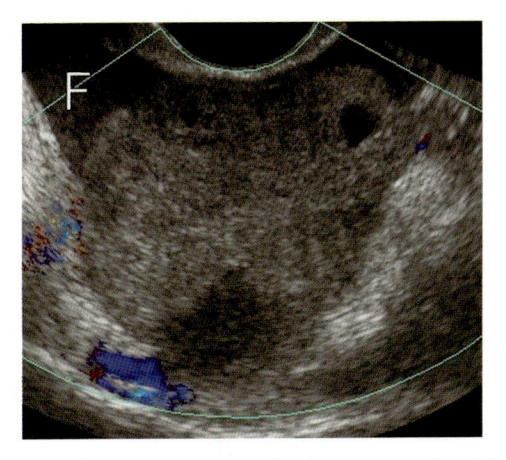

Color Plate 6 Ovarian torsion. Doppler image of an enlarged (7 cm) ovary with abnormal echogenicity and no blood flow. Note the small amount of free fluid adjacent to the ovary (F) (see Figure 5.25).

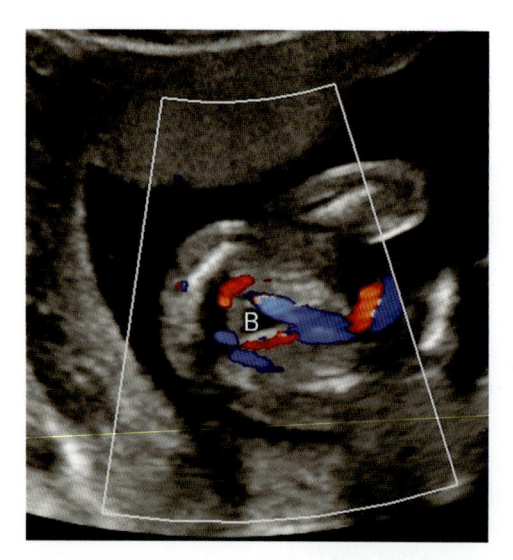

Color Plate 7 Axial image of the fetus at the level of the urinary bladder (B). Presence of a normal three-vessel (two arteries and one vein) umbilical cord can be confirmed using color Doppler. If there are two vessels (e.g., umbilical arteries) coursing around the bladder as seen in this case, then a three-vessel umbilical cord is present. Two-vessel umbilical cord (one artery and one vein) may be associated with chromosomal abnormalities, other fetal structural abnormalities, and IUGR (see Figure 5.36).

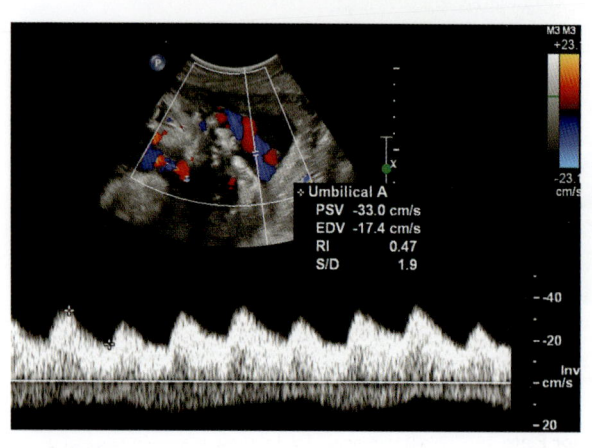

Color Plate 8 Normal UA Doppler showing measurement of the resistive index (RI) (see Figure 5.37).

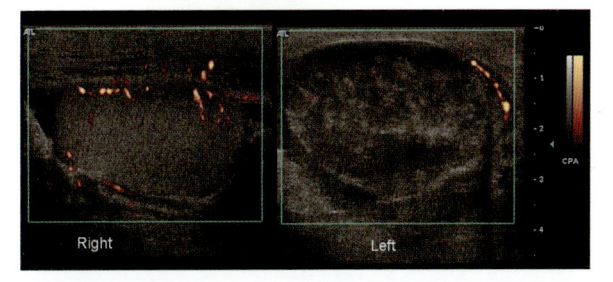

Color Plate 9 Testicular torsion. Sagittal images of the normal right testis and torsed left testis showing abnormal heterogeneous echogenicity of the left testis with absent Power Doppler flow and normal vascularity on right (see Figure 5.39).

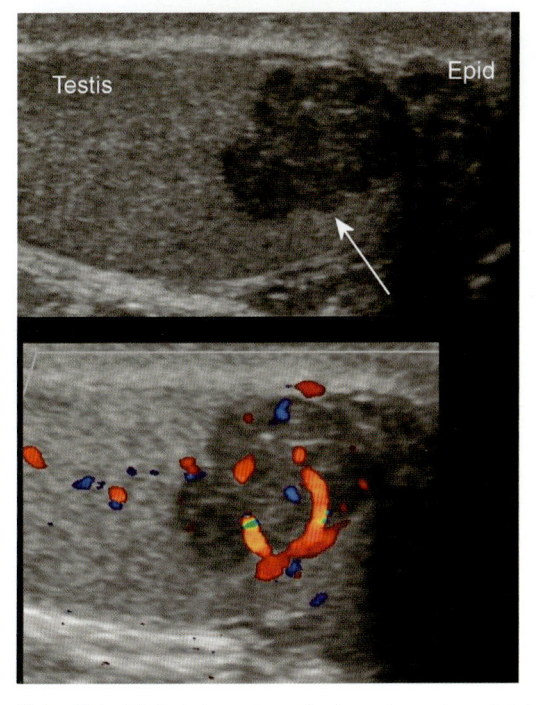

Color Plate 10 Testicular seminoma. Top image shows a hypoechoic lobular mass (arrow) in the inferior testis. Color Doppler (bottom) shows increased blood flow in this mass (see Figure 5.40).

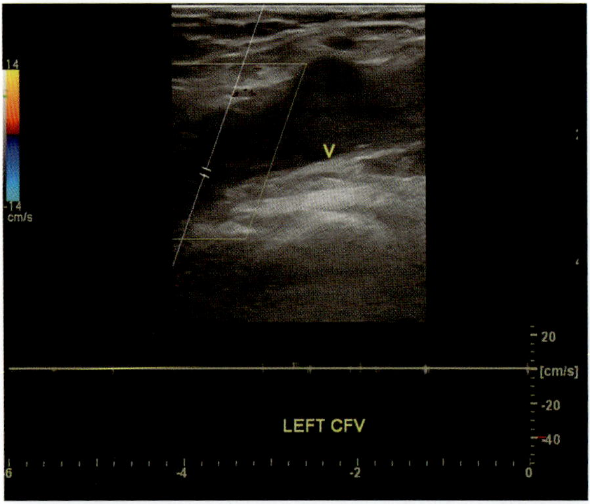

Color Plate 11 Common femoral vein thrombosis. Longitudinal image of the common femoral vein showing absent color and spectral Doppler waveforms. Also note the echoes seen in the vein (see Figure 5.44).

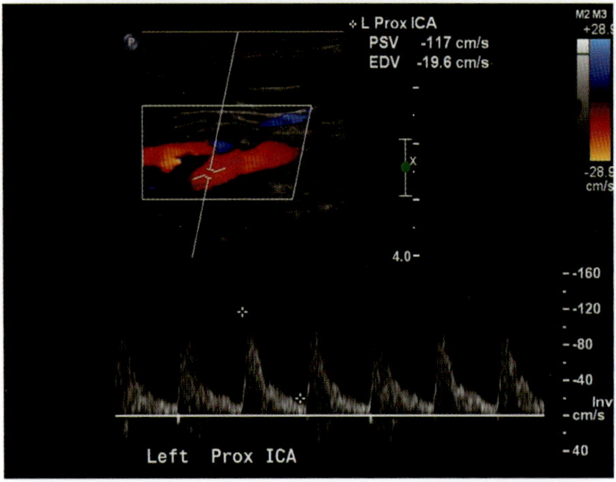

Color Plate 12 Normal left internal carotid artery Doppler color flow and Doppler spectral waveform (see Figure 5.45).

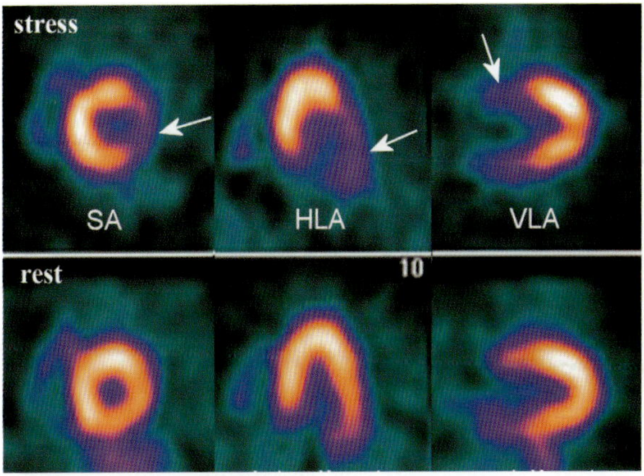

Color Plate 13 Coronary ischemia. Myocardial perfusion scan performed on a patient with chest pain. Decreased blood flow in the lateral wall on stress (arrows) that is normal at rest. Cardiac catheterization confirmed stenosis of the left circumflex coronary artery (see Figure 9.9).

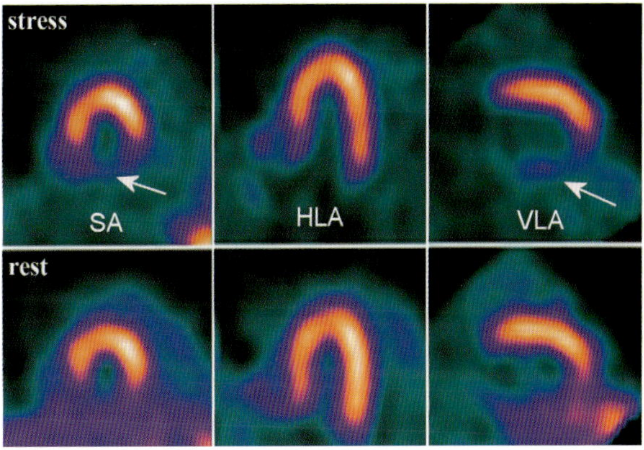

Color Plate 14 Myocardial infarct. Myocardial perfusion scan performed on a patient with a history of MI and dyspnea. Fixed defect in the inferior wall indicating infarction (arrow). No ischemia detected (see Figure 9.10).

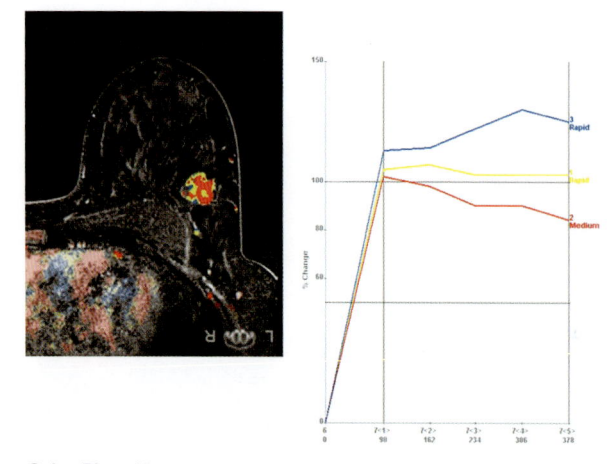

Color Plate 15 Computer assisted analysis of breast MRI contrast kinetics. Left image is an invasive ductal carcinoma showing 'malignant' or rapid wash out of contrast (red). Right image demonstrates the typical contrast washout curves for benign (blue), malignant (red) and indeterminate (yellow) processes (see Figure 11.14).

- Diffuse thickening of the bowel *may* be seen on ultrasound such as in Crohn disease, ischemia, or intussusception.
- May be used in children to reduce radiation exposure.

Luminal dilatation

Many conditions that present as dilatation of hollow organs can be imaged by ultrasound, e.g., hydronephrosis, biliary dilatation, hydrops of the gallbladder, and endometrial cavity distention.

- In many cases, there are normal standards for luminal diameter, and luminal dilatation can be assessed both subjectively and objectively (e.g., normal appendiceal transverse diameter should = 6 mm or less).

If bowel loops are filled with fluid (e.g., in the fetus, but sometimes in babies and children), bowel dilatation can be detected by ultrasound.

Organ enlargement

There are ultrasound-derived normal age-related ranges for many of the solid organs that allow us to compare measurements to determine if an organ is too small or too large. This is particularly true in the pediatric population. Liver, kidneys, spleen, testicular and ovarian volume are commonly referenced.

Abdomen

Ultrasound is generally an excellent way to image the abdomen, although it is both patient and operator dependent. Given that it uses no ionizing radiation, it is particularly useful as the first step in evaluating possible abdominal pathology in children.

What examination should I order and how is it performed?

There are several abdominal ultrasound examinations that can be performed (see Table 5.2). Which one you choose depends on the clinical question you want answered.

How is the patient positioned?

Most commonly, the patient is positioned supine with ultrasound probe placed on the abdomen anteriorly or laterally, with an intercostal or subcostal approach.

Alternatives:
- Decubitus position with probe placed between the ribs. Used for:
  - Gallbladder and kidneys in particular.
  - To see if gallstones are mobile.
- Prone position, sometimes helps visualizing the kidneys better, particularly in young children.

Usually a combination of these positions is needed to obtain satisfactory images. Patient cooperation is also necessary:
- Patient is often instructed to take a deep inspiration to try to move a particular organ away from another or from under the ribs or move the bowel.
- With Doppler imaging, patient must be able to suspend respirations for imaging to be successful.

CHAPTER 5 Ultrasound

Table 5.2

Exam	Organs imaged	Typical indication
RUQ	Gallbladder, liver/bile ducts, pancreas, right kidney	Liver/gallbladder pathology (gallstones, cholecystitis, elevated liver function tests), biliary ductal dilatation
Complete abdomen	All preceding plus spleen, left kidney, abdominal aorta and IVC	Survey of the entire abdomen for abdominal pain/hepatosplenomegaly
Complete abdomen with duplex Doppler of the liver	All preceding plus evaluation of blood flow in the portal and hepatic veins and hepatic artery	Cirrhosis and hepatitis C, surveillance for hepatocellular carcinoma, portal hypertension; TIPS shunt patency
Limited abdomen	All four quadrants of the abdomen looking for free fluid/ascites	Ascites assessment, is volume enough for paracentesis?
Renal ultrasound	Kidneys and bladder	Hydronephrosis, cortical scarring, interval growth (pediatric patients), renal stones, bladder pathology including ureterocele, wall thickening, measurement of post void bladder residual, post surgical follow-up
Abdominal aorta	Abdominal aorta and proximal common iliac arteries	Screening for abdominal aortic aneurysm

Patient preparation

With all abdominal ultrasounds (RUQ, complete abdomen), patients must have nothing by mouth (NPO) for preferably at least 8 hours. This allows for maximum distension of the gallbladder and reduces the presence of bowel gas peristalsis from a recent meal, which can obscure organs.

Normal anatomy

The following four figures (Figures 5.8–5.11) are normal ultrasound images of selected abdominal organs. All organs are imaged in both long and short axis (roughly sagittal and axial depending on organ orientation).

Liver and gallbladder

Normal liver size <15 cm cranial-caudal in mid-clavicular line with homogenous echogenicity slightly greater than kidney.
- Portal vein tributaries have echogenic walls (if no fatty infiltration), hepatic veins do not.
  - Portal venous flow is hepatopetal (toward liver).
  - Hepatic venous flow is hepatofugal (away from liver—see Color Plate 3).
- Intrahepatic biliary system not visible.
- Gallbladder should have thin wall <3 mm, and no intraluminal masses.
- Usually <10 cm but will vary with fasting level (↑with prolonged fasting).

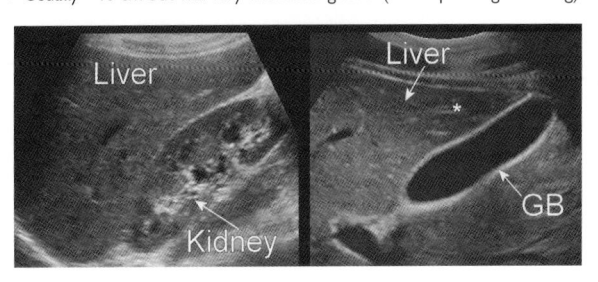

Figure 5.8 Left: sagittal image showing normal liver and right kidney. Right: normal gallbladder * = echogenic portal vein branches.

Kidney

Normal kidney size in an adult ≈10–13 cm (usually within ≈1 cm of each other). Kidneys should be homogenous, and slightly less echogenic than the liver with smooth or mildly lobulated contour.
- Normal renal cortical thickness ≈1 cm.
- In children and young adults, the pyramids may appear relatively hypoechoic, however in older patients, this would be a sign of *cortical* echogenicity (usually medical renal disease).
- A little fluid in the pelvis, or an extra-renal pelvis is normal.
  - Color Doppler helps distinguish fluid from vessels.
- Calyces should not be dilated or the ureter seen.

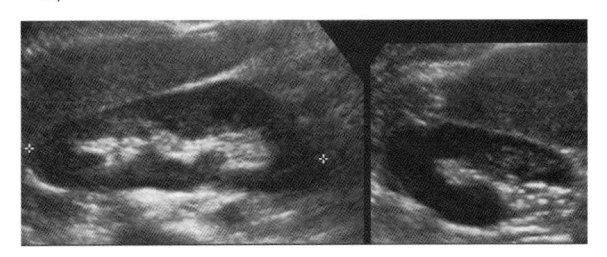

Figure 5.9 Normal long axis (left) and short axis (right) kidney.

Pancreas

Visualization of the pancreas is highly variable due to overlying bowel gas, and in obese patients may be very limited, especially the tail.
- The pancreas is relatively hypoechoic in the young and becomes more echogenic with age.
- Landmarks to help localize the pancreas are the portal vein-splenic vein confluence and splenic vein.

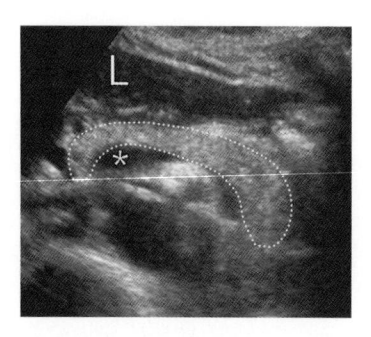

Figure 5.10 Transaxial scan of pancreas (dotted lines). L = liver, * = portal vein-splenic vein confluence.

Aorta

Visualization of the aorta and branches will depend on patient size, dense wall calcifications, and presence of bowel gas. Normal size ≈ 2 cm.

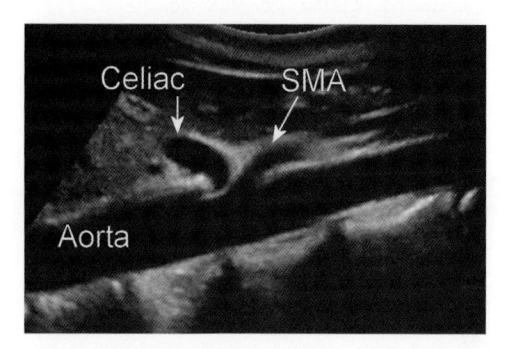

Figure 5.11 Sagittal image of the abdominal aorta. The origins of the celiac trunk and superior mesenteric artery (SMA) are also shown.

Spleen
- Normal size ≤13 cm cranial-caudal.
- Homogenous echogenicity greater than liver and adjacent kidney.
- No focal masses, smooth contour.

Common conditions

Cholelisthiasis
Ultrasound is the imaging test of choice for gallstones. They appear echogenic, show posterior shadowing, and are mobile unless wedged in the neck of the gallbladder.
- Shadowing of the posterior part of the stone and structures behind it makes large stones appear as echogenic crescents (only the anterior part is seen).
- Size, number, and mobility of stones can be assessed.
- A contracted gallbladder filled with gallstones is seen as two adjacent echogenic curvilinear structures: The first is the wall of the gallbladder and the second the multiple gallstones with posterior shadowing. This sometimes can be mistaken for bowel gas.

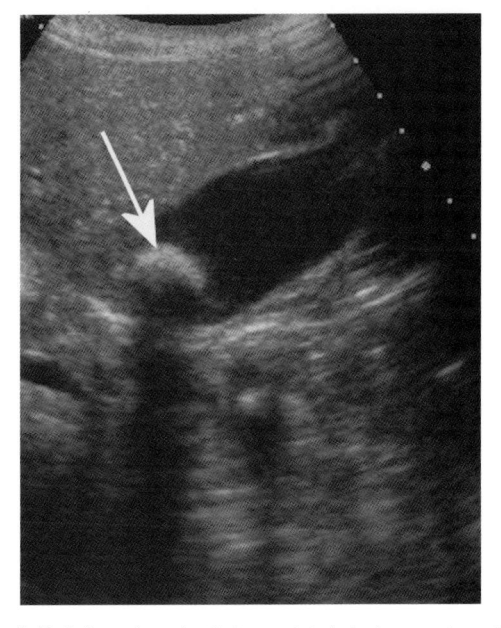

Figure 5.12 Gallstone (arrow) with characteristic shadowing posterior to the echogenic stone.

Cholecystitis—acute and chronic
Acute cholecystitis
The presence of a sonographic Murphy's sign (pain when the ultrasound transducer is specifically placed over the gallbladder and pressure applied) with cholelithiasis has a greater than 90% positive predictive value for acute cholecystitis. Other findings of acute cholecystitis:
- Peri-cholecystic fluid.
- Gallbladder wall thickening (wall thickness > 3 mm).
  - Diffuse gallbladder wall thickening in itself is nonspecific and can be seen in hypoproteinemia, hepatic dysfunction, chronic cholecystitis, adenomyosis, ascites, HIV, and CHF.
- Sometimes non-shadowing echoes are seen in the gallbladder lumen due to sludge, which can coexist with gallstones and cholecystitis, or it can be due to prolonged fasting, e.g., in ICU patients (see Figure 5.6).

A nuclear medicine hepatobiliary scan is a more specific test for diagnosing acute cholecystitis (p. 442)

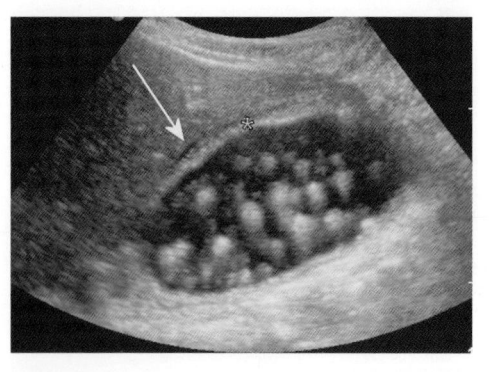

Figure 5.13 Acute cholecystitis. There are multiple gallstones, gallbladder wall is thickened (*) with pericholecystic fluid (arrow).

Chronic cholecystitis
In chronic cholecystitis the gallbladder may:
- Appear normal.
- Contain stones.
- Have diffuse or focal wall thickening.
- A hepatobiliary (nuclear) scan may reveal an abnormal gall bladder ejection fraction.

Fatty liver

Many causes of fatty liver infiltration, including alcohol, NASH (nonalcoholic steatohepatitis), obesity, Type II diabetes, and certain drugs.

Steatosis on ultrasound is seen as diffusely increased echogenicity of the liver with poor penetration of the sound waves, as evidenced by poor visualization of the diaphragm and posterior structures. The right kidney appears relatively hypoechoic.

- May be focal, seen as geographic areas of increased echogenicity (common near the falciform ligament) representing focal fatty infiltration.

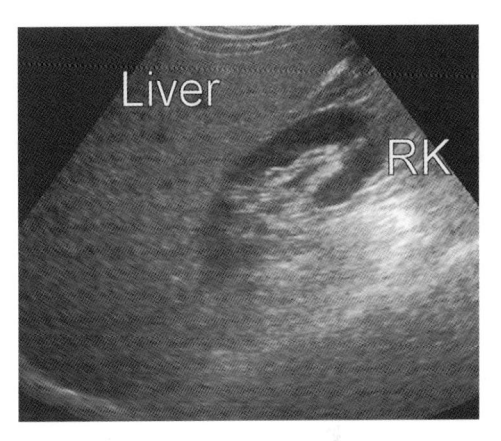

Figure 5.14 Fatty liver. The liver has diffusely increased echogenicity as compared to the normal right kidney (RK). Notice how the normally bright walls of the portal veins do not stand out as usual.

Ascites

Ultrasound is an excellent modality for evaluation of free fluid within the abdomen.

- A targeted ultrasound exam may be performed in which all four quadrants of the abdomen are examined for the presence of free fluid.
- Fluid may be simple (see Figure 5.5) or contain echoes (e.g., hemoperitoneum) As discussed later, ultrasound may also be used to guide paracenteses (p. 450 and 471).

> **FAST Exam (Focused Assessment with Sonography for Trauma)**
> - A rapid ultrasound exam performed at the bedside in trauma, specifically looking for intraperitoneal hemorrhage and pericardial tamponade.
> - Four targeted areas scanned:
>   - Perihepatic and hepatorenal (Morrison's pouch).
>   - Perisplenic.
>   - Pelvis/cul-de-sac.
>   - Pericardium.
> - Although it can be performed rapidly and at the bedside, FAST ultrasound diagnostic accuracy is dependent on both the patient (e.g., lower sensitivity in obesity) and the experience of the operator.

Liver masses

Frequently require further characterization by CT or MRI as ultrasound findings are often nonspecific, with the exception of cysts.
- <u>Solid masses:</u> Are often hypoechoic with increased blood flow. These findings are not specific. Ultrasound has lower sensitivity than CT/MRI for detection of liver metastasis but is widely used worldwide for hepatocellular carcinoma screening.
- <u>Cysts:</u> Simple and complex cysts in the liver follow the ultrasound criteria for simple and complex cysts seen elsewhere.
- <u>Hemangiomas:</u> Have a characteristic appearance on ultrasound:
  - Typically well circumscribed mass of uniformly increased echogenicity, with posterior acoustic enhancement.
  - If there are multiple echogenic masses, further imaging by CT or MRI may be needed, as certain malignancies such as renal-cell carcinoma can present with hyperechoic metastases.

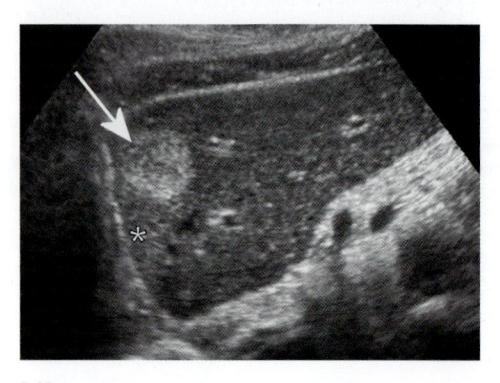

Figure 5.15 Liver hemangioma. A well circumscribed hyperechoic hepatic mass (arrow) with increased posterior sound transmission (*), characteristic of a hemangioma.

ABDOMEN

Biliary obstruction
Extrahepatic biliary ductal dilatation
Is usually easily seen on ultrasound (see Figure 5.16), except for the distal common bile duct (CBD), which may be obscured by bowel gas.

> **CBD size**
> - In an adult, CBD diameter of >6 mm is considered dilated.
> - For each decade > 50 years of age, add 1 mm to the maximum CBD duct diameter of 5 mm. (for an 80 year-old patient, max CBD diameter = 8 mm).
> - Postcholecystectomy, these measurements do not apply, and CBD diameters up to 10 mm may be normal.

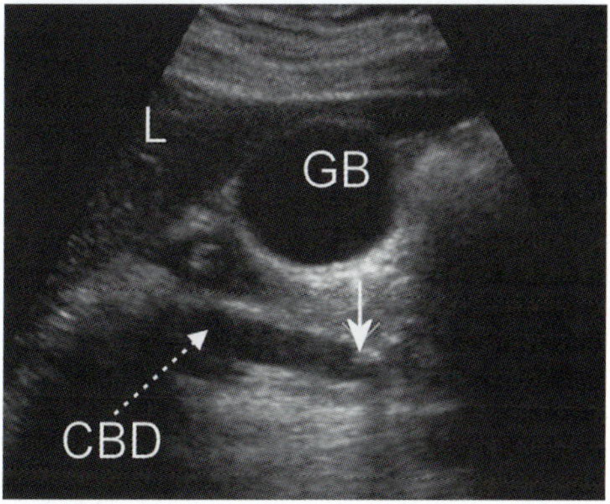

Figure 5.16 Dilated common bile duct due to a stone in the distal portion of the duct (arrow). L = liver, GB = gallbladder, CBDs = common bile duct. Note the increased sound transmission posterior to the gallbladder.

Intrahepatic biliary ductal dilatation
Can be more difficult to demonstrate on ultrasound depending on patient body habitus and the degree of dilatation.
- Diagnosis made if there is so-called "tram tracking," where the parallel echogenic walls of the bile ducts become prominent alongside the portal vein branches; both of a similar caliber. (see Color Plate 4).

The cause of biliary obstruction may be difficult to diagnosis by ultrasound. Small ampullary/pancreatic head cancers and CBD stones may be missed due to bowel gas and/or limited evaluation secondary to patient body habitus.

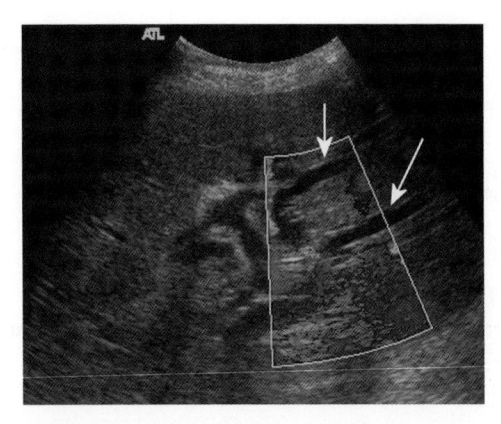

Figure 5.17 Intrahepatic biliary ductal dilatation. Dilated intrahepatic bile ducts (arrows). Note how the color Doppler distinguishes these from vessels. See Color Plate 4.

Pancreatic abnormalities
The sensitivity of ultrasound for pancreatic pathology is low. The pancreas is often difficult to visualize on ultrasound due to overlying bowel gas. CT and MRI are superior to ultrasound for evaluating the pancreas.

Appendicitis
Ultrasound has a high sensitivity and specificity in the detection of appendicitis (~90%), comparing favorably to that of CT. The primary advantage of ultrasound is the lack of ionizing radiation.

Limitations:
- Patient body habitus; difficult to detect in obese patients.
- Bowel gas can obscure appendix.

A normal appendix is usually not seen on ultrasound. Thus, if the ultrasound findings are equivocal coupled with a non-definitive clinical exam, further evaluation with CT may be indicated.

Imaging findings:
- Dilated (>6 mm in diameter), non-compressible, blind-ending tubular structure.
- +/– Shadowing calcification in the appendiceal lumen (appendicolith).
- +/– Associated hypervascularity on color/power Doppler.
- If perforation has occurred, a peri-appendiceal fluid collection/abscess or free fluid may also be seen.

Abdominal aortic aneurysms
Ultrasound is a good screening and follow-up test in patients with suspected or known abdominal aortic aneurysms, depending on the patient's body habitus. An AP measurement ≥3 cm is considered aneurysmal (see Figure 5.18).

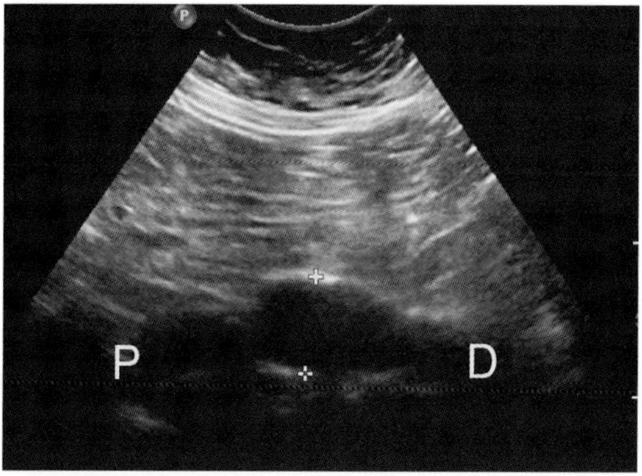

Figure 5.18 Sagittal image of the abdomen showing a 3.5 cm mid aortic aneurysm (+-+). P = proximal D = distal aorta.

- In patients who are significantly obese, CTA is probably the better modality of choice to screen and/or follow-up suspected abdominal aortic aneurysms.
- Aortic measurements and involvement of vessel ostia are more accurately obtained on CTA than by ultrasound, especially for pre-operative planning.
- Ultrasound may be used in the emergency setting to diagnose/exclude a ruptured aneurysm in patients who are too unstable to have CT.

Renal calculi

- Renal calculi are echogenic and, if large enough, will show posterior acoustic shadowing on ultrasound.
- Small calculi, those less than 5 mm or so, may be below the resolution of the ultrasound machine.
- On color Doppler imaging, renal calculi (or any other calcified structure) may show a "twinkle" artifact, which refers to an artifactual mixture of color behind the stone, which helps confirm the diagnosis (see Figure 5.19).

Renal cysts and masses

Cysts

Most renal cysts can be confidently diagnosed by ultrasound.

- Renal cysts are similar to cysts elsewhere—round or oval, anechoic, smooth posterior border, with posterior acoustic enhancement.
- Some complex cysts contain echoes and cannot be distinguished from solid masses. These indeterminate lesions will need follow-up or further imaging with enhanced CT or MRI.

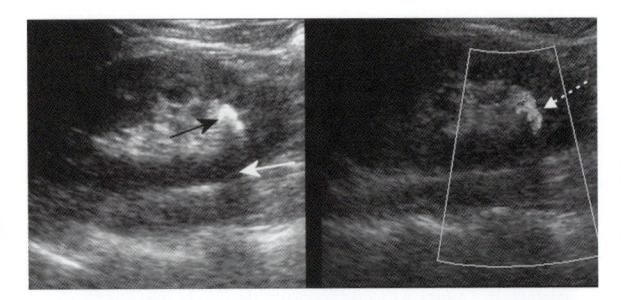

Figure 5.19 Renal calculus. Sagittal image of the kidney on grey scale (left) and color Doppler (right) shows a small echogenic stone in the lower pole (black arrow). Note the posterior shadowing (white solid arrow) and twinkle artifact (white dashed arrow). See Color Plate 5.

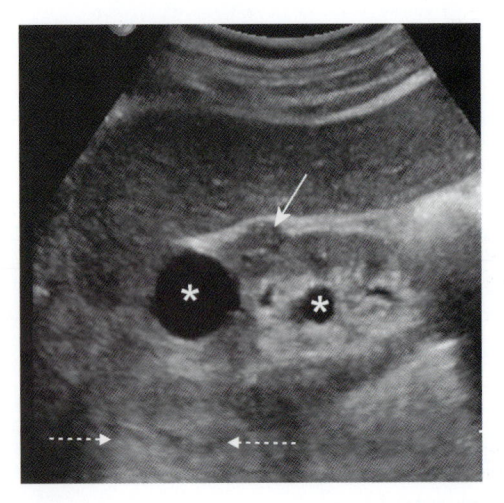

Figure 5.20 Long-axis view of right kidney showing 2 simple cysts (*). Note the increased through transmission (arrows) behind the larger cyst. There is also a small solid mass (arrow), found to be a small renal cell carcinoma.

Masses
- May be hyoechoic, echogenic, or heterogeneous.
- Doppler can be used to identify internal vascularity.
- Solid masses may require biopsy/excision, as renal cell carcinoma, oncocytoma, lymphoma, and other solid masses cannot be distinguished.

Hydronephrosis

Dilatation of the renal collecting system is diagnosed on ultrasound by fluid distending the renal calyces, which all connect to a dilated renal pelvis (also called pelvicaliectasis).

- If the level of obstruction is at the level of the ureter, a dilated ureter may also be visualized.
  - Normally the ureter is not visualized on ultrasound.
- Evaluation of the bladder for the presence or absence of ureteral jets on color Doppler imaging (urine passing from the ureter into the bladder identified as a linear jet of color on color Doppler) is helpful.
  - If a ureteral jet is visualized in the setting of a dilated collecting system, this means a complete obstruction is not present.
  - Useful in the evaluation of pregnant patients presenting with flank pain to help determine if the dilated collecting system is due to physiologic dilatation from pregnancy or an obstructive process.

<u>Pitfall</u>: Parapelvic cysts can be mistaken for hydronephrosis, but cysts cannot be connected together as the pelvicalyceal system does.

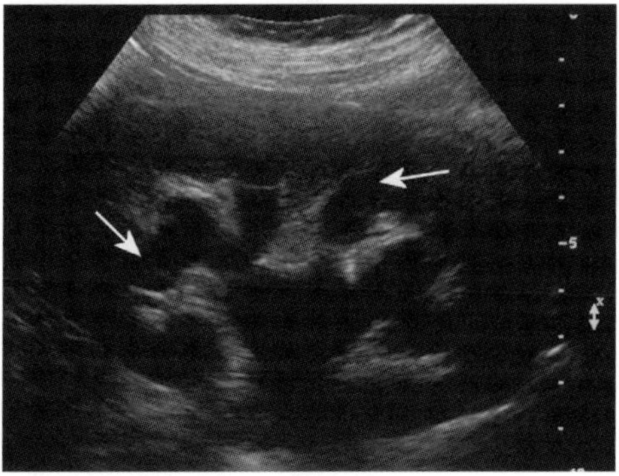

Figure 5.21 Hydronephrosis of the right kidney. Note the dilated calyces (arrows).

Pelvis

Ultrasound is the imaging modality of choice for the female pelvis. The gynecologic indications include workup for pelvic pain, ovarian torsion, fibroids, ovarian masses, dysfunctional and post menopausal bleeding, amenorrhea, pelvic inflammatory disease, and evaluating position of intrauterine devices. In certain instances, MRI is indicated to provide additional diagnostic information, such as the location of multiple fibroids, characterization of a complex ovarian mass, and confirmation of adenomyosis suspected on ultrasound.

What examination should I order and how is it performed?

A standard pelvic ultrasound provides sagittal and transverse images of the uterus, endometrium, cervix, ovaries and adnexae, and cul-de-sac. Ultrasound of the pelvis may be performed transabdominally or endovaginally.

Protocols

Transabdominal
- Images obtained with the ultrasound probe placed on the skin surface of the lower abdomen/pelvis, using a full bladder as the sonographic window.
- Used in pre-sexual teens and children, men, and sometimes for imaging larger pelvic masses or high ovaries, as well as bladder lesions.

Transvaginal
- Images obtained with placement of an endovaginal probe within the vagina.
- In contrast to the transabdominal approach, the bladder should be empty.
- Provides considerably better images of the uterus and ovaries and is performed whenever possible in adult women or sexually active teenagers.

Sonohysterography/Hysterosonography
- Small-caliber catheter is inserted through the endocervical canal, into the uterus.
- Fluid instilled into the endometrial cavity during the acquisition of ultrasound images using a transvaginal probe (see Figure 5.28).

Transrectal
- Prostatic ultrasound in men for diagnosis and guided biopsies.
- Postpartum evaluation of poorly healed ano-rectal tears in women.

Normal Anatomy

Uterus
The normal uterine myometrium is uniformly hypoechoic. The endometrium has a variable appearance in premenopausal women dependent on the menstrual cycle (see Figure 5.22 and discussion p. 267).

Ovaries
The normal ovaries contain small follicles, seen as round hypo or anechoic structures. Ovaries are commonly measured in three planes, and a volume is calculated (see Figure 5.23).
- Average adult premenopausal ovarian volume is $\approx$4–5 cm^3.
- Varies with age, menstrual status, and within the menstrual cycle (e.g., a prominent follicle or corpus luteum will increase the volume.

PELVIS 263

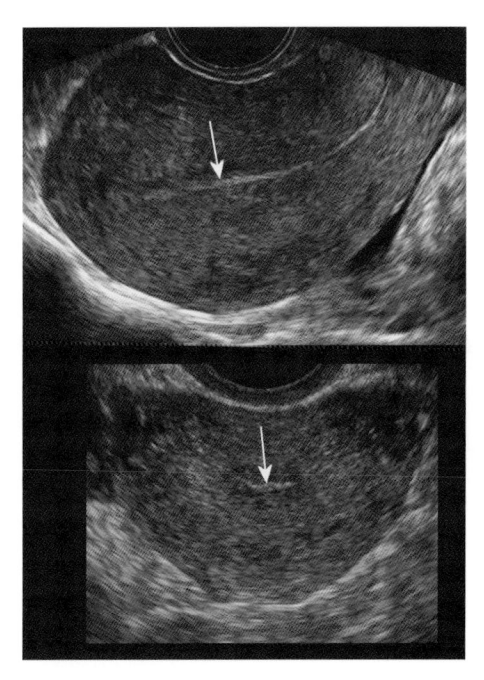

Figure 5.22 Sagittal (top) and axial (bottom) images of a normal uterus. Note the uniform echogenicity of the myometrium of the uterus and the thin echogenic endometrium (arrow).

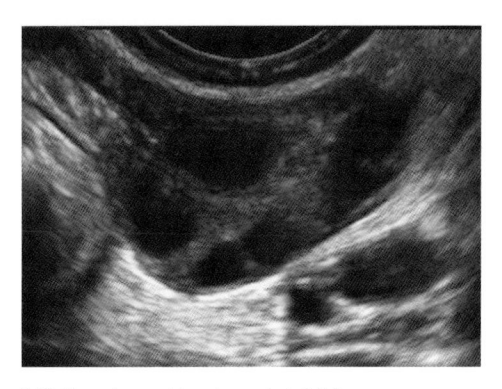

Figure 5.23 Normal ovary. Note the anechoic follicles.

Common conditions

Ovarian cysts
- Ovarian cysts are classified as simple or complex.

Simple cysts
Simple cysts are very common. Most cysts are physiological and resolve in a menstrual cycle or two. Simple cysts meet the ultrasound criteria for simple cysts and appear similar to simple cysts shown elsewhere (see p. 247, "Patterns of Disease").
- Extremely unlikely to be malignant:
  - 100% simple cysts in pre-menopausal women are benign and 95% in post menopausal women are benign.
- In premenopausal women, cysts <3 cm are considered normal and do not require follow-up.
  - US follow-up for larger cysts will depend on size and patient's symptoms.
- In postmenopausal women, cysts >3 cm should be followed by US, and CA 125 levels may be measured.

Complex cysts
Cysts that contain internal echoes, septations, mural nodules, blood flow, or a combination.

<u>Etiologies:</u> A hemorrhagic corpus luteum (benign) is the most common complex ovarian cyst. Other etiologies include endometrioma (so called "chocolate" cyst) and ovarian malignancies.

<u>Management:</u> In premenopausal women with a complex cyst >5 cm suspected of being a hemorrhagic cyst, a follow-up ultrasound in 6–12 weeks is suggested to confirm resolution and exclude other etiologies.

In post-menopausal women, a complex ovarian cyst warrants close serial sonographic follow-up, characterization by alternative imaging such as MRI, and/or consideration of laparoscopy.

Solid ovarian masses
Solid ovarian masses may be benign or malignant.
- With cystic masses that contain solid components with blood flow, the suspicion of malignancy is high. Correlation with other findings such as presence of ascites and elevated CA-125 may be helpful.
- Ovarian dermoid (benign cystic teratoma) can have a variable appearance on ultrasound.
  - The diagnosis can be made with high confidence if there is a cystic mass with an echogenic mural nodule (dermoid plug) (see Figure 5.24) or a predominantly echogenic mass with ill-defined posterior acoustic shadowing due the presence of fat and calcifications.

Ultrasound is not reliable in differentiating benign from malignant solid ovarian masses and in many instances, surgery is indicated.

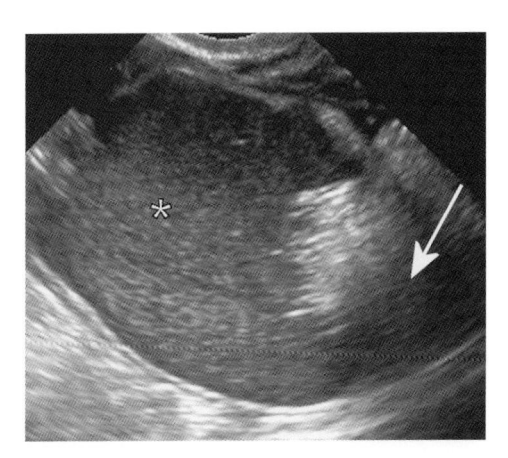

Figure 5.24 Transverse image of the ovary shows a complex cystic mass with fine echoes (*) and an echogenic mural nodule with posterior shadowing (arrow). Mature cystic teratoma confirmed by pathology.

Ovarian torsion

This is one of the most common indications for a pelvic ultrasound in a female presenting with acute pelvic pain. Ultrasound is the imaging modality of choice in the evaluation of ovarian torsion.

Ultrasound findings

- Enlarged heterogeneous ovary that is often more anteriorly located in the pelvis than usual.
- Peripheral location of follicles due to edema.
- A coexistent mass such as a hemorrhagic cyst or dermoid may be present.
- The twisted vascular pedicle may also be seen.
- Doppler imaging:
  - May show absence of all blood flow to the ovary.
  - May show only arterial and no venous blood flow (important to document pulsed Doppler waveforms).

Remember that ovaries may torse and detorse, so the presence of blood flow at the time of imaging only indicates no current evidence of torsion.

Endometriosis

Condition in which endometrial cells of the uterus implant outside the uterus. The ovary is most common site. Clinical presentation includes dyspareunia, infertility, and pelvic pain that may be exacerbated during menses.

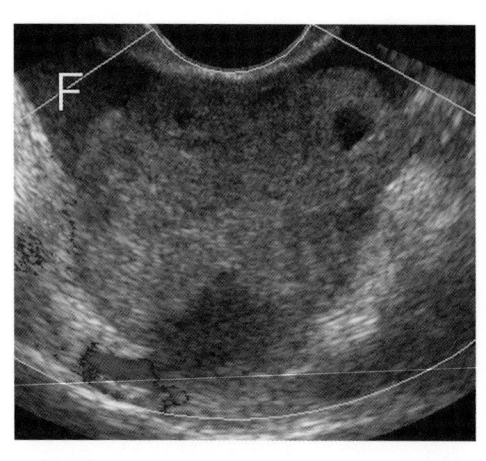

Figure 5.25 Ovarian torsion. Doppler image of an enlarged (7 cm) ovary with abnormal echogenicity and no blood flow. Note the small amount of free fluid adjacent to the ovary (F). See Color Plate 6.

Ultrasound findings
- Classic appearance is a complex adnexal cystic mass containing low-level echoes.
- The primary differential consideration is a functional hemorrhagic ovarian cyst. A follow-up ultrasound can help in differentiating the two, because a hemorrhagic cyst will resolve, whereas an endometrioma will persist.

Uterine fibroids
Most common uterine "mass."

Ultrasound findings
- Usually hypoechoic relative to myometrium, although can have variable appearances.
- May contain calcifications or cystic areas of degeneration.
- Described with respect to location in the uterus.
  - Intramural (within the myometrium).
  - Submucosal (extending into the endometrial cavity).
  - Subserosal/exophytic (arising from the surface of the uterus).
  - Pedunculated (on vascular pedicle separate from uterus).

Subserosal fibroids can sometimes mimic an adnexal or ovarian mass. With fibroids, vessels can be seen connecting the mass and the uterus and the ovaries may be identified separately. If findings are equivocal → MRI.

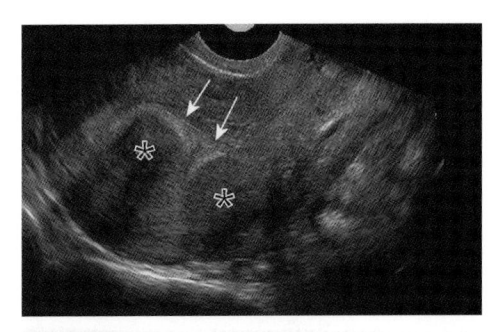

Figure 5.26 Sagittal transvaginal ultrasound shows two submucosal fibroids (*) protruding into the endometrial cavity (arrows).

Endometrial thickening—benign and malignant
Ultrasound is the most appropriate imaging test for abnormal vaginal bleeding both in pre- and postmenopausal women.

The normal premenopausal endometrium
- The endometrial thickness and echogenicity vary according to the stage of the menstrual cycle.
- <u>Proliferative phase</u>: Is the time immediately after the woman has finished her period.
  - Best phase to evaluate the endometrium as the endometrium is the thinnest, especially during early proliferative phase.
  - The endometrium has a trilaminar appearance (hypoechoic-echogenic-hypoechoic).
- <u>Secretory phase</u>: Is the second half of the menstrual cycle, from the time of ovulation to the time of menses.
  - The endometrium is uniformly hyperechoic and is maximally thickened during this phase. Thickness up to 15 mm is normal.

The normal postmenopausal endometrium
The normal value of endometrial thickness is dependent on whether or not the woman is on hormone replacement therapy (HRT).
- If not on HRT, endometrium should measure < 5 mm.
- If on HRT, endometrium should measure < 8 mm.

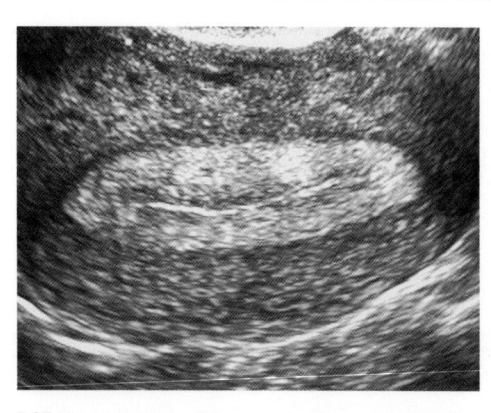

Figure 5.27 Transverse image of the uterus showing normal echogenic endometrium (measuring 12 mm) in the secretory phase of the menstrual cycle.

Benign causes of endometrial thickening
- Physiologic (related to menstrual cycle).
- Hyperplasia.
- Polyp.
  - May be suspected if there is focal thickening with associated vascularity.
- Submucosal fibroid.
- Tamoxifen.
  - Tamoxifen can cause endometrial thickening and cystic changes. Endometrial biopsy is often needed to exclude malignancy.

Malignant causes of endometrial thickening
- Endometrial cancer.

Sonohysterography
In some cases, further imaging by sonohysterography may be helpful in the evaluation of endometrial thickening and differentiating polyps from submucosal fibroids.

Hydrosalpinx
- Dilatation of the fallopian tube secondary to tubal occlusion, most commonly by pelvic inflammatory disease, endometriosis, or adhesions form prior surgeries. Infertility may result.
- Tube may be filled with fluid ("hydrosalpinx"), blood ("hematosalpinx"), or pus ("pyosalpinx").

Ultrasound findings
Tubular cystic adnexal structure of variable diameter. Located adjacent to the ovary. May contain echoes if blood or pus is present.

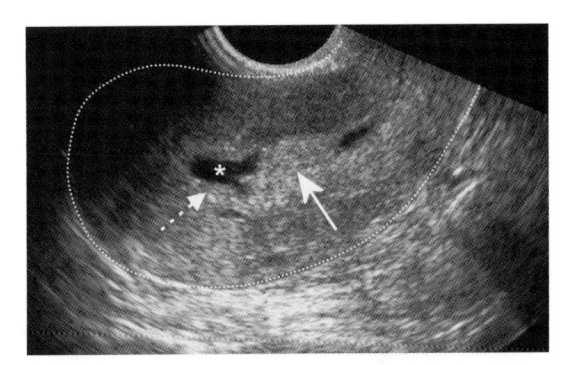

Figure 5.28 Long-axis view of sonohysterogram of an endometrial polyp (arrow), identified as an intracavitary hyperechoic mass surrounded by the injected saline (*). Dashed arrow = normal endometrium, uterus is shown by dotted lines.

Prostate

Ultrasound of the prostate is performed with a transrectal probe and usually done in the clinical setting of an elevated prostatic specific antigen (PSA).

- Most cancers of the prostate appear as hypoechoic areas and about two-thirds originate in the peripheral zone of the prostate gland, but the findings are often non-specific.
- Tumors in the central zone cannot be distinguished from hyperplasia.
- Ultrasound is very helpful in guiding the urologist or radiologist in biopsying the suspicious lesions, or performing random biopsies in the patient with elevated PSA and no focal lesions.

Reproduction

Pregnancy
Ultrasound is the imaging modality of choice used to evaluate the fetus throughout pregnancy.

Infertility
Ultrasound plays an important role in women with infertility problems who are trying to conceive. A baseline scan may be performed to exclude anatomical problems. Ultrasound is used to monitor the number and size of ovarian follicles in women on fertility drugs, to determine when to retrieve the follicles and to guide placement of fertilized embryos during in vitro fertilization.

First trimester pregnancy
When do I need to do an ultrasound in early pregnancy?
- Dating (unknown dates).
- Viability (bleeding, history of miscarriage, infertility Rx).

- Nuchal translucency measurements (see p. 271).
- Possible multiple gestations (infertility Rx, hyperemesis, family history, abnormally raised beta human chorionic gonadotropin [βhCG]).

How early can I diagnose an intrauterine pregnancy?
- By 5.5-weeks post last menstrual period (LMP).
- An intrauterine gestational sac that contains a yolk sac is diagnostic of intrauterine pregnancy, rather than an ectopic pregnancy.
- Viability cannot be assessed before 6-weeks post LMP.

Early pregnancy findings on transvaginal ultrasound
- Gestational sac is not seen before 5-weeks post LMP at the earliest.
- Yolk sac should measure <7 mm at any gestation.
- When an embryo is identified, cardiac activity is usually seen at same time.
  - Cardiac activity should be seen when an embryo measures >5mm in crown-rump length (CRL).
  - Heart rate should be >100 bpm.
  - Heart rate < 100 bpm have a poor prognosis and a follow-up ultrasound should be performed 7–10 days later.

How accurate is dating?
The earlier the ultrasound is done, the more accurate is the dating; accuracy declines later in pregnancy.
- Ultrasound in the first trimester of pregnancy is preferred and the CRL measurement is used for determining the estimated date of delivery (EDD).
- ≥ 12 weeks post LMP, dating is based on fetal measurements including head circumference, biparietal diameter of the fetal head, abdominal circumference, and humerus and femur lengths. At this stage, measurement accuracy is on the order of plus or minus 7–10 days.
- In the third trimester, dating accuracy falls to on the order of ±14–21 days.

Anatomy on the early OB ultrasound

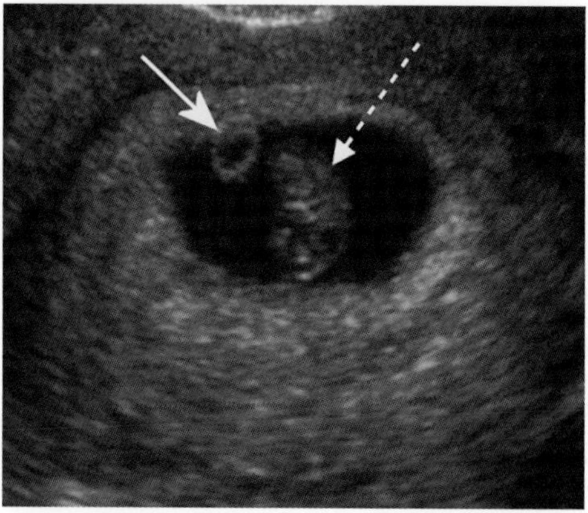

Figure 5.29 Normal structures seen in a 6–7 weeks pregnancy. The fluid filled gestational sac is anechoic (black), and contains the yolk sac (solid arrow) and the embryo (dashed arrow).

> **Embryonic structures appear in a specific order, which allows accurate dating.**
>
> | Structure visible on TV ultrasound | Weeks post LMP |
> |---|---|
> | Intra-uterine gestational sac | 5 |
> | Yolk sac | 5.5 |
> | Embryo | 6 |
> | Cardiac activity | 6+ |

Common conditions

First trimester aneuploidy screening

Nuchal translucency screening

Measurement of the nuchal translucency was introduced in the 1990s as a tool for aneuploidy risk assessment.

- The hypoechoic space at the back of the fetal neck (nuchal translucency) is measured transabdominally.
  - >3.5 mm is definitely abnormal, but the normal value increases with embryonic age.
  - Larger the value, greater the risk of a fetal anomaly.
  - If the risk assessment for a chromosomal abnormality is higher than expected, diagnostic procedures such as chorionic villus sampling or amniocentesis should be offered.
- Abnormal values associated with:
  - Chromosomal problems—for example, trisomy 21 and 18.
  - Structural heart defects.
  - Genetic disorders.
  - Poor pregnancy outcome.
  - Normal finding (see next).
- Fetus must measure between 45 and 84 mm (CRL) at the time of the screening ($\approx$ 11th to 14th weeks of pregnancy).
- Measurement correlated with the mother's age and mother's serum blood levels of two proteins, plasma protein-A (PAPP-A) and human chorionic gonadotropin (hCG) and the risk of aneuploidy is calculated.
  - This combination screening identifies $\approx$81–90% of Trisomy 21 fetuses with a false positive rate of $\approx$ 3–5%.

Spontaneous abortion

Potential ultrasound findings

- May have an embryo with no recordable heart rate measuring less than dates ("missed abortion").
- No intra-uterine gestational sac seen with the endometrial cavity filled with blood.
- May be suspected if there is a low position of the intra-uterine gestational sac within the lower uterine segment or near the cervix as sac is being expelled.
  - Normally the intra-uterine gestational sac implants near the fundus of the uterus.

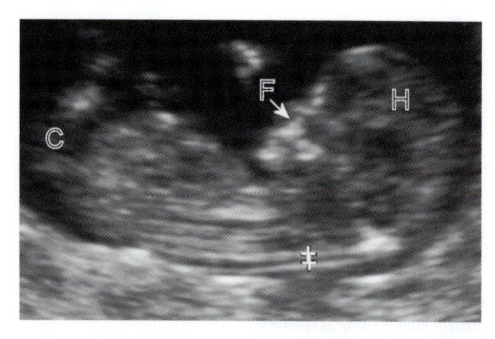

Figure 5.30 Sagittal image of a normal fetus showing where the nuchal translucency measurement is made (+). H = head, F = face, C = caudal end embryo

- Correlation with clinical history, most importantly date of LMP, is needed. Management may be conservative, or involve either medical or surgical completion (D&C).
- Usually clinicians will follow serial serum βhCGs to ensure that these decline and approach zero.

> **Diagnosing abortion or anembryonic pregnancy**
> This can be challenging for the radiologist. Accurate dates or correlation with βhCG or urine pregnancy test is often key:
> - May need delayed scan 7–10 days to distinguish between very early pregnancy and a failed pregnancy:
>   - Provided no suggestion of ectopic pregnancy.
> - Should see fetal heart when embryo is > 5 mm by transvaginal US.

Ectopic pregnancy
Ectopic pregnancy refers to a fertilized egg that has implanted outside the uterus, most commonly in the fallopian tubes, but also can occur in the ovaries/adnexa, cervix, or abdomen.
- These are non-viable pregnancies and can pose serious medical problems to the mother, including pain, bleeding, and death if rupture.
- Very rarely, intra-uterine pregnancy and an ectopic pregnancy co-exist (heterotopic pregnancy). More commonly seen in women who are undergoing infertility treatments.

Ultrasound findings
- Extra-uterine location of gestational sac with yolk sac + embryo (see Figure 5.31). If you see this, the diagnosis of ectopic pregnancy can be made with confidence.
- "Adnexal tubal ring sign"
  - Adnexal/ovarian ectopic pregnancy presenting as a mass with peripheral vascularity.
  - May or may not see yolk sac or embryo.

- Pseudogestational sac: fluid or blood in the uterine cavity that can be mistaken for a gestational sac.
  - Note, >99% of the time, a round fluid-filled area in the endometrium of a pregnant patient *is* a gestational sac.
- Hemoperitoneum
  - Consider a ruptured ectopic pregnancy if you see complex free fluid in the pelvis.
  - May also track up into the flanks, so scan Morrison's pouch for fluid transabdominally if you see fluid in the pelvis.

If an intra-uterine pregnancy cannot be confirmed (= a gestational sac containing a yolk sac) when a woman has a positive beta βhCG, an ectopic pregnancy cannot be excluded. In these clinical situations, monitoring serial serum quantitative βhCGs and follow-up ultrasound imaging is indicated.
- Should see a gestational sac when serum βhCG >1000 mIU/mL.

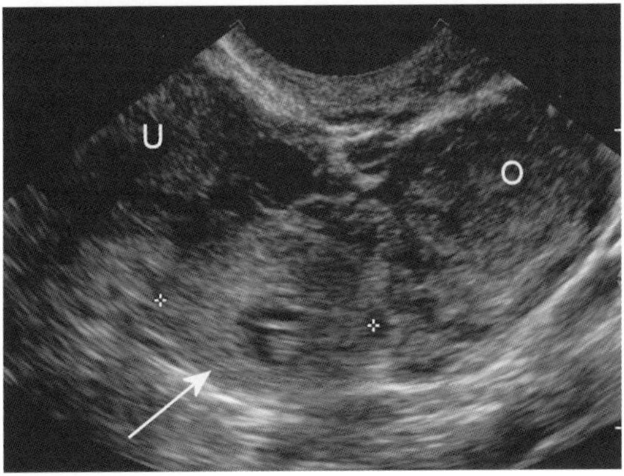

Figure 5.31 Ectopic pregnancy in the left adnexa. A gestational sac (arrow) containing a live embryo (seen real-time) is seen. U = uterus. O = ovary.

Multiple pregnancies

The incidence of multiple pregnancies increases in women who are receiving fertility drugs or assisted reproductive technology. Ultrasound scanning early in multiple pregnancies is important, as the chorionicity and amnionicity, important prognostic factors, are best evaluated in the first trimester.
- <u>Chorionicity</u> refers to the number of chorionic sacs.
- <u>Amnionicity</u> refers to the number of amnions present within each chorion.

Twin pregnancies
- Dichorionic, diamniotic (DC/DA)—two chorions and two amnions, two placentas or a single fused placenta (see Figure 5.32).
- Monochorionic, diamniotic (MC/DA)—one chorion and two amnions, single placenta.
- Monochorionic, monoamniotic (MC/MA)—one chorion and one amnion, single placenta.
- Dizygotic twinning accounts for 69% twin pairs; monozygotic 31%.
- MC/DA twins share vascularity with a common chorionic plate and have greater risk of potential complications such as twin-twin transfusion compared to DC/DA twins.
- MA/MC twins have the highest risk of complications.

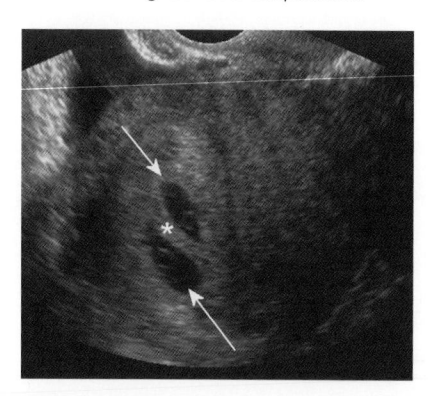

Figure 5.32 Transvaginal US of early dichorionic, diamniotic twin intra-uterine pregnancy. Two amniotic cavities (arrows), each with a yolk sac separated by thick echogenic chorion (*). A monochorionic pregnancy would only have a very thin sheet of amnion between the two sacs.

Second and third trimester pregnancy
The most common indication for ultrasound in the second trimester is screening the fetus for structural abnormalities.

When do I need to do an ultrasound?
- Fetal morphology screening, usually performed mid-second trimester
- Follow-up of:
  - Fetal anomalies, such as ventriculomegaly, pelvicaliectasis.
  - Fetal growth, fluid and umbilical artery Doppler in patients deemed high risk or with multiple gestations.
  - Placental position if earlier in pregnancy it was low-lying or previa.
- Size > dates or size < dates by clinical evaluation.
- Preterm labor.
- Premature rupture of membranes.
- Vaginal bleeding.
- Assessment of fetal position and presentation in third trimester.

Aneuploidy and anomaly screening
- A fetal anatomic morphology screening ultrasound is typically performed between the 18th to 20th weeks of gestation.
- Consists of a detailed fetal anatomic survey, which includes intracranial, facial, cardiac, and spinal fetal anatomy as well as evaluation of the abdomen, kidneys/bladder, and extremities.
- Multiple measurements are obtained and compared to normal values.

Major congenital abnormalities
The fetal morphology scan can detect major anomalies of the heart, brain, abdomen, lungs, kidneys, bladder and skeleton. See p. 281 for a more detailed discussion by organ system. Some of these anomalies are highly associated with aneuploidy, whereas others are isolated abnormalities.
Fetuses with aneuploidy have a very high rate of major congenital anomalies.
- The incidence of aneuploidy with a specific major anomaly is highly variable.
  - E.g., Omphalocele >> gastrochisis.
- Amniocentesis is often recommended if these are detected (e.g., omphalocele, cardiac anomalies).

Minor congenital abnormalities
There are several sonographic "minor markers" (minor changes that have been shown to be associated with increased risk for aneuploidy) that can be seen at this time. Likelihood ratios (LR) of the risk of trisomy 21 have been calculated; three most common are shown in following box. (These LRs have to be combined with the patient's baseline risks [e.g., age, serum markers]).

Sonographic Marker	LR if Isolated Marker*
Absence nasal bone	15.0
Nuchal thickening	11.0
Hyperechoic bowel	6.7

*N.B. A single minor marker is commonly encountered for 22.6% fetuses with trisomy 21 and 11.3% euploid fetuses.

Biometric measurements
Various fetal measurements are also obtained for dating and compared to previous ultrasounds to determine if appropriate fetal growth has occurred. These are:
- Head circumference and biparietal diameter.
- Abdominal circumference.
- Humerus and femur lengths.
- (Cerebellar diameter and other extremity measurements may be used on occasions).

Size/date discordance
- Early pregnancy (first trimester) ultrasound or accurate menstrual/conception dating is key to determine later fetal growth.
- Clinical assessment with uterine fundal height is also important.
- If there is a discrepancy between fetal size/dates, an ultrasound is often performed to evaluate fetal growth and to check amniotic fluid volume.

CHAPTER 5 Ultrasound

Bleeding

Vaginal bleeding in the second and third trimesters of pregnancy may indicate:
- An impending miscarriage.
- A problem with the placenta.
  - Placenta is too close to the cervix (placental previa see p. 278).
  - Subchorionic hemorrhage (also seen in first trimester).
  - Placental abruption (see p. 279).

Normal Anatomy

Shown below are selected images of normal fetal anatomy at 18–20 weeks. The extensive discussion of fetal anatomy is beyond the scope of this book. Some important areas for which images are obtained are shown in Figures 5.33–5.36:

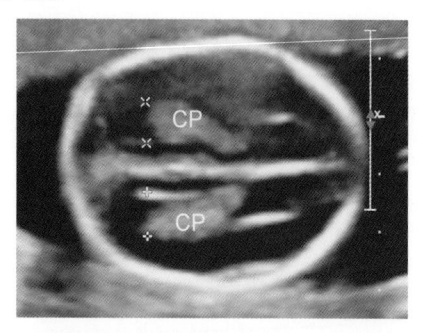

Figure 5.33 Axial image of the fetal head showing normal-size lateral ventricles (measured by the calipers) containing normal echogenic choroid plexus. Note the choroid plexus completely fills the lateral ventricle. Lateral ventricles should measure less than 10 mm in diameter.

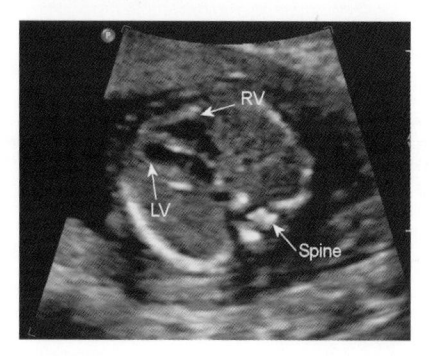

Figure 5.34 Axial image of the fetus at the level of the heart, showing a normal four-chamber heart view. Both four-chamber view and views of the left and right ventricular outlets are routinely taken. LV = left ventricle, RV = right ventricle.

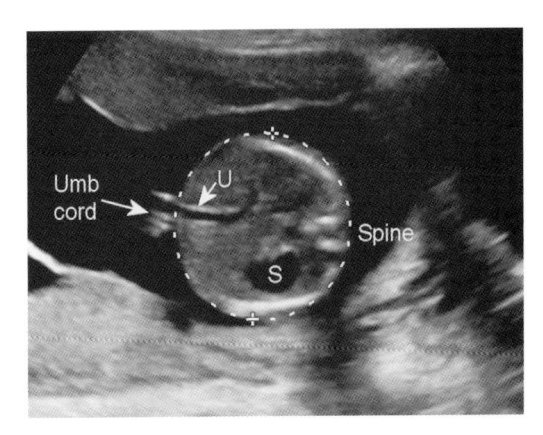

Figure 5.35 S=Fetal stomach. U=umbilical vein. + – + shows the measurement of the abdominal circumference. The stomach should be present and not enlarged. Both kidneys should be seen with no pelvicaliectasis (<4 mm at 18–20 weeks).

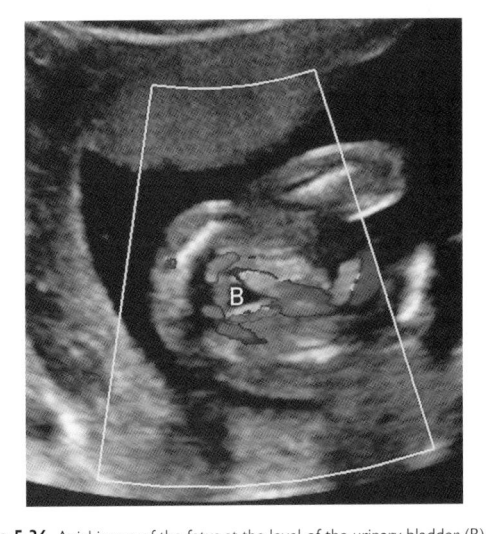

Figure 5.36 Axial image of the fetus at the level of the urinary bladder (B). Presence of a normal three-vessel (two arteries and one vein) umbilical cord can be confirmed using color Doppler. If there are two vessels (e.g., umbilical arteries) coursing around the bladder as seen in this case, then a three-vessel umbilical cord is present. Two-vessel umbilical cord (one artery and one vein) may be associated with chromosomal abnormalities, other fetal structural abnormalities, and intra-uterine growth restriction (IUGR). See Color Plate 7.

Hand and forearm
- We want to see the hands open as certain chromosomal abnormalities present with clenched hands.

Foot
- Looking for club-foot anomalies.

Face
- Looking for cleft lip/palate and to measure the nasal bone (NB).
  - Short (<2 mm)/absent nasal bone can be associated with trisomy 21.

Common conditions

Growth disorders

Clinical concern for fetal growth problems arise when ultrasound measurements of the fetus are discordant with those expected for the estimated gestational age. The fetus can be too small (SGA) or too large for gestational age (LGA).

SGA fetus—IUGR

Defined as a fetal weight that is less than the 10th percentile for expected gestational age. There are two general types of IUGR:
- <u>Symmetric</u>—all fetal measurements (head, abdomen, etc.) are small
  - Usually result of an insult early in pregnancy, such as chromosomal abnormalities, in utero infections, and severe alcohol abuse.
- <u>Asymmetric</u>— the abdominal measurement is small, but the head and limb measurements are normal.
  - Typically presents in the third trimester due to placental problems, smoking.

LGA fetus

- Defined as a fetal weight greater than the 90th percentile for gestational age.
- Diabetic mothers are at risk of having LGA fetuses.
- Increased risk for peri-partum complications such as shoulder dystocia, failure to progress.

Placental disorders

When you evaluate the placenta, there are several important things you want to evaluate:
- Where is the placenta located in relation to the cervix?
- How many lobes of the placenta are there?
- Where does the umbilical cord insert into the placenta?
- Is there hemorrhage behind or superficial to the placenta?

Placental location

If there is suspicion of a placental previa or low-lying placenta on standard transbdominal imaging, endovaginal scanning is indicated.
- <u>Complete placenta previa:</u> the placenta crosses the internal cervical os.
  - Important to diagnosis because a vaginal delivery is not possible because this would result in maternal hemorrhage.
- <u>Marginal palcenta previa:</u> the placenta abuts the cervix and/or partially covers the os.
- <u>Low-lying placenta:</u> the placenta lies within 2 cm of the internal os

Low lying, marginal, and even complete previas may not persist into the third trimester because there is differential growth of the lower portion of the uterus relative to the fundus.
- A follow-up ultrasound in the late second trimester or early third trimester is performed to see if the placenta has "moved up" from the cervix.

> **Pitfalls in determining placental position**
> Remember that a full bladder, uterine contractions, and/or transabdominal scanning can falsely make a placenta appear low lying or cross the internal cervical os.
> - To minimize this, make sure the patient's bladder is empty, and try to wait for the uterine contraction to pass before assessing the relationship of the placenta to the cervix.

Accessory lobes of the placenta
- Usually there is only one placenta in singleton pregnancies.
- Sometimes the placenta can have accessory lobes, called succenturiate lobes.
  - These are typically smaller than the main placenta.
  - They are connected to the main placenta by blood vessels.
- Potential complications:
  - <u>Vasa previa:</u> the fetal vessels cross the internal cervical os, which increases the risk of fetal hemorrhage because they can be torn during delivery.
  - <u>Postpartum bleeding:</u> if the succenturiate lobe is not delivered at the time of the main placenta and remains in the mother.

Placental cord insertion of the umbilical cord
- Normally the umbilical cord inserts into the middle of the placenta.
- Can insert anywhere from the center to the periphery of the placenta.
- <u>Velamentous cord insertion:</u> The umbilical cord inserts beyond the border of the placenta, onto the chorioamniotic membranes (uncommon).
  - Risk of fetal hemorrhage and possible death.
  - Association with growth disorders.
  - Can also result in vasa previa.

Placental abruption
Echogenic fluid (blood) collection acutely (becomes hypoechoic with age), between the placenta and the uterine myometrium.

Umbilical artery Doppler (see Figure 5.37)
Pulsed Doppler of the umbilical artery may be used as a measure of potential placental insufficiency, particularly in IUGR. The normal resistive index (RI) is between 0.6–0.8, and falls in later pregnancy.
- Increasing values are abnormal.
- Lack of diastolic flow or reversed diastolic flow (away from placenta) is a worrisome sign.

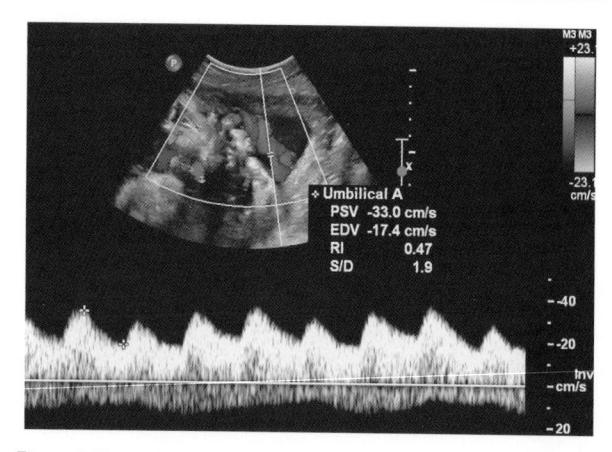

Figure 5.37 Normal UA Doppler showing measurement of the resistive index (RI). See Color Plate 8.

Amniotic fluid abnormalities
The fluid surrounding the fetus is important for development of the fetal lungs, kidneys, and gastrointestinal tract, and also serves to protect the fetus in utero. Too little or too much fluid may indicate significant problems with the fetus.

Amniotic fluid index (AFI)
- Calculated by summing the measurements of the deepest fluid pocket in all four quadrants of the uterus.
- The normal values vary according to the age of the fetus (normal value tables exist).
- In multiple pregnancies, single deepest pocket is used.

A general rule of thumb is that the AFI is usually between 10 and 20 cm after the 20th week of pregnancy.

Oligohydramnios (too little fluid):
- AFI of less than ≈10 cm.
- Can result in pulmonary hypoplasia and limb deformities.
- Causes of oligohydramnios include genitourinary tract anomalies, IUGR, premature rupture of membranes, and post-date pregnancy. In monochorionic-diamniotic twin pregnancies, twin-twin transfusion can also result in oligohydramnios of the donor twin.

Hydramnios (too much fluid):
- Previously called "polyhydramnios."
- AFI of greater than ≈20 cm.
- Can result in premature delivery.

- Causes of hydramnios include fetal swallowing problems (CNS related, esophageal/GI tract abnormalities), maternal diabetes, maternal-fetal blood incompatibilities, and in monochorionic-diamniotic twin pregnancies, the recipient twin in twin-twin transfusion.

Biophysical profile (BPP)

If there are concerns about the fetal well being, a "biophysical profile" may be obtained at ultrasound. Each element is scored 0 or 2 (normal) for a total of 10 points.

This includes assessment for a 30-minute period:
1. Fetal breathing (presence for at least 30 secs = 2/absence = 0).
2. Fetal tone (normal hand flexion-extension = 2/absence = 0).
3. Fetal movements (presence of at least 3 gross = 2/absence = 0).
4. Amniotic fluid volume (normal = 2/abnormal = 0).
5. Fetal heart rate variability on non-stress test (normal = 2/abnormal = 0)

Multiple pregnancies

In multiple pregnancies, ultrasound follow-up is routinely performed in the second and third trimesters due to the need to monitor closely the growth of each fetus and the amniotic fluid volume.

Major anomalies

A complete discussion about fetal anomalies is beyond the scope of this chapter. Table 5.3 gives a cursory overview of the major anomalies that we routinely screen for.

Table 5.3	
	What fetal anomalies are we looking for?
Head	Hydrocephalus; Chiari malformation; cysts in the choroid plexus; thickened nuchal fold
Face	Cleft lip & palate; short nasal bone
Heart	Congenital heart defects (ventricular, atrial and endocardial cushion defects, transposition of the great vessels, hypoplastic left heart)
Chest	Masses, size
Diaphragm	Presence of diaphragm (excludes diaphragmatic hernia)
Abdomen	Abdominal wall defects (omphalocele, gastroschisis); echogenic bowel, absent stomach, dilated bowel, calcifications, heterotaxy
Genitourinary	Hydronephrosis; absent kidneys; posterior urethral valves
Spine	Neural tube defects (myelomeningocele); vertebral body anomalies
Limbs	Short or missing limbs/digits; clubbed feet; clenched hands
Umbilical cord	3 (normal) or 2 (abnormal) vessels

Imaging guidance for procedures
Ultrasound is commonly used to guide interventions in pregnancy, including choriovillous sampling, amniocentesis, fetal blood transfusions and blood sampling and fetal reductions.

Scrotal ultrasound

Scrotal ultrasound is commonly used to evaluate a palpable testicular mass, scrotal pain, and is also used in the evaluation of suspected hydroceles and varicoceles.

Anatomy on the testicular ultrasound

Scrotal ultrasound evaluates the testes both in gray-scale and color Doppler imaging. Testicular volumes can be calculated.

Testicles
The testes should have uniform echogenicity. In the mid portion of the testis is a normal echogenic band called the mediastinum, which may contain small cystic structures that are called rete testis (which should not be mistaken for a mass). On color Doppler imaging, the testes have symmetric blood flow.

Epididymis
The epididymides are also homogenously echogenic with symmetric blood flow, and they consist of a head (superior, largest portion), body and tail (inferior).

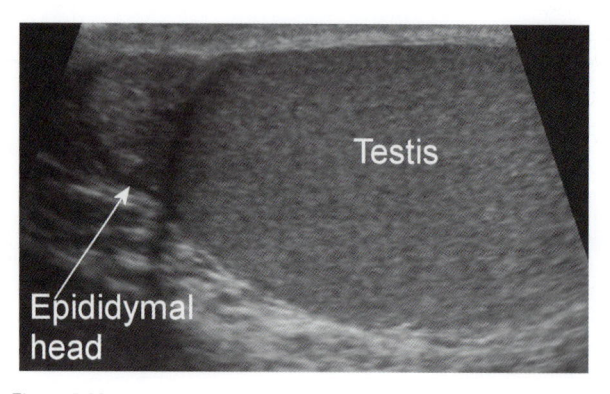

Figure 5.38 Normal anatomy of the testis (inferior portion not imaged in its entirety here) and epididymal head.

Common conditions

Testicular torsion
Timely diagnosis is imperative, because the likelihood that the testis is salvageable is time dependent. Ultrasound is the principle imaging modality to diagnose testicular torsion.

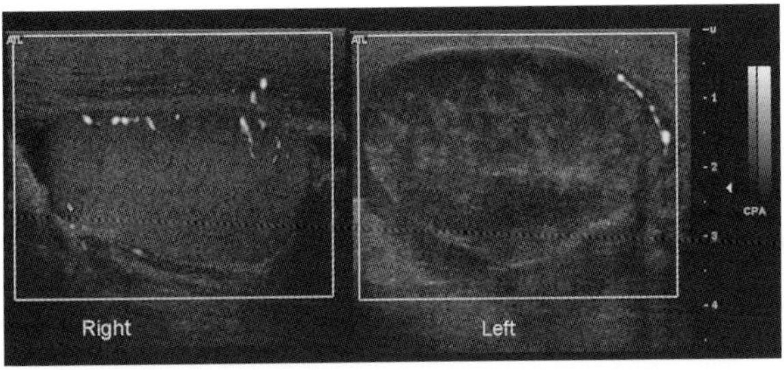

Figure 5.39 Testicular torsion. Sagittal images of the normal right testis and torsed left testis showing abnormal heterogeneous echogenicity of the left testis with absent Power Doppler flow and normal vascularity on right. See Color Plate 9.

Ultrasound findings
- Testis is enlarged, swollen, hypoechoic, or heterogenous.
- Color Doppler and spectral Doppler imaging show absence of blood flow.

Epididymitis/orchitis
This is very common in males, and presents with testicular pain.

Ultrasound findings
- Color Doppler shows increased blood flow in the affected epididymis and/or testis, both may be diffusely enlarged, sometimes simulating a mass.
- Occassionally a follow-up ultrasound after clinical therapy is needed to ensure that the sonographic findings have resolved and that there is no underlying lesion in the testicle.

Hydroceles
Hydroceles are extra-testicular collections of fluid in the scrotal sac. May be comprised of simple fluid or contain blood or pus in the setting of trauma or infection, respectively.

Ultrasound findings
- Anechoic fluid surrounding the testicle (simple).
- Hypoechoic fluid surrounding the testicle (complex). Usually can see particles moving in the fluid.
- Variable in size, can be large such that on clinical exam, a testicular mass is suspected.

Inguinal hernias
Common finding in adults and occasionally babies. Imaging is done when diagnosis is in doubt (e.g., cause of groin or scrotal mass).
- May contain bowel (with peristalsis unless incarcerated), or omental fat.
- May require valsalva maneuver or imaging patient upright.

Testicular trauma
Testicular trauma can cause hematoceles and intratesticular or subcapsular hematomas.

Ultrasound findings
- Hematoma may have variable echogenicity and cystic-appearing component depending on the time since the trauma (due to evolution of the blood products).
- Sometimes possible to see a fracture of the testis (hypoechoic line through the testis).
- Hematocele appears as a complex hydrocele (see p. 283).

Testicular masses
Ultrasound is the imaging modality of choice to evaluate a palpable testicular abnormality.

An intra-testicular mass is malignant until proven otherwise.

Ultrasound findings: see Figure 5.40.
- Testicular neoplasms are often hypoechoic with increased vascularity and may have ill-defined borders.
- Focal inflammation/infection should be also be considered in the appropriate clinical setting.
- There is a controversial association between testicular microlithiasis (multiple tiny testicular calcifications) and testicular tumors.
  - Testicular ultrasound monitoring may be recommended in some men with extensive microlithiasis.

Other small parts ultrasound

Thyroid ultrasound
There are two main indications for thyroid ultrasound:
- Evaluation of a palpable abnormality; either enlargement of the gland or a discretely palpable nodule.
- Further characterization of a nodule seen on other imaging modalities such as CT or PET.

Ultrasound findings
There are some ultrasound characteristics of thyroid nodules that are suspicious for malignancy. However, there is considerable overlap with benign nodules. Suspicious features include:

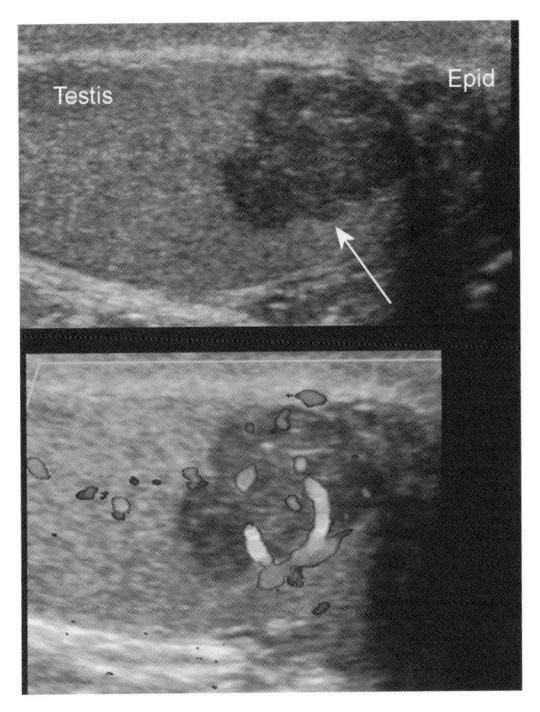

Figure 5.40 Testicular seminoma. Top image shows a hypoechoic lobular mass (arrow) in the inferior testis. Color Doppler (bottom) shows increased blood flow in this mass. See Color Plate 10.

- "Taller-than-wide" shape.
- Marked hyopechogenicity (but not anechoic).
- Spiculated or ill-defined borders.
- Microcalcifications.
- Hypervascularity on color Doppler.

Although ultrasound is excellent in characterizing a nodule as being cystic, solid, or mixed cystic/solid, it cannot reliably distinguish between benign and malignant solid thyroid nodules.

Often the next step in management of an indeterminate or suspicious thyroid nodule is biopsy, which can be done under ultrasound guidance.

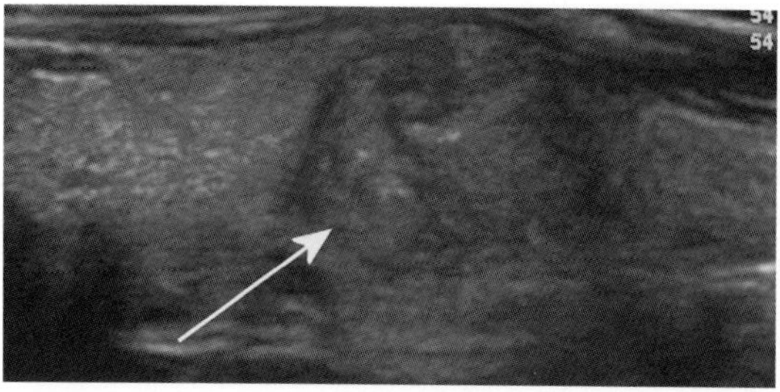

Figure 5.41 Sagittal image of left lobe of thyroid showing 15 mm heterogeneous solid round mass (arrow) containing small echogenic calcifications. There was flow within the mass on color Doppler imaging (not shown). Papillary carcinoma was diagnosed on biopsy.

Find the foreign body
Ultrasound may be used to localize foreign bodies. Radiographs are the primary modality for metallic bodies and most gravel (although these, too, will be seen on US) (see Figure 4.11).
- US detects most wood, glass (some leaded glass is radiopaque) and plastic foreign bodies that may not be radiopaque on radiographs.
  - Appear as echogenic foci, often with shadowing.
- US can identify abscesses caused by the foreign body.
- A high resolution linear transducer should be used +/- standoff pad.
  - US can be used to guide the incision.

Vascular ultrasound

Vascular ultrasound uses high frequency linear transducers, and may be performed by radiology or vascular surgery.

Venous ultrasound
Venous ultrasound may be used for:
- Identifying venous thrombosis in the extremities.
- Identifying venous organ thrombosis (e.g., renal, splenic, hepatic veins, portal vein).
- Identifying venous flow abnormalities (e.g., in cirrhosis).
- Evaluating venous shunt graft patency such as dialysis grafts.
- Evaluating TIPS patency and stenoses.
- Evaluating vascular anomalies such as peripheral arteriovenous malformations (AVMs).

Peripheral venous thrombosis
Ultrasound is an excellent non-invasive means for evaluating for thrombosis in the upper and lower extremities. It is the modality of choice in patients presenting with signs of a deep vein thrombosis. Sonographic evaluation

consists of gray-scale imaging, color Doppler, and Doppler spectral waveform analysis.
- A systematic approach starting proximally and scanning distally is usually applied.

Gray-scale imaging
- Non-compressibility of the vein (most specific finding). The vein should normally compress (flatten, with apposition of front and back walls) when pressed on by the transducer. Thrombosis prevents the vein from compressing.
- Arteries do not change in diameter with moderate compression.
- Distended vein with internal echoes (thrombus).

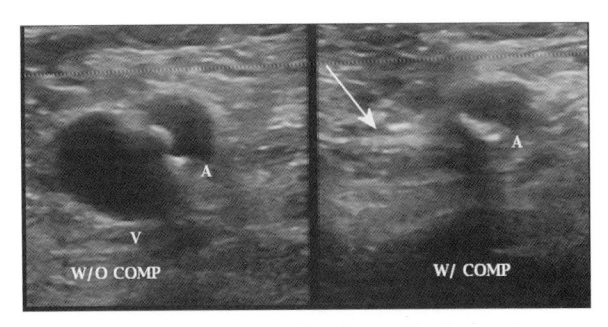

Figure 5.42 Transverse images of a normal common femoral vein without (left) and with compression (right). Arrow indicates compressed vein.

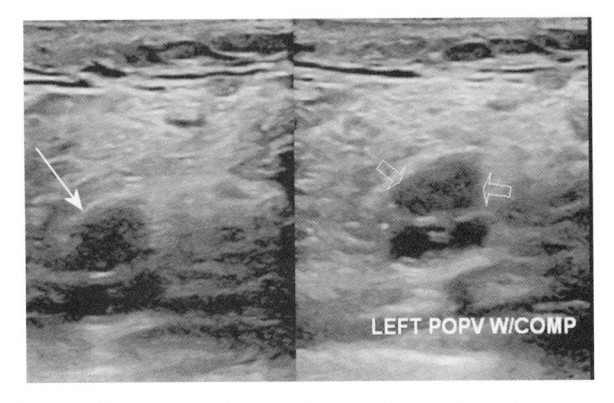

Figure 5.43 Popliteal vein thrombosis. Transverse images of the popliteal vein without (left) and with compression (right). The popliteal vein (arrows) does not compress (open arrows). Note the two small arteries posterior to the popliteal vein on both sets of images.

Color Doppler and Doppler spectral imaging

Complete thrombosis
Absent color flow and Doppler venous waveforms (see Figure 5.44).

Non-occlusive thrombus
Color flow present with Doppler waveforms but the color flow does not fill the entire lumen of the vein.

Central thrombosis
Involvement of central venous structures (IVC, iliac vessels) can sometimes be inferred by lack of enhancement of pulsed Doppler waveforms by the valsalva maneuver.

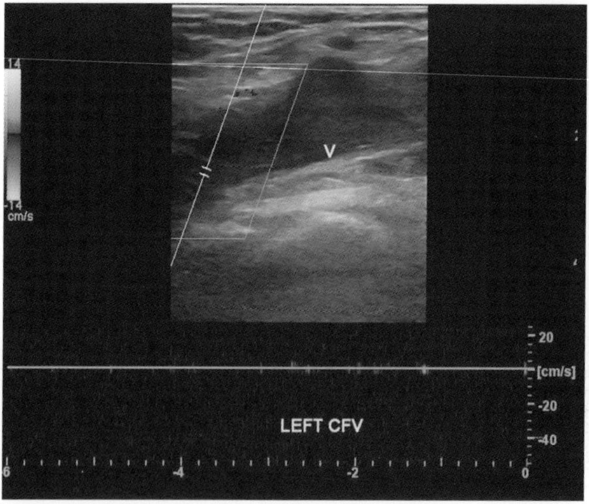

Figure 5.44 Common femoral vein thrombosis. Longitudinal image of the common femoral vein showing absent color and spectral Doppler waveforms. Also note the echoes seen in the vein. See Color Plate 11.

Arterial ultrasound

A complete discussion of arterial ultrasound is beyond the scope of this book. Some applications have already been mentioned. Indications include:
- Identifying vascular stenoses, for example:
  - Renal arteries in hypertensive patients.
  - Superior mesenteric artery in patients with abdominal angina.
  - Anastomotic stenoses after transplants.
  - Carotid arteries.

- Identifying end-organ disease by the presence of abnormal wave forms and resistive indices (see p. 244), for example:
  - In renal and liver transplants.
  - In the placenta (umbilical artery).
  - In fetal brain (middle cerebral artery [MCA] Doppler).

Carotid artery ultrasound

Ultrasound is the modality of choice to screen for atherosclerotic plaques in the carotid arteries (see Figure 5.45).
- It can determine if the stenosis caused by the plaque is hemodynamically significant by comparing the velocities in the arteries to standard reference tables.

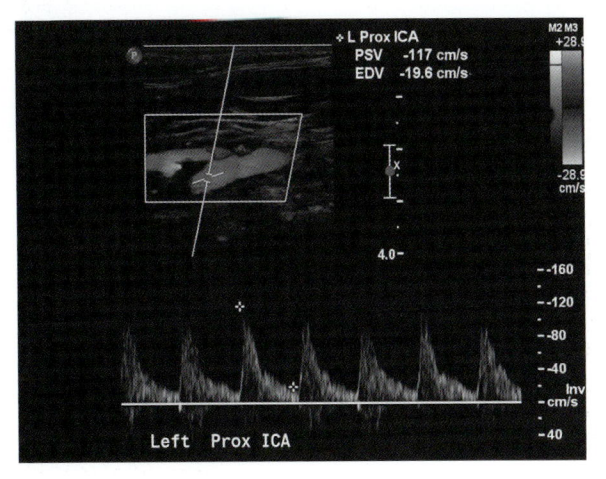

Figure 5.45 Normal left internal carotid artery Doppler color flow and Doppler spectral waveform. See Color Plate 12.

Ultrasound guided procedures

When can ultrasound help me with procedures?

The portability of ultrasound, lack of radiation, real-time imaging, and flexibility of imaging planes makes it an ideal modality to guide many procedures. There are some technical challenges, however, and there is a significant learning curve to develop the hand-eye coordination required.

See chapter 10 "Interventional Radiology," p. 450 for complete discussion.

Other applications of ultrasound

Other applications of ultrasound not discussed here include: endoluminal ultrasound, in which small probes are combined with endoscopic units to image the bowel or bronchial walls; and endovascular ultrasound, in which tiny US probes can be inserted into vessels as small as coronary arteries, during angiography to image wall plaque and dissections.

References

Introduction to obstetrical ultrasound from ob-ultrasound.net http://www.ob-ultrasound.net/

Middleton WD, Kurtz AB, Hertzberg BS. *Ultrasound: The Requisites*. Maryland Heights, Missouri: Mosby, 2004.

University of Virginia Emergency Ultrasound http://www.med-ed.virginia.edu/courses/rad/edus/

Chapter 6

Pediatrics

Michael A. DiPietro, MD

Why is imaging in babies and children different? *286*
Imaging in neonates *287*
  Lines and tubes in neonates and infants *288*
  Neonatal chest radiographs *289*
  Neonatal abdominal radiographs *293*
  Neonatal GI tract fluoroscopy *297*
  Neonatal neuroimaging *298*
Older infants and children *299*
  Normal CXR *300*
  Common chest conditions *300*
  Common GI conditions *304*
  Patterns of fractures specific to children *309*
  Developmental dysplasia of the hip *315*
  Transient synovitis of the hip *317*
  Legg-Calve-Perthes disease *317*
  How to evaluate the young child with hip/leg pain or a painful limp *317*
Child abuse *318*
Don't miss diagnoses *322*
References *322*

CHAPTER 6 **Pediatrics**

This chapter aims to describe the specific pediatric conditions and imaging in children that is not covered in other chapters.

Why is imaging in babies and children different?

There are a number of factors that affect how and when imaging is performed in the pediatric population compared to adults. These factors also vary with age, from premature neonates to adolescents.

Radiation exposure
Babies and children are much more sensitive to the effects of radiation; the younger the child, generally the more sensitive (see Essentials p. 22). The thyroid gland and female adolescent breasts are particularly sensitive to radiation. This means that:
- Imaging should only be performed when truly needed.
  - Will the imaging affect clinical management?
- Ultrasound and MRI should be used where possible, that is, when they provide comparable or near comparable information to tests using ionizing radiation.
- Only image the area needed.
  - Cone images when possible.
  - Don't do "babygrams" (that is, total baby image in 1 exposure).
  - Do include a joint above and below the area of concern because pain is poorly localized in children.
- Specific pediatric imaging protocols should be used.
  - CT specific pediatric low dose protocols.
  - Single rather than multiphase CT imaging protocols.
  - Pulsed digital fluoroscopy with use of fluorostore images (see Fluoroscopy p. 330).
  - Lower-dose digital radiography.
- Lead or bismuth shielding whenever possible of pelvis, thyroid, and breasts.

Size and age
The size of the child will also affect image resolution, which is less in small babies/children. The age (developmental stage) may affect what technique can be used.
- Ultrasound can often be used in children for locations and indications where it cannot be used in adults:
  - For appendicitis and hip effusions.
  - Intracerebral and spinal cord imaging in neonates.
- As the child ages, techniques change.
  - US can be used in babies up to about 6 months to exclude developmental dysplasia of the hip, but radiographs needed later on.
  - MRI will be needed as fontanelles close to assess for hydrocephalus or for spinal cord tethering.

Cooperation
Kids often don't cooperate with you! This means that:
- Movement on images may impair interpretation.
- Breath holding is often not possible in smaller children for CXR or CT.
- The child may need to be held by an adult during imaging.
- Sedation may be required for CT, MRI, nuclear medicine, and sometimes fluoroscopic studies.
- Short imaging protocols (e.g., fast brain MRI, short CT scans) may be required to avoid sedation.

Fear and embarrassment
Imaging can be very scary to kids. This means that:
- Sedation may be needed.
- Child-friendly rooms should be used. DVDs and such may help distract children.
- Technologists and radiologists need expertise in dealing with frightened children and concerned parents.
  - Simple, age appropriate explanations of procedures should be used.
- Parents may be allowed to stay during procedures.
- Adolescents may be very embarrassed during procedures that involve exposure of breasts or genitals.
- Recently potty-trained children may be very resistant to voiding on instruction during voiding cystourethrograms (VCUGs).

Imaging in neonates

Radiographic views

Chest
- Obtained supine (AP).
- The upper third or so of the abdomen is often also included.

Abdomen
- Includes the entire abdomen. Obtained supine.

Chest/abdomen
- If both chest and abdomen are needed, a single supine radiograph is usually obtained.

Supplemental views
To look for air (e.g., pneumothorax or pneumoperitoneum) or layering liquid (e.g., gas fluid levels in bowel), obtain a radiograph with a horizontal x-ray beam:

Cross table lateral chest or cross table lateral abdomen:
- Baby is supine, x-ray beam enters the side of the patient. Often adequate in neonate.

Lateral decubitus chest or lateral decubitus abdomen:
- Baby is lying on side, right side up for free air.

Lines and tubes in neonates and infants
Central vascular catheters, PICC lines, and feeding tubes are used in children as in adults, and their proper positioning is discussed in the chapter 2, Chest Imaging, p. 52.

Endotracheal tubes (ETT)
Very short tracheas in neonates, so only tiny adjustments in position needed.
- Aim for position between thoracic inlet and carina.
- As chin goes down, tube goes down further, so keep above carina.

Umbilical artery catheters (UACs)
Normal course (see Figures 6.1, 6.4, 6.5, and 6.7):
Umbilical artery→ internal iliac artery→ to common iliac artery→ aorta.

On radiographs:
Recognized by their descent from the umbilicus into the lateral pelvis prior to their ascent up the aorta.
- Tip position away from the origin of the renal arteries (L2) to prevent catheter tip microthrombi from embolizing into a kidney. Usually placed midthoracic or below L2.

Umbilical venous catheters (UVCs)
Normal course (see Figure 6.1):
Umbilical vein (very superficial in anterior abdomen)→ dives posteriorly→ into the left portal vein→ductus venosus→IVC.

On radiograph:
Ascends directly from the umbilicus →medial RUQ →dome of the liver →right atrium.
- Optimally tip near the IVC—right atrial junction or in right atrium.
- If the liver is shifted in the abdomen (e.g., congenital diaphragmatic hernia), the UVC course will shift with it.

Aberrant positions:
As a UVC is sometimes used for infusion of blood, large fluid volumes and medications, aberrant UVC positions must be recognized and corrected.
- Right or left portal vein (most common).
- Into the SVC (or above).
- Across the foramen ovale into the left atrium and out a pulmonary vein.
- Down the IVC.
- Down the main portal vein into the superior mesenteric or splenic vein.

As the UVC is very superficial. lateral rotation of the patient will project the UVC in that direction.

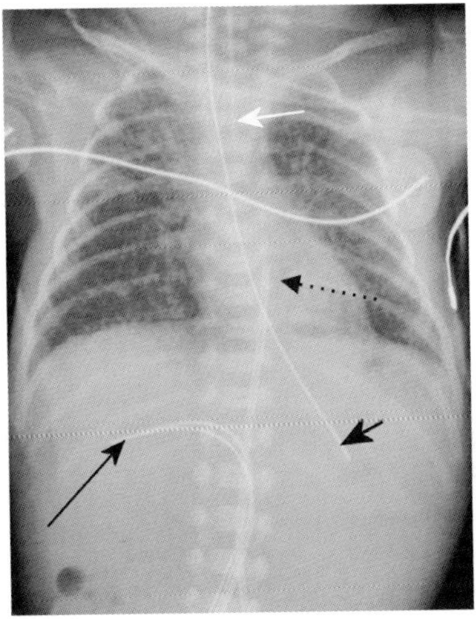

Figure 6.1 AP supine chest and abdomen in a premature neonate. ETT tip (white arrow) is just above the carina. UAC tip is at T7–T8 (dashed black arrow). 2 UVCs (long black arrow) extend aberrantly into the right portal vein. Gastric tube is in the stomach (short black arrow). See also Figures 6.4 and 6.5.

Neonatal chest radiographs

Normal film
See Figure 6.2.

Cardiothoracic ratio

The normal cardiothoracic ratio (see Chest p. 53) is usually ≤ 0.5, although in otherwise normal small for dates infants it can be 0.6.

Thymus

The newborn thymus is visible as a density in the upper mediastinum.
- It can appear quite large in proportion to the chest.
- It may be asymmetrical.
- As the thymus is located anteriorly it can project far to the right or left with even slight rotation of the patient.

Mediastinum

The normal thymus usually obscures visualization of the aortic arch, and so aortic sidedness must be determined by the position of the thoracic trachea.
- Left (normal) sided arch: trachea deviated to the patient's right.
- Right sided arch: trachea deviated to the patient's left.

Lungs

- A diaphragm height at the ninth posterior rib is generally considered adequate expansion.
  - Angulation of the x-ray beam may preclude accurate evaluation.
- Diaphragms that are high and convex usually indicate shallow inspiration.
- Diaphragms that are low and flat usually indicate hyperexpanded lungs.

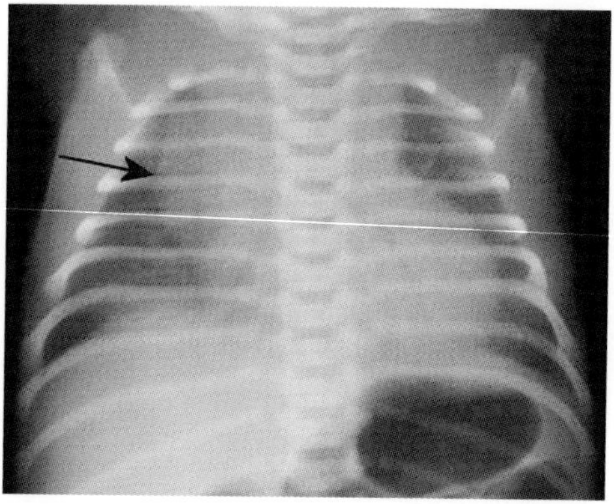

Figure 6.2 Normal AP CXR on supine 1 day old term newborn. The lungs are normal. Normal prominent thymus is in the upper mediastinum (arrow). Infants often have a lot of air in the stomach.

Pneumothorax and pulmonary interstitial emphysema

Pneumomediastinum or pneumothorax can occasionally occur in an otherwise healthy term newborn following delivery and is usually self limited. More significantly, mechanical ventilation in premature neonates, (especially if high ventilation pressures are necessary), may cause symptomatic pneumothoraces (PTX) or pulmonary interstitial emphysema (PIE).

Pneumothorax

Radiographic findings:
- Most conspicuous on a *cross table lateral* projection.
  - Free air is anterior.
- *Lateral decubitus* free air is against the "up" chest wall.
- *AP supine view*:
  - "Deep sulcus sign" (p. 70): deep, lucent costophrenic sulcus.
  - Heart border appears too distinct because pleural air rather than hazy lung is next to it.
  - More lucent hemithorax due to the anterior pleural air. Look for collapsed lung.
  - Visualization of visceral pleural edge.

- Tension pneumothorax (see Figure 6.3):
  - Mediastinal shift toward the opposite side
  - Flattening or inversion of the ipsilateral hemidiaphragm.

NOTE – since the lung might be stiff with poor compliance (producing the need for high ventilator pressures), the lung might not be collapsed in a tension pneumothorax.

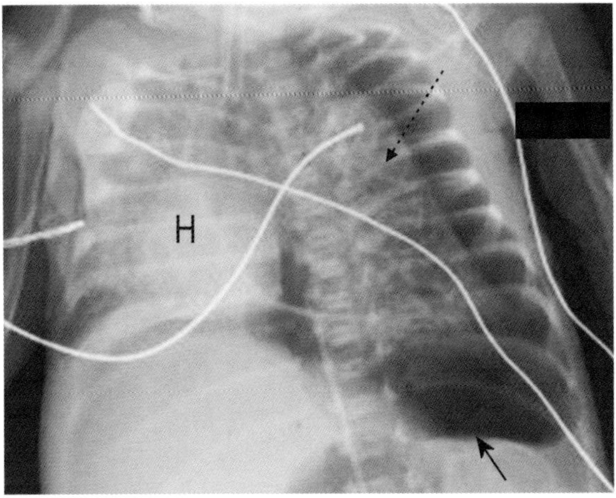

Figure 6.3 Supine chest shows hyperlucent left hemithorax, inverted left hemidiaphragm (solid arrow) and mediastinal shift to the right (H = heart), consistent with tension pneumothorax in this mechanically ventilated premature infant. Also note the bubbly lungs due to PIE (dotted arrow). The left lung is stiff and has not collapsed.

Pulmonary interstitial emphysema (PIE)

PIE is tracking of air in the bronchovascular interstitium, which can occur in any portion of the lung. The baby is almost always on high-pressure mechanical ventilation.

<u>Radiographic findings:</u>
- Linear or bubbly lucencies in a lung or portion of a lung along the interstitium.
- More coarse and heterogeneous than the fine air bronchograms of surfactant deficient.
- Hyperinflation—focal or diffuse. Can produce tension with mediastinal shift.

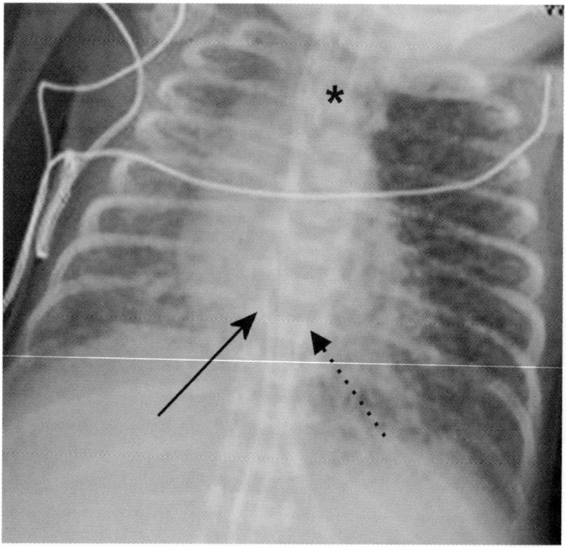

Figure 6.4 Left lung PIE —Linear bubbly lucencies radiate out from the left hilum. They are coarser and more radiolucent than air bronchograms in the right lung. Left lung is hyperexpanded compared to right. Normal UAC (dashed arrow), UVC (solid arrow) and ETT (*)positions

Surfactant deficiency

Formerly referred to as hyaline membrane disease (HMD), it affects premature babies whose surfactant production is inadequate to keep alveoli open during expiration.

Radiographic findings:

- Diffuse fine granular or "ground glass" appearance of the lungs, caused by diffuse alveolar collapse (see Figure 6.5).
- Air bronchograms.
- Reduced lung volumes, consequent to the alveolar collapse.

Transient tachypnea of the newborn (TTNB)

Also known as retained fetal lung liquid. More common in Caesarean section babies, especially if the mother never went into labor.

Radiographic finding:

- Streaky opacities radiating out from the hila.
- Interstitial prominence (occasional Kerley B lines)+/–fluid in the fissures.
- Generally well expanded lungs.
- Looks similar to interstitial pulmonary edema in adult.

As the name implies, tachypnea and the radiographic abnormalities usually resolve in 24 hours.

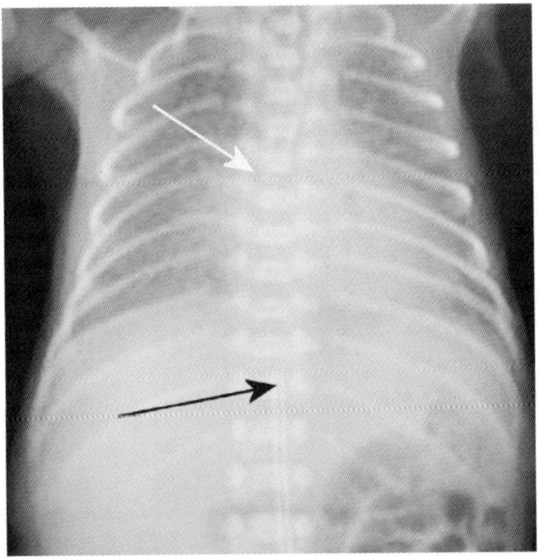

Figure 6.5 Premature infant, 1-hour old (hence paucity of bowel gas) with surfactant deficiency. Lungs are granular with air bronchograms indicative of hyaline membrane disease. ET tip is just entering the right main bronchus (white arrow). UVC tip (black arrow) is superficial and inferior, just entering the liver.

Congenital thoracic abnormalities

These include:
  Congenital diaphragmatic hernia (CDH)—most common of these.
  Congenital pulmonary airway malformation (CPAM, formerly termed CCAM).
  Pulmonary sequestration.
  Congenital hyperinflated lung (includes what was formerly called congenital lobar emphysema).
- All can be detected on prenatal imaging, and so may be known at birth.
- All these abnormalities will be fluid filled at birth and hence radiopaque on radiographs until air replaces the fluid.

Congenital diaphragmatic hernia (CDH)

Bowel herniates into the thorax via a diaphragmatic defect, most commonly the postero-lateral foramen of Bochdalek (lumbocostal triangle) (see Figure 6.6).
- The bowel occupies space in the hemithorax which contributes to an ipsilateral hypoplastic lung.
- CDH is diagnosed more often on the left (80%) than on the right (20%). (The liver may occlude a hole in the right hemidiaphragm).

<u>Radiographic findings:</u>
- Air filled tubular structures (bowel) in one hemithorax.
- Opaque hemithorax if bowel loops are fluid filled, rather than air filled. This may occur if newborn was intubated prior to breathing and swallowing air.

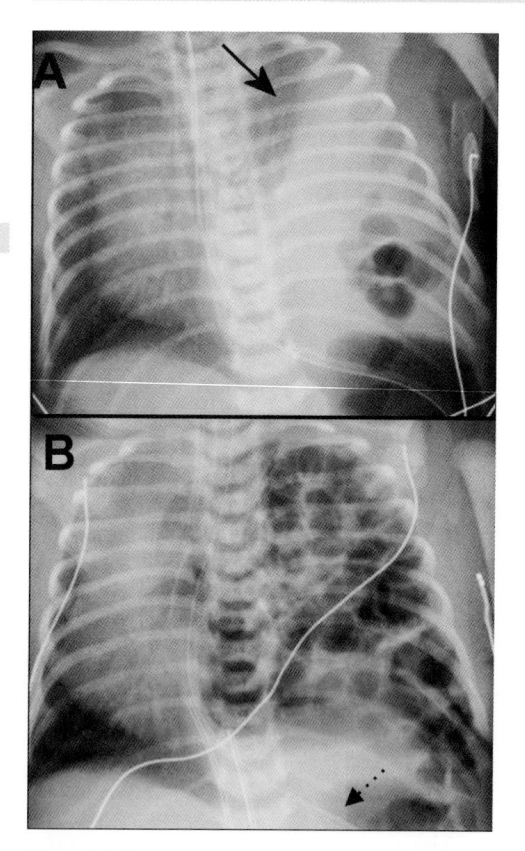

Figure 6.6 Newborn with left CDH. (a) Almost immediately after birth when the herniated bowel is still fluid filled, hypoplastic left lung (arrow) is clearly seen. (b) 1 hour later, air has replaced fluid in the bowel, obscuring the hypoplastic aerated left lung. An esophagogastric tube (dotted arrow) extends into the stomach, beneath the diaphragm. In other cases the stomach is also intrathoracic.

Neonatal abdominal radiographs

Normal film

Stomach

Look for a left sided gastric bubble. A midline stomach or a stomach on the patient's right could indicate situs ambiguous (heterotaxy syndrome) or situs inversus. A full discussion of this is beyond the scope of this book. However, both can be associated with congenital heart disease.

Bowel gas pattern

<u>First few postnatal hours:</u>
- Limited bowel gas, bowel filled with swallowed amniotic fluid.

<u>Normal neonatal pattern:</u>
- As the newborn swallows air, the bowel loops look like numerous thin walled, faceted, small polygons dispersed throughout the abdomen.

<u>Should there be gas in the rectum?</u>
- Lack of gas in the rectum can be normal in the supine neonate as the rectum is most dependent. Placing the baby prone for the radiograph elevates the rectum and allows gas to enter it.

> To interpret the bowel gas pattern correctly, you must know the age of the baby, and position of baby for the radiograph.

Calcifications
All calcifications in the newborn abdomen or pelvis are abnormal.
- In utero bowel perforation can spill meconium into the peritoneal cavity. The meconium can calcify, causing "meconium peritonitis."
- Ovarian mass (teratoma) or infarcted torsed ovary can calcify.
- Gallstones and urolithiasis are rare at this age.

Pneumoperitoneum
Free air in the neonatal abdomen almost always indicates bowel perforation, a surgical emergency.

Radiographic findings

<u>Supine view</u> (see Figure 6.7):
- Increased lucency over the upper abdomen caused by anteriorly layering air.

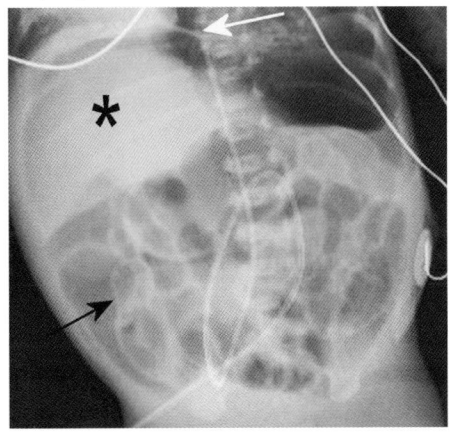

Figure 6.7 Pneumoperitoneum due to necrotizing enterocolitis. Large amount of free air seen over liver (*) and between bowel loops (arrow). Note the normal course and position of the UAC with tip at ~ T9 (white arrow).

- Distinctly visible falciform ligament may be seen, rendered visible because it is surrounded by air.
- Visualization of both sides of the bowel wall (Rigler sign).

Left lateral decubitus view:
Air collects lateral (i.e., superior) to the right lateral liver edge.

Cross table lateral view:
Air collects in the anterior, upper abdomen.

Necrotizing enterocolitis
Necrotizing enterocolitis (NEC) can develop as early as the first postnatal week. Multifactorial and variable causes including: infection; hyperosmolar intestinal load; hypotension, and interruption of mesenteric blood flow→ bowel ischemia → bowel wall necrosis →radiographic findings.

Radiographic findings
(In increasing order of severity—not all may be present)
- Segmental bowel dilatation +/– bowel wall thickening.
  - May look like small lucent "sausages."
- Pneumatosis intestinalis: linear or bubbly gas in bowel wall (see Figure 6.8).
  - Produced as the bowel wall breaks down and gas enters.
- Portal venous gas: branching lucencies over RUQ.
  - From gas entering the mesenteric venous system.
- Pneumoperitoneum (see Figure 6.7).
  - From bowel necrosis.
  - Infant usually critically ill at this point with peritonitis.

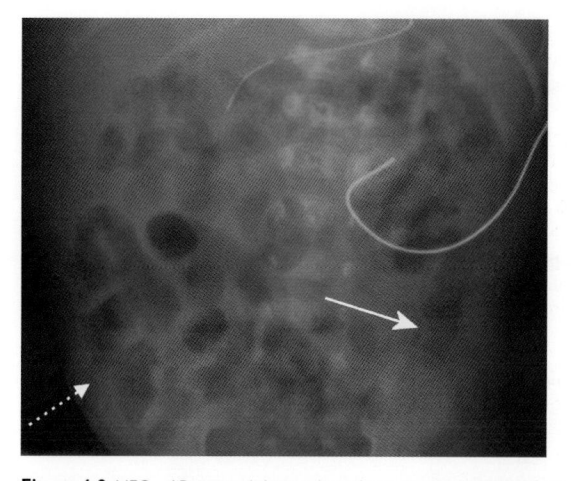

Figure 6.8 NEC – AP supine abdomen shows linear pneumatosis intestinalis (solid arrow) along the left lateral abdomen, likely in descending colon. Typical 'sausage like' segmental bowel dilatation and wall thickening in RLQ (dotted arrow).

Pneumatosis intestinalis, portal venous gas and pneumoperitoneum may also be recognized incidentally on ultrasound.

The sequelae of NEC can present in later infancy with colonic obstruction due to post NEC strictures.

Bowel obstruction: radiography

The radiograph can help to determine the site of obstruction: gastric outlet (rare in newborn), in the duodenum (duodenal atresia, duodenal stenosis, malrotation), in the small bowel (atresia, meconium ileus, malrotation with volvulus, internal hernia, mass), or in the colon (meconium plug, Hirschsprung disease, imperforate anus).

Depending on the clinical scenario and the likely site of obstruction, an upper GI series (for high obstruction or suspected malrotation) or a contrast enema (for low obstruction) might be indicated.

How to assess for bowel obstruction on the radiograph

- How much bowel gas is present?
- How far distally does bowel gas extend?
  - Not far = high or proximal obstruction.
  - Far distally = low or distal obstruction.
  - Is there gas in the rectum?
- Are there dilated loops of bowel?
  - Where are the bowel loops dilated?
  - Are there localized areas of bowel distension?

Pitfalls

- In neonates, especially in premies, colonic haustra are poorly developed, which impedes differentiating dilated colon from dilated small intestine.
- Absence of rectal gas can merely be a function of the supine posture!

Duodenal obstruction:
- "Double bubble" sign, that is, air in stomach (bubble 1) and proximal duodenum (bubble 2) but no bowel gas distally.
- Indicative of total duodenal obstruction, usually duodenal atresia.
- Duodenal atresia is frequent in babies with trisomy 21 (Down syndrome).

Malrotation/midgut volvulus:
- In proximal obstruction, UGI series often indicated, especially if malrotation is possible.

See p. 311 "malrotation" for more information.

The neonate with bilious vomiting requires an emergent UGI study to rule out malrotation and midgut volvulus.

Neonatal GI tract fluoroscopy in obstruction

Whether an upper GI series or a contrast enema should be performed is determined by the clinical scenario (e.g., bilious vomiting) and the appearance of the radiograph (likely site of obstruction). Often both are needed.

Neonatal UGI (See p. 311)
- Indicated when proximal obstruction is suspected.
- Neonatal UGIs are performed with single contrast technique. This may be with thin barium or with non-ionic water soluble contrast.
- Some institutions may strap the infant onto a board to facilitate a quick, accurate study with lowest radiation dose possible.

Neonatal contrast enemas
- Indicated when distal obstruction (multiple gas filled loops) is likely.
- Water soluble contrast typically utilized, but could be barium.

Normal sized colon
- Occurs with proximal small bowel obstruction.
- Allows succus entericus to pass to colon and distend it normally.
- Can occur with late gestational distal small bowel obstruction.

"Micro-colon" or "unused colon"
- Very narrow caliber colon.
- Colon has not had material passing through it.
- Ileal atresia.
- Meconium ileus (may be initial presentation of cystic fibrosis). Inspissated thick meconium collects in the terminal ileum causing distal small bowel obstruction. The meconium can sometimes be washed out with water soluble contrast enemas, relieving the obstruction.

Meconium plug syndrome (aka "small left colon" and "colonic inertia")
Note: NOT related to meconium ileus or cystic fibrosis.
Seen in infants of diabetic mothers or when the mother had been on medication such as MgSO4 to prevent premature labor.
- Small left colon with mildly dilated transverse/ascending colon containing filling defects (the meconium plugs).
- Water soluble contrast enema can be therapeutic and help the newborn to pass the impacted meconium plug.
- Can co-exist with Hirschprung disease and biopsy or close follow-up required.

Colonic aganglionosis or Hirschprung disease
Failure of a newborn to pass meconium within 24–48 hours of birth could indicate colonic aganglionosis.
- Aganglionosis occurs in the rectum and extends a variable distance proximally. Rarely involves entire colon.
- Aganglionic segment remains contracted and obstructs colon.
  - Colon distended above aganglionic segment.
  - Small bowel may also become dilated.

<u>Enema findings:</u>
- Small caliber rectum +/− sigmoid colon with dilated colon proximally.
- Findings can be very subtle and biopsy needed for definitive diagnosis.
- Total colonic aganglionosis can have a variable appearance on contrast enema, including essentially normal.

Neonatal neuroimaging

Two modalities are typically used for neuroimaging in neonates—US and MRI. US can be performed via the open fontanelles, and is the modality of choice for diagnosing hydrocephalus and intracranial hemorrhage due to prematurity.

- US can also be used in neonates and young infants to assess spinal cord abnormalities such as tethered cord before the posterior spinal elements ossify completely.
- MRI is needed in older infants and for more complex neurological disorders.

Intracranial hemorrhage (ICH)

Intracranial germinal matrix hemorrhage is common in premature infants and may lead to significant neurological consequences. Premature neonates are usually screened with cranial ultrasound.

US findings

Blood appears echogenic.
- ICH is graded I–IV, with increasing severity and worsening prognosis:
  - **I**: hemorrhage only in germinal matrix (caudothalamic groove).
  - **II**: hemorrhage into normally sized ventricles (see Figure 6.9).
  - **III**: hemorrhage distends ventricles.
  - **IV**: hemorrhage into brain parenchyma.
- Follow-up of hemorrhage is to assess for progression and complications such as hydrocephalus.
- Periventricular leukomalacia, a result of ischemia producing cysts or cavities in the periventricular white matter, can occur with or without ICH.

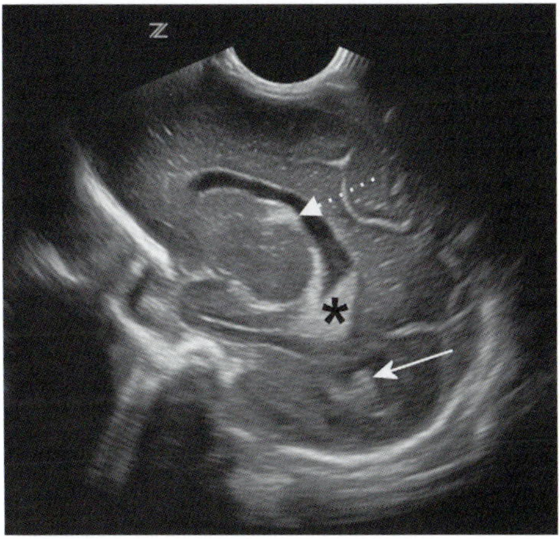

Figure 6.9 Sagittal ultrasound image in a premature neonate with a Grade II bleed on the right. Blood is seen in the atrium of the left ventricle (*), caudothalamic groove (dashed arrow) and occipital horn of the lateral ventricle (solid arrow).

Older infants and children

Chest
Views (see also chapter 2, Chest Imaging, p. 41)
In babies and young children, AP views are typical (supine in younger children). In older children, PA views can be obtained. Lateral views may be cross-table, or upright (older children). Lateral decubitus studies are obtained for similar reasons as in adults (see p. 42).
- Studies should always be marked by the technologist with the projection and patient's position.
- Some radiology departments use a specialized "baby holder" to position a baby upright for frontal and lateral CXRs.

Normal CXR
Use the same search pattern of the chest radiograph as with adults (see p. 52)
- The thymus remains prominent in young children, but gradually comprises a smaller proportion of the cardiomediastinal contour as the child ages. The normal thymus is soft and will not move or compress adjacent structures such as the trachea.
- Always identify the side of the aortic arch.
  - A right aortic arch could indicate a vascular ring anomaly and is identified by tracheal deviation to the patient's left.

Common conditions
Bronchiolitis and reactive airways disease (RAD) (aka asthma)
Both can have a similar radiographic appearance. Clinical signs of viral bronchiolitis include: tachypnea, hyperinflation, and wheezing in addition to cough and fever. In both diseases, the chest radiograph is performed to exclude a consolidation, which could indicate additional bacterial pneumonia.
- Inflammation of the small bronchiolar walls → close on expiration → air trapping → hyperinflation and wheezing.
- Older children and adults, peripheral airways are larger and stay open.

The wheezing toddler
"All that wheezes is not asthma." Inspiratory and expiratory radiographs might be needed to rule out focal air-trapping, usually from foreign body aspiration. See p. 307.

Radiographic findings of bronchiolitis and RAD:
Study can be normal.
- Bilateral perihilar peribronchial thickening.
- Bilateral hyperinflated lungs.
  - Best seen by flattened hemidiaphragms on lateral study.
- Focal opacities may be due to focal atelectasis or pneumonia.
  - Atelectasis very common with RSV and can be lobar or segmental.
  - Atelectasis may change rapidly between studies.
- Coarse bronchovascular markings with perihilar peribronchial thickening without consolidation in a setting consistent with viral pneumonia is sometime called bronchopneumonia.
  - The term *bronchiolitis* is usually reserved for infants (see Figure 6.10).

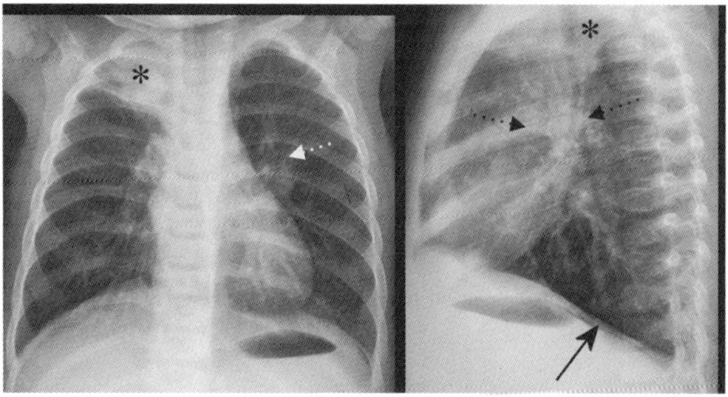

Figure 6.10 RSV bronchiolitis in a one-year-old. Peribronchial thickening (dotted arrows), hyperinflation (flattened hemidiaphragms, solid arrow) and associated RUL collapse (*).

Foreign body aspiration

Foreign bodies may be aspirated into a major airway of young children (most commonly) or in adults (e.g., catching tossed peanuts).
- A foreign body may produce a "ball-valve" type obstruction, allowing air in but not out, and hyperinflating the ipsilateral lung.
- Over time, the bronchus may become completely obstructed and the lung gradually collapses, producing a low volume ipsilateral lung.

Diagnosis:
Inspiratory CXR: patient MUST NOT be rotated.
- Look for hyperinflation of one lung relative to other.
- Mediastinal shift away from more inflated lung.
- The foreign body is rarely seen.

Expiratory CXR: will make the shift and asymmetry more apparent.
- Helpful in adults, difficult to obtain in young children.

Decubitus views (bilateral):
- A normal dependent lung will collapse relative to the "top" lung.
- A lung or lobe with a major bronchial obstruction will not collapse.

Fluoroscopy:
- Brief chest fluoroscopy will show a "swinging" mediastinum if one lung is not inflating and deflating as well as the other.

Round pneumonia

Bacterial pneumonia in children can sometimes develop as a round or spherical opacity and be mistaken for a mass. The signs and symptoms must be considered in the interpretation of the CXR (see Figure 6.11).

Radiographic findings:
- Round opacity.
- Slight indistinctness of the margins.
- Usually resembles a more typical pneumonia after a few days of antibiotic treatment.
  - Follow up CXR in a few days will confirm this change in shape which will not happen with a true mass.

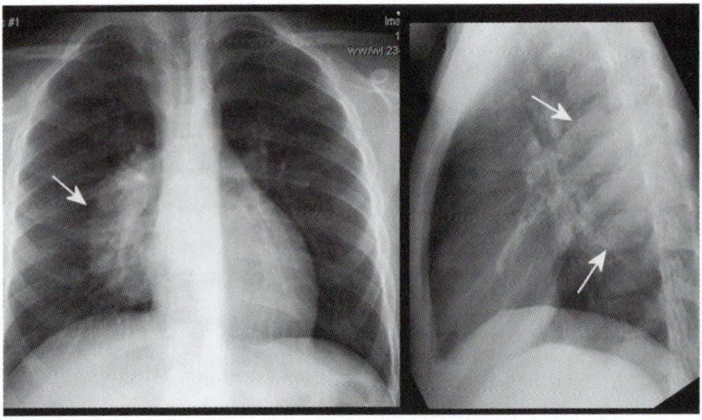

Figure 6.11 Round pneumonia. AP and lateral views of round pneumonia (arrows) in the superior segment of the RLL.

Airway

Views
The airway is evaluated by AP and lateral views, both should be performed upright, and obtained with phonation to appose the cords to demonstrate the normal subglottic shoulder (AP).
- These are SOFT TISSUE radiographs of the neck, not CXRs or C-Spine studies.

Common conditions
Croup
Croup, typically of viral origin, presents in infants and pre-schoolers with inspiratory stridor and the characteristic "barking" cough as might epiglottitis/supraglottitis (see below). Management differs markedly. Occasionally an airway radiograph is obtained (see Figure 6.12).

Radiographic findings:
AP view: an elongated narrowed subglottic trachea, with loss of the normal subglottic shouldering, called the "steeple sign." Caused by subglottic edema.

> Both AP and lateral views should be obtained if airway radiographs are requested. Epiglottitis occasionally has subglottic extension, which might suggest croup on an AP only study. This could be a fatal mistake.

Epiglottitis (aka supraglottitis)
Clinical presentation can mimic croup. It is an emergency and is treated markedly differently than croup. Prevalence is lower than 20 years ago due to the H. flu vaccine. However, there have been outbreaks among non-immunized children.

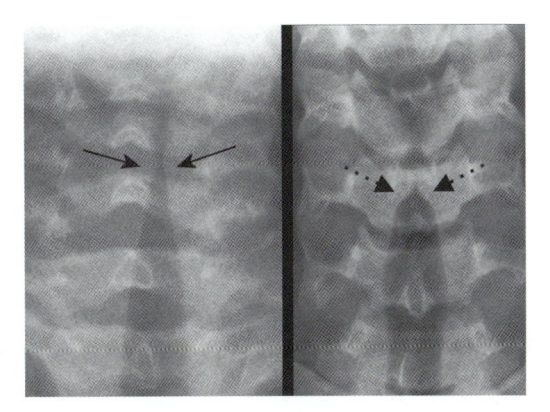

Figure 6.12 Croup, with narrowing and "steeple configuration" of the subglottic trachea (arrows). A comparison normal airway is shown on the right with normal subglottic "shoulders" (dotted arrow).

- Children present with fever, dysphagia, stridor, and fever.
- Drooling and difficulty swallowing, which might falsely suggest a pharyngeal problem rather than an airway problem.

> ### Suspected epiglottitis
> Keep child calm and upright, do not attempt to visualize pharynx (no tongue depressors). A team adept at difficult intubation should stay with the child at all times.
> - AP and lateral upright radiograph of soft tissue neck is obtained expeditiously, without aggravating the child, and interpreted STAT.
> - In most major pediatric centers, direct expert laryngoscopic visualization is performed and no imaging is obtained. However, supraglottitis can occasionally be an unexpected radiographic finding, which must be recognized and treated immediately.

Radiographic findings (see Figure 6.13):
- Effacement of the valleculae.
  - Follow the base of the tongue inferiorly to the air filled valleculae at the level of the hyoid bone.
- Thickened epiglottis and aryepiglottic folds.
  - Normal epiglottis usually no more than ~3 mm thick.

Tracheoesophageal fistula (TEF)

TEFs are usually diagnosed soon after birth when the esophagus is atretic (most common) or when a large fistula is present. Small "H"-type fistulae might not be diagnosed until late infancy or childhood.
- Patient may have recurrent aspiration pneumonia.
- Diagnosed with an esophagram (non-ionic water soluble).

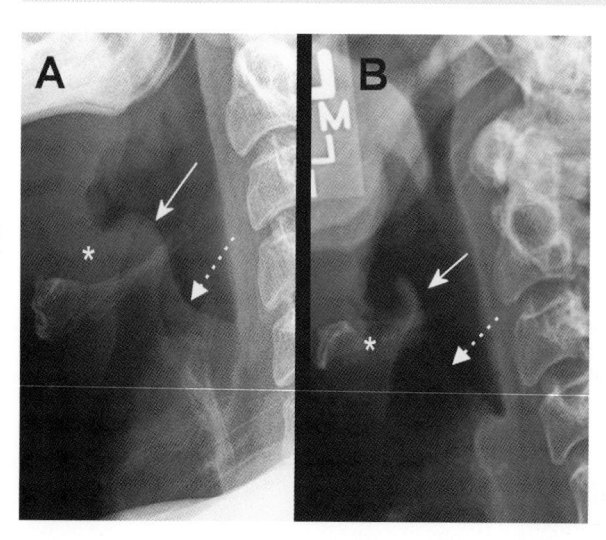

Figure 6.13 Upright lateral views of (A) epiglottitis and (B) normal pharynx. (A) Shows thickened epiglottis (arrow) and aryepiglottic folds (dashed arrow) compared to (B). Aryepiglottic folds are normally very thin and barely visible. Note that the vallecula anterior to the epiglottis is obliterated by supraglottic swelling (*). Air in the vallecula should normally extend to the hyoid bone (* on B).

Gastrointestinal system

Common conditions

Gastroesophageal reflux (GER)

GER is very common in children, especially in neonates and infants. Silent GER can result in chronic stridor or aspiration. Depending on age and clinical presentation, imaging might not be indicated.

Upper gastrointestinal (UGI) fluoroscopy:
- Child might or might not exhibit GER during the study.
  - Cannot be used to exclude reflux.
- Often done to exclude anatomical problems, for example, hiatal hernia or other causes of vomiting; GER then a diagnosis of exclusion.

Radionuclide gastric emptying study or a radionuclide milk scan:
- Monitors for GER over a longer time period and can provide quantitative information about frequency of reflux and gastric emptying.
- Delayed imaging can show aspiration if radiotracer seen in lungs.

Hypertrophic pyloric stenosis (HPS)

Cause of non-bilious vomiting at 4–6 weeks of age. Most common in male first born infants.
- The hypertrophied pyloric muscle is sometimes palpable as a pyloric "olive".

Radiographic findings:
Ultrasound
The imaging modality of choice. Scan the baby in RPO position, so gastric fluid accumulates in the antrum. Thick, elongated hypertrophied pyloric muscle is seen (see Figure 6.14).
- A persistent single wall thickness of >4 mm (i.e., over a few minutes of sonography; transient thickness is due to pylorospasm).
  - Early or mild HPS could be 3–4 mm.
- A persistent pyloric channel length >17 mm.
- A little fluid passing through the pylorus might be seen ("string sign") but does not exclude HPS as long as the pyloric muscle does not thin and the channel "open up" while observing for several minutes.

Upper gastrointestinal (UGI) fluoroscopy
Performed to evaluate vomiting when HPS is thought to be unlikely on the basis of clinical presentation or age, or performed occasionally in a borderline case on US (but repeat US in a few days preferred).
- Narrowed, elongated pyloric channel ("string sign").
- Poor flow into duodenum.

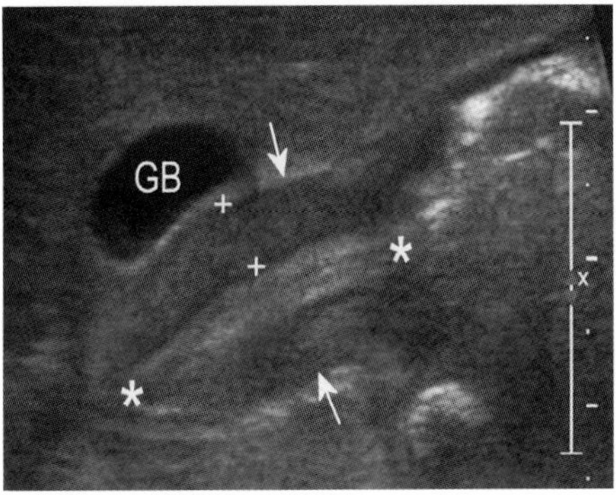

Figure 6.14 Ultrasound of hypertrophic pyloric stenosis. Elongated pyloric channel (echogenic mucosa measured from *→*). Hypoechoic hypertrophic pyloric muscle (arrows) measured 4 mm thick (between +_+). GB = Gallbladder.

Malrotation

Usually discovered in neonates and infants, however, can present at any age, even adult.
- Malrotation can result in obstruction from either midgut volvulus or Ladd bands.
- *Midgut volvulus* is a fatal condition when missed. Usual presentation is <u>bilious</u> vomiting since the volvulus occurs beyond the duodenal ampulla.
- Volvulus can be intermittent, and might not be present on UGI at the time of the study. However, the malpositioned duodenal-jejunal junction will be identified (see Figure 6.15).

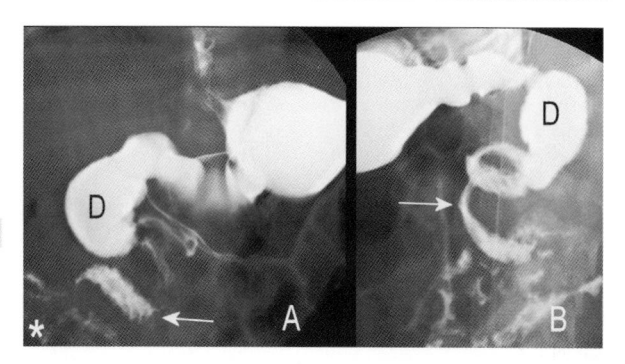

Figure 6.15 (A)AP and (B) lateral views from an UGI showing malrotation. Arrows in both views show the likely DJ junction, which is too inferior, too midline, and too anterior to have a normal ligament of Treitz. There is no volvulus, but the proximal duodenum (D) is dilated, possibly due to crossing Ladd bands. Jejunum is in the right upper quadrant (*)

Diagnosis

> The critical finding on a neonatal or infant UGI study to exclude malrotation is identifying a normally positioned duodenal-jejunal (DJ) junction.

Normal position of the DJ junction:
1. To the left of the spine (AP view).
2. At the same height as duodenal bulb/pylorus (AP view).
3. Posterior to the duodenal bulb (lateral view).

Normal DJ junction position indicates that there is a ligament of Treitz (supensory ligament of duodenum) and no malrotation. In malrotation the position of the DJ junction varies.

UGI:

Intermittent imaging is performed while the patient drinks dilute barium. The course of the duodenum must be documented in both AP and true lateral projections. All 3 of the preceding criteria should be met to exclude malrotation, and normal jejunum should also be seen in the left upper quadrant (LUQ).
- If volvulus has occurred, the distal duodenum or jejunum is obstructed in a "beak-like" configuration.

What are Ladd bands?

Ladd bands are fibrous peritoneal bands that attach the cecum to the abdominal wall. In malrotation, the abnormal position of the bowel can lead to these crossing the duodenum.
- May lead to complete or partial mid-duodenal obstruction
- This does not typically have a beak-like configuration, as volvulus does.

Intussusception

"Telescoping" of distal ileum into cecum and colon produces intermittent crampy abdominal pain in children, sometimes accompanied by bloody "currant jelly" stools. 80% occur under 24 months of age.

<u>Etiology:</u>
- Post neonatal period to age 1 5 years: usually idiopathic, typically intestinal or mesenteric lymphatic tissue.
- Neonates and older children/adolescents: idiopathic is less likely; usually pathologic lead point, for example:
  - Lymphoma, Meckel diverticulum, ileal enteric duplication cyst, bowel wall hematoma or thickening.

<u>Diagnosis:</u>
Ultrasound
Sensitive technique. Seen as a multi-layered cylindrical mass produced by one bowel loop being within the other like a collapsed telescope.
- The inner bowel loop (intussusceptum) might be accompanied by mesenteric fat and lymph nodes inside the outer bowel loop (intussuscipiens).
- Looks like a "target" in short axis, and a "pseudo kidney" in long axis (see Figure 6.16).
- Reduction with saline enema under ultrasound is popular in Europe, and its use will likely increase in the USA.

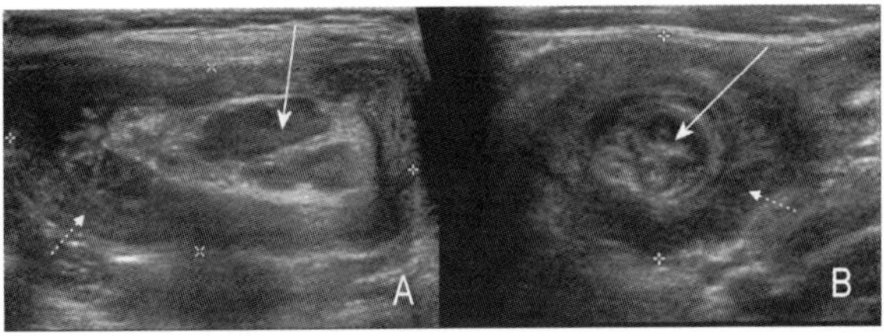

Figure 6.16 Intussusception on ultrasound. A = long axis B = short axis. The intussuscepiens (dashed arrow) contains the intussusceptum, lymph nodes and echogenic mesenteric fat (solid arrow).

Radiography
Not sensitive. May show the soft tissue mass of the intussusceptum if the intussuscipiens contains enough gas in its lumen to outline it.
- It is sometimes seen better in upright, lateral decubitus, or prone positions than when supine.

Air enema
Both diagnostic and therapeutic (see Figure 6.17).
- Air is gently pumped by hand into the rectum under fluoroscopic guidance. The air fills the colon and outlines the intussusceptum. Increasing the air pressure (monitored via a gauge) will reduce the intussusceptum in $\cong$ 85–90% cases.

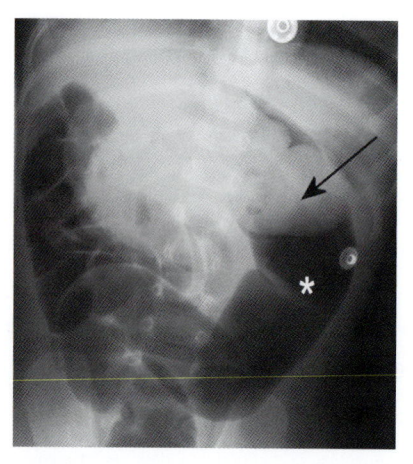

Figure 6.17 Air enema in intussusceptions. Air in the descending colon (*) outlines the large intussusceptum "mass" (arrow). Two metallic objects on right are EKG electrodes.

- Air must be seen to bubble into the distal ileum to confirm successful reduction.
- Contraindicated by peritonitis, free air, or clinical instability.
- If repeated attempts fail, then usually surgery is required.
- Occasionally reoccurs in next 24–48 hours, enema can be repeated.

Genitourinary system

Vesicoureteral reflux (VUR)

Reflux of urine from the bladder up one or both ureters, which can occur with bladder filling or during emptying (voiding). Diagnosed with a voiding cystoureterogram (VCUG).

Indications for voiding cystoureterogram (VCUG)
- Dilation of the urinary collecting system.
- Urinary tract infection (see also p. 38 "Algorithms").

Diagnosis

Fluoroscopic VCUG:
- For more details and image see chapter 7, Fluoroscopy, p. 329.

Radionuclide cystogram/VCUG:
Radiotracer is dripped into the bladder via a catheter and VUR is detected with a gamma camera. See chapter 9, Nuclear Medicine, p. 431.

Advantages:
- Radiation dose is less than fluoroscopic VCUG.
- Continuous imaging, so quite sensitive to detecting VUR.
- Useful for follow-up of VUR or screening siblings for VUR.

Disadvantages:
Low anatomic detail, cannot assess urethra (e.g., boys for posterior urethral valves) or morphology of duplicated collecting systems.

Additional imaging
- To assess for scarring from reflux, a renal US is commonly performed.
- Nuclear Tc-99m dimercaptosuccinic acid (DMSA) scan (with SPECT) is sometimes used, which also allows assessment of differential function.

Musculoskeletal system

Normal variants
The ends of children's bones vary in appearance during growth and development and can manifest many normal anatomic variants.
- Consult an Atlas of Normal Variants (e.g., Keats).
- Obtain a matching view of the same portion of the contralateral normal extremity for problem solving.

Patterns of fractures specific to children
Salter-Harris classification of fractures
Children have unfused growth plates (physes), which, if injured, can lead to premature fusion and growth arrest of that portion of bone.
- If the entire width of the physis is destroyed, there is no further growth and that limb may end up short if child is young.
- If part of physis is destroyed, uneven growth may occur (in only the intact portion), which can lead to crooked bones and later joint deformities.

Fractures involving the growth plates have a special classification system: "Salter-Harris Classification" (see Figure 6.18 and Table 6.1).
- The higher the Salter-Harris number, the more likely the possibility of growth disturbance at that end of the bone.

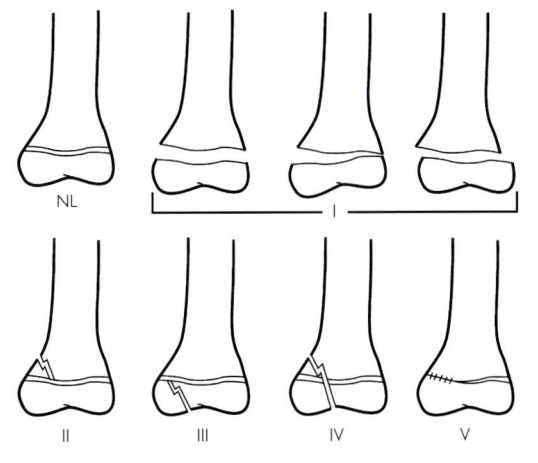

Figure 6.18 Diagram illustrating Salter-Harris classification of pediatric fractures.

Table 6.1

Salter Harris Classification		
I	**S**ame	Physis is widened, symmetric, or asymmetric. Epiphysis can be distracted (pulled away), displaced (slipped), tilted (angled), or a combination, from the metaphysis.
II	**A**bove	A fracture line extends from the metaphysis into the physis.
III	be**L**ow	A fracture line extends from the epiphysis into the physis.
IV	**T**ogether	A fracture line extends through the physis and both the metaphysis and epiphysis.
V	c**R**ushed	The physis is entirely or partially crushed.

Incomplete or "greenstick" fractures

In general, pediatric bones are less brittle than adult bones and might respond to trauma as incomplete cortical breaks, often on one side, causing bone to bend like a "young sapling." Incomplete fractures are common (see Figure 6.19).

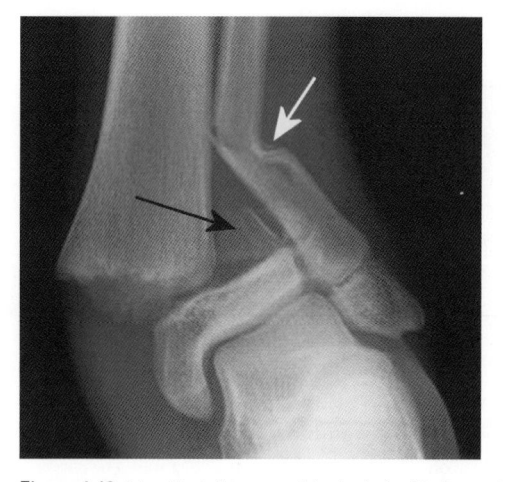

Figure 6.19 Salter Harris II fracture of the distal tibia (black arrow) with lateral displacement and valgus (lateral) angulation of the distal fragments relative to the proximal fragment. Incomplete (greenstick) fracture of the fibula (white arrow) with distal valgus angulation.

Torus or buckle fractures (see Figure 6.20)

Another type of incomplete fracture. Portion of cortex is partially compressed and trabecula are warped creating a focal buckling of cortex.
- Can occur in any long bone, for example, radius and ulna.
- Subtle torus fractures can occur in the metacarpals and fingers with falls.
- Children jumping from moderate heights (e.g., upper bunk) incur metatarsal greenstick and torus fractures from the sudden dorsi-flexion of the feet upon landing.

Avulsion of secondary ossification centers/apophyses

As well as epiphyseal injuries, secondary ossification centers can be avulsed +/− displaced with trauma (see Figure 6.21).
- May be acute (e.g., elbow trauma).
- May be chronic due to overuse (e.g., "Little league elbow," pelvic apophyseal avulsions in young athletes).

Knowledge of the normal apophyseal development patterns is key to interpreting radiographs (see Keats' reference).

Common fractures specific to the pediatric population
Slipped capital femoral epiphysis (SCFE)

A Salter I fracture of the proximal femoral physis, which presents with pain as the femoral head slips on the physis relative to the femoral neck.
- Most cases are idiopathic. However, any process that weakens the physis can lead to SCFE, for example, hypothyroidism, external beam radiation.

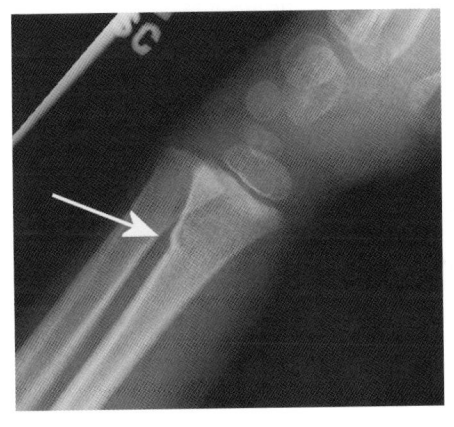

Figure 6.20 Buckle or torus fracture of the distal radius (arrow). This was only seen on this lateral view.

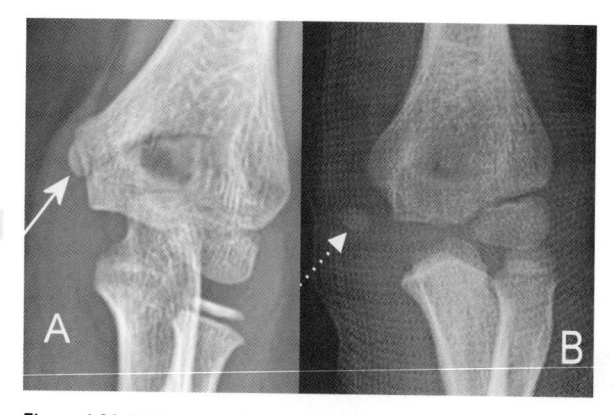

Figure 6.21 (A) Normal medial epicondyle apophysis of distal humerus. (B) Acutely avulsed medial epicondyle (patient in a cast).

SCFE patients tend to be:
- Late grade school to early high school.
- Obese.
- Near a growth spurt.

Radiography (see Figure 6.22):
- AP and frogleg views.
- Look for the epiphysis (femoral head) slipping off the femoral neck, much like a scoop of ice cream slipping off its cone.
- Might be better seen on abducted (frog leg) views.
- A line drawn along the lateral aspect of the femoral neck should intersect a portion of the femoral head (see Figure 6.22).
  - If this line passes lateral to the femoral head, SCFE is likely.

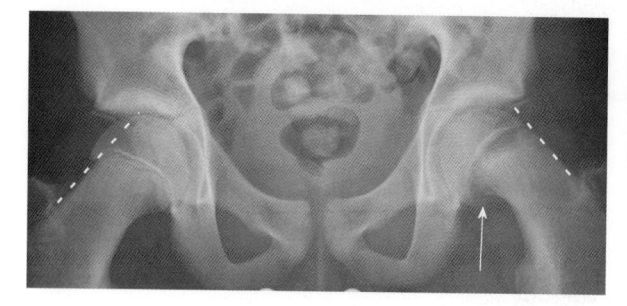

Figure 6.22 13-year-old boy with left SCFE. AP radiograph of the hips shows widening of the left proximal femoral physis, the head is slipped medially (arrow), and the lateral femoral neck line (dotted) does not intersect the femoral head. (Note normal intersection of the femoral neck line in the normal right hip).

Findings can be subtle, so always obtain views of the asymptomatic contralateral hip for comparison.
- Physis is often widened on abnormal side.
- One epiphysis appears "larger" than the other.

Toddler's fracture (see Figure 6.23)

Consider in the 18-month to 4-year-old who won't walk.

The toddler is still relatively new at walking, is unstable, and may fall while the foot is planted and the leg twists during the fall.
- Sudden or insidious onset.
- Child otherwise in no distress, just unwilling to walk.
- The fall is often not witnessed.

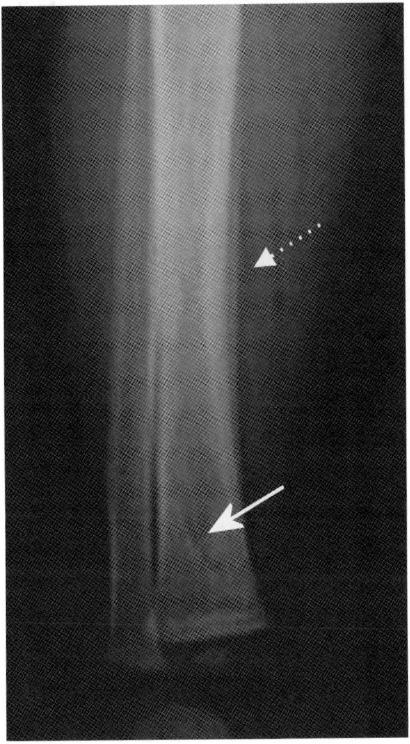

Figure 6.23 Healing toddler fracture, occult on first study. Fracture line (solid arrow) is only partially seen, and spirals superiorly. There is associated periosteal reaction (dotted arrow).

CHAPTER 6 **Pediatrics**

Radiographic findings:
- A hairline, oblique, or spiral fracture of the tibial diaphysis.
- May be occult on initial radiographs.
  - Leg might be splinted or casted for comfort regardless of whether the fracture is identified.
  - If pain persists, follow-up views in 2 weeks—look for a sclerotic edge or periosteal new bone.

Less commonly, the toddler can fracture the calcaneus, cuboid., or metatarsals and present in a similar manner.
- In a puzzling case, where a "wait and see" approach seems inappropriate, consider a radionuclide bone scan.

Distal humeral supracondylar fracture

This is the most common elbow fracture in a child and can be subtle (see Figure 6.24).
- Fracture might be occult although accompanied by a joint effusion.
- Look for displacement of the distal humerus relative to the anterior humeral shaft.

In a pediatric patient with upper extremity trauma and with no apparent fracture on a radiograph, if an elbow joint effusion is present, assume a supracondylar fracture and treat expectantly. Re-image in 7–10 days.

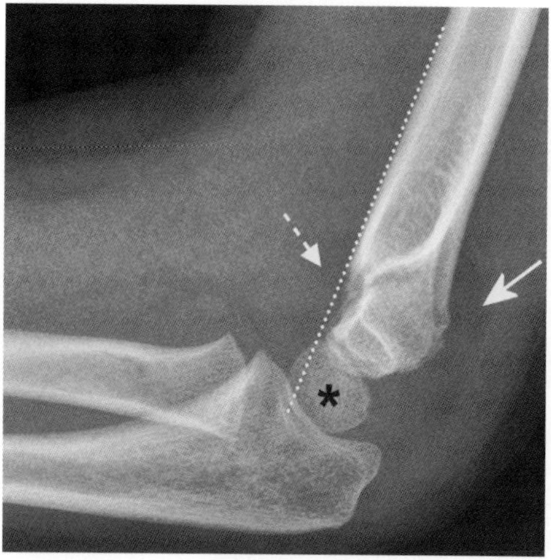

Figure 6.24 Subtle supracondylar fracture. Note the anterior humeral line (dotted line) does not pass through the middle of the capitellum epiphysis(*) as it should, due to posterior displacement of the distal humerus fracture fragment. Posterior fat pad sign (solid arrow) and anterior fat pad (sail) sign (dotted arrow) indicate the joint effusion.

Buckle/torus fracture of the distal radius (see Figure 6.20)
Very common especially in the spring when children return to playing outside, riding bicycles, and so forth.
- These can be very subtle and might be seen only on one view.
  - Obtain three views and treat any "wrinkle," angulation or step-off in the cortex as a fracture.

Radial head dislocation
Also known as "nursemaid' elbow." Due to the relative ligamentous laxity in children, the radial head can dislocate out of the annular ligament. Usually when the arm is tugged or pulled violently, but can be by a fall.
- Unusual >5 years other than from severe trauma.

<u>Radiographic findings:</u>
AP and lateral elbow studies show mal-alignment of the radial head with the capitellum.
- Can spontaneously reduce, so radiograph may be normal.

Other common pediatric musculoskeletal problems
Developmental dysplasia of the hip (DDH)
Incidence 1:1000.

<u>Risk factors include (but aren't limited to):</u>
- Breech presentations that result in ligamentous laxity.
- Abnormally shallow acetabular roof.

The femoral head is not tightly held in the acetabulum and does not develop properly. In severe cases it will sublux or even dislocate.

<u>Clinical presentation:</u>
- Neonates/ young infants: excessive laxity on exam or a palpable clunk during Barlow and Ortolani maneuvers, respectively.
- Older children: may present with a dislocated hip, limited hip abduction, delayed walking, or a limp (functionally "short leg").
- Delayed diagnosis can lead to severe hip arthritis.

<u>Diagnosis:</u>
From 0–6 months: hip ultrasound
- Shallow angle of the acetabular roof.
  - Normal α angle acetabular roof >60° (see Figure 6.25).
- Coverage of the femoral head
  - Normal >90° femoral head covered by the total acetabulum; ossified roof should cover at least 50% of head.
- Stress is applied to hip joint to assess for subluxation.

After~ 6 months: radiographs (see Figure 6.26).
The femoral head ossification hinders good visualization by ultrasound. Radiographs are performed in neutral and abducted positions.
- Assess for symmetry of femoral head ossification and position.
- Measure acetabular roof angles.
- The steep acetabular roof is abnormal. The "steep" roof has a low angle on US and a high angle on radiographs since different baselines are used to measure the two methods. Just remember—"steep is bad."

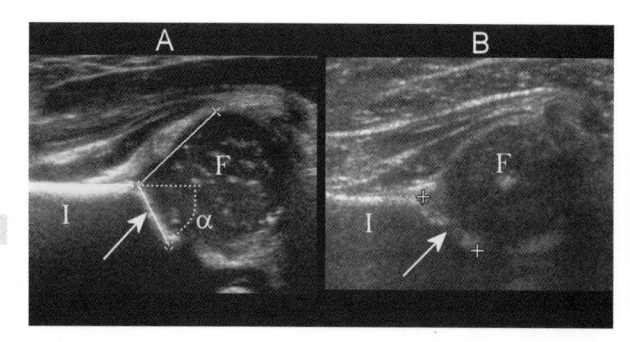

Figure 6.25 Ultrasound of the hips (coronal plane) showing measurement of the acetabular roof angle. F-femoral head, I-ileum, arrow-acetabular roof. (A) Normal study with deep acetabulum (alpha angle 65), (B) DDH with a shallow acetabulum and a steep roof (alpha angle 44). For orientation, in your mind rotate each US view 90 degrees clockwise and think of it as an AP radiograph of a left hip.

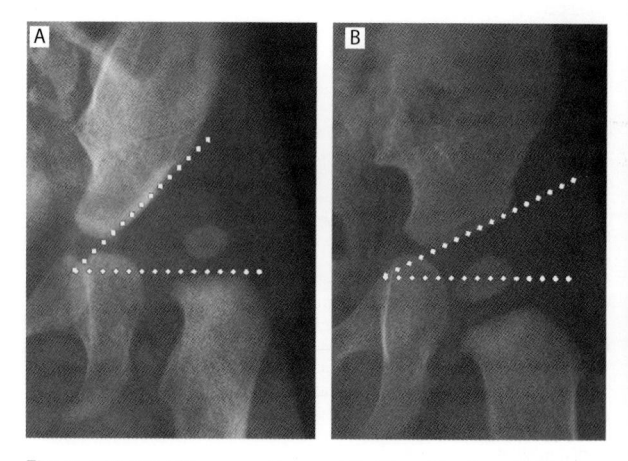

Figure 6.26 DDH (A) compared to normal hip (B) on AP radiograph. Note steep acetabular roof in A (dotted line) and left femoral head is slightly laterally subluxed.

Transient synovitis of the hip

Most common cause of acute hip pain in children age 3–10 years. Approximately half have a history of a recent respiratory tract infection, and some may have a fever.

- Ultrasound shows a hip joint effusion that can be indistinguishable from septic arthritis. Aspiration with analysis of the fluid is needed to completely exclude septic arthritis (see Figure 6.27).

How do I diagnose a hip joint effusion?

<u>Radiography:</u>
Obtain AP neutral and abduction lateral views of BOTH hips to allow comparison to the normal contralateral hip.
- Mostly performed to check for other causes of hip pain.

<u>Ultrasound:</u>
Accurate to detect joint effusion but cannot distinguish the nature of the effusion, for example, septic arthritis versus sterile transient synovitis.
- High resolution linear transducer should be used, looking for >2 mm fluid distending the hip joint capsule.
- Aspiration can be performed under ultrasound guidance if an effusion is seen.

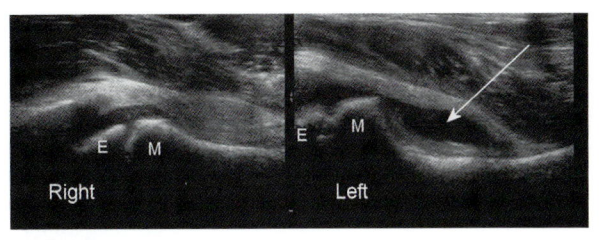

Figure 6.27 Sagittal US of normal right hip and abnormal left hip obtained over the femoral neck. The femoral head is on the left side of each image (M = metaphysis, E = epiphysis). The black convexity (arrow) is the left hip joint distended with fluid.

Legg-Calve-Perthes disease ("Perthes")

This is a form of idiopathic ischemic necrosis (AVN) that affects one or both femoral heads and may result in femoral head deformity and premature hip arthritis if untreated.
- Pre-school to grade school age.
- Can be detected on radionuclide bone scan or MRI, whereas radiograph is still normal or subtly abnormal.

See "Musculoskeletal Imaging," p. 219 for imaging findings of AVN.

How to evaluate the young child with hip/leg pain or a painful limp
The pain cannot be localized
Broad differential, including inflammation, infection, fracture or neoplasm anywhere from the vertebral column (e.g., discitis) to the foot (occult calcaneus, cuboid or metatarsal fracture).

Radiographs:
Should be the initial exam: hip→foot.

Consider a bone scan:
- Helps to locate the site of pain when physical exam is non-localizing.
- Images the entire skeleton.
- Does result in significantly more total radiation exposure than radiography.
- More expensive than radiography.

Pain localizes to hip

Differential diagnosis (for more details see separate sections):
- Hip joint effusion—septic arthritis, transient synovitis.
- Psoas irritation—abscess, pyomyositis (usually requires CT or MRI).
- Osteomyelitis (see chapter 4, p. 206).
- Perthes disease.
- Slipped capital femoral epiphyses (SCFE).

Child abuse

(Aka non-accidental injury (NAI), Syndrome X)

There are reports of 1,200–1,500 pediatric abuse related deaths (approximately 1.7 per 100,000 children) and 140,000 pediatric abuse related injuries each year, likely under-reported. If you work in pediatrics, you will likely encounter a case of child abuse.

Its radiologic manifestations can be diagnostic or at least highly suspicious, so familiarity with these findings is important.

When to think of child abuse

Radiological evidence of trauma that is inappropriate for the patient's age or non-concordant with the alleged history.
- Posterior rib fractures.
- Any fracture in an infant.
- Any metaphyseal corner fracture or "bucket handle" fracture.
- Multiple fractures, especially of various ages.
- Retinal hemorrhages.
- Subdural effusions, especially of varying age and without skull fracture (shaken baby).
- Internal visceral injuries, for example, pancreatic pseudocyst, duodenal hematoma.

Reporting suspected abuse

If you suspect child abuse based on a radiographic finding, the referring clinician must be notified immediately. In many hospitals there is a Child Protection Team that can be notified immediately. The goal is to remove the child from possible further harm. **Radiographic findings that are even just suspect for possible child abuse warrant notification and action.**

CHILD ABUSE

How to image suspected child abuse
When it has been determined that child abuse might have occurred, screening the child for other injuries must be performed. A key finding is multiple fractures of varying ages; this confirms multiple traumatic episodes over time.

Radiographic skeletal survey
Comprised of multiple radiographs ($\cong 24$).
- <u>Skull and spine</u>: AP and lateral views.
- <u>Ribs</u>: AP view +/− bilateral obliques (may increase conspicuity of rib fractures).
- <u>Extremities</u>: AP views of proximal arms and legs; distal arms; and legs, hands, and feet.
  - If physical examination or initial AP view is positive or suspicious, additional lateral or focused views may be warranted.

Do NOT do a "babygram" (single film of whole baby) as the image quality is insufficient to visualize subtle fractures.

Radionuclide bone scan
Bone scans have some limited use in challenging child abuse cases. They may be more sensitive for posterior rib fractures. Fractures appear "hot."

Disadvantages
<u>Time</u>: Sedation is often needed due to the time needed to obtain the images, as motion impairs image quality.
<u>Radiation dose</u>: The radiation exposure from a bone scan is significantly more than from skeletal survey.
<u>Insensitive for skull fractures.</u>
<u>Growing physes are "hot"</u>: Both metaphyseal fractures and the normal physis are "hot," so asymmetric uptake at the physes is the key sign.
- Careful attention to positioning is crucial to prevent incorrect interpretations.

Dating the fractures
Dating the age of fractures is far from an exact science, but it is probably more accurate by radiography than radionuclide bone scan.
- The length of time that a fracture is "hot" (i.e., active) on a radionuclide bone scan varies by patient age due to differences in bone turnover.
  - Infant fractures might be hot for weeks→ few months.
  - In older child, they may be hot for months→ a year.
- It takes 7 to 14 days for periosteal new bone to develop following fracture, although the exact onset is variable. However, it is not seen in the first few days.
- If multiple fractures in a child are of various ages, this indicates more than a single traumatic episode. This can be diagnosed when the fractures differ from each other in regard to:
  - The presence of periosteal new bone.
  - The degree or maturity of the callus.

Head CT or MRI

CT
- High specificity and sensitivity for detecting intracranial hemorrhage (see Figure 6.28).
- Usually, the most expedient modality in an acute situation that might require immediate neurosurgical attention.
- Does involve radiation exposure, but that is usually outweighed by benefits.

MRI
- Provides the highest sensitivity and specificity for intracranial injury.
- Long scan duration often requires sedation; not optimal in the critical setting.
- MRI can be useful following a positive CT scan to assess for more subtle intracranial changes and after a negative CT scan if there is still clinical concern about possible intracranial injury.

Pathognomonic findings
Neurological
Subdural hemorrhage
- Diagnosed on MRI or CT.
- Multiple layers of variable ages, very suspicious for abuse.

Unexplained skull fracture
- Best identified on CT.

Beware: Significant CNS damage from abuse can occur WITHOUT incurring a skull fracture.

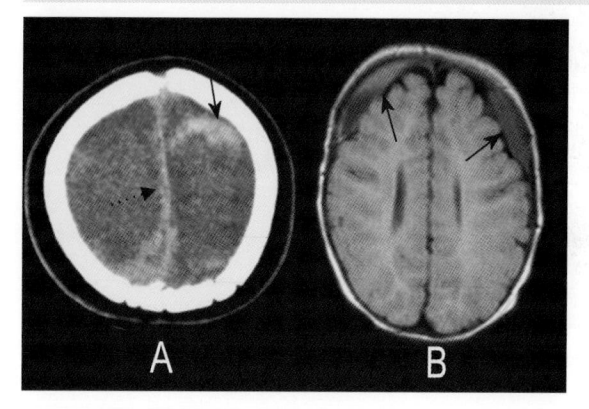

Figure 6.28 Child abuse. (A) CT scan shows high attenuation over the left parietal convexity (solid arrow) and along the interhemispheric fissure (dotted arrow). (B) T1 weighted MRI in a different patient shows bilateral frontal subdural hematomas (arrows). The different signal intensities (right frontal) indicate different age subdural hematomas.

CHILD ABUSE

Musculoskeletal
Multiple fractures of variable ages.
- Acute: lucent fracture line, displacement.
- Subacute: periosteal new bone formation.
- Old: callus formation.

Corner fractures, "bucket handle" fractures
- Tugging and twisting the ends of long bones pulls periosteum and portions of cortex off the metaphysis.
- When it pulls straight off the end of the metaphysis, the avulsed fragment looks like a "bucket handle" (see Figure 6.29).

Rib fractures
- Multiple of varying ages as shown by varying degrees of healing callus (see Figure 6.30).
- Commonly posterior ribs: any part of a rib can fracture, but the posterior-medial portion of the rib breaks when the chest is squeezed, crushing the rib against the adjacent transverse process of the vertebra.
  - The transverse process acts as a fulcrum, and the rib cracks there.

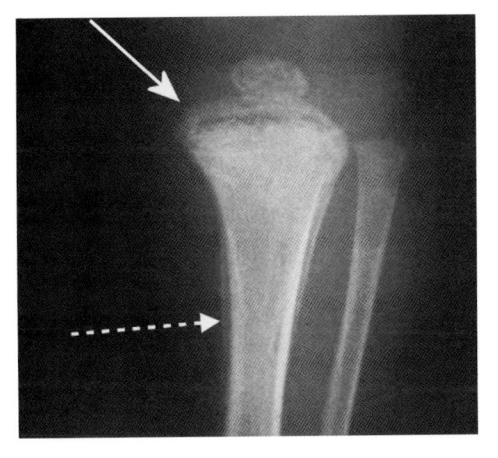

Figure 6.29 AP view of left leg shows bucket handle fracture of proximal left tibia (solid arrow) and periosteal thickening (dotted arrow).

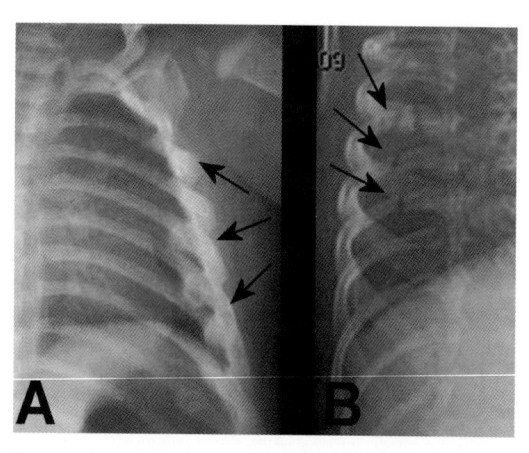

Figure 6.30 (A) AP chest shows bulky callus about the lateral aspects of multiple left ribs, consistent with old fractures. (B) In another patient, LPO view of ribs shows acute vertical fractures of the postero- medial aspects of several adjacent ribs.

Don't miss diagnoses

Epiglottitis/supraglottitis
- Airway can suddenly close – manage expectantly with appropriate level of anesthesia support available.

Intestinal malrotation
- Can lead to midgut volvulus and dead bowel.

Pneumoperitoneum
- Can indicate bowel perforation and subsequent peritonitis.

Child abuse
- Consider on EVERY study, for example, always look for rib fractures on CXRs.
- If unrecognized, child is subject to further, even fatal, injury.

References

American Academy of Pediatrics. Policy Statement diagnostic imaging of child abuse. *Pediatrics* 2009; 123:1430–1435. Also found at: *http://aappolicy.aappublications.org/cgi/reprint/pediatrics; 123/5/1430.pdf*

Keats T.E., Anderson M.W. *Atlas of Normal Roentgen Variants That May Simulate Disease.* Philadelphia, PA: Saunders-Elsevier 2006.

Lonergan GJ, Baker AM, Morey MK, Boos SC. From the archives of the AFIP – Child abuse: Radiologic-pathologic correlation. *RadioGraphics* 2003; 23:811–845. http://radiographics.rsna.org/content/23/4/811.full.pdf+html

www.virtualpediatrichospital.org Curated by Drs. Donna M D'Alessandro, and Michael P D'Alessandro.

Chapter 7

Fluoroscopy

Jocelyn D. Chertoff, MD

How are images acquired? *324*
Patterns of disease *327*
　Lesion Localization *327*
　Strictures and obstructions *329*
　Leaks *330*
　Motility disorders *330*
　Fold thickening *331*
Upper GI tract fluoroscopy *332*
　Patient preparation *332*
　What examination should I order and how is it performed? *334*
　Anatomy on upper GI fluoroscopic studies *335*
　Postsurgical Anatomy *337*
　Common conditions evaluated with UGI/SBFT *337*
Lower GI tract fluoroscopy *345*
　What examination should I order and how is it performed? *345*
　Colonic anatomy on lower GI fluoroscopic studies *347*
　Postsurgical Anatomy *347*
　Common conditions on lower GI fluoroscopic studies *349*
GU tract fluoroscopy *354*
　Voiding cystourethrogram (VCUG) *354*
　Cystogram *354*
　Retrograde urethrogram (RUG) *355*
　IVP *355*
　Hysterosalpingogram (HSG) *356*
　What exam should I order? *357*
　Common conditions evaluated with GU fluoroscopy *358*
Tube studies *361*
　What examination should I order and how is it performed? *361*
　Feeding tubes *361*
　T-tube cholangiogram *361*
　Drain injections *362*
References *362*

How are images acquired?

Fluoroscopy is the process of viewing x-ray examinations in real time. With fluoroscopy, the radiologist usually controls and operates the equipment. Fluoroscopy is not only used by radiologists doing barium studies, but also by interventional radiologists, vascular surgeons, cardiologists, orthopedic surgeons, and gastroenterologists, among others, for real-time imaging in the operating room.

Technology

All modern fluoroscopy units are digital. The components of modern fluoroscopy are:

Under the table and the patient:
- The x-ray generator produces either continuous or pulsed electricity.
- The x-ray tube converts that electricity into x-rays.
- The collimator limits the x-ray beam to the area of interest and reduces exposure.

Above the table and the patient:
- The image intensifier absorbs the transmitted x-ray beam and converts x-ray photons into light (luminescence).
- It amplifies the signal, which makes the image brighter.
- The optical coupler sends the light image to a video camera and to recording devices.
- The video camera converts the light image to a voltage signal.
- The monitor receives the signal and displays the image.
- Images can be captured on film and/or sent to a PACS workstation.

Display

- The image is displayed with high density structures (bone, barium) black on the TV monitor but can be printed black on white or white on black, depending on the operator's preference.
- Static images can be acquired either by:
  - Taking a "fluoro-spot," which is a screen capture of the current image (no additional radiation). Lower resolution.
  - Taking a dedicated radiograph (additional radiation). Higher resolution.

Radiation risk

Although the radiation exposure for a second of fluoroscopy is about 20 times less than a comparable exposure time for a radiograph, fluoroscopy is performed for longer durations, and radiation exposure is a significant issue for the patient as well as for other people in the room.
- Fluoroscopy requires that the operator is aware of radiation dose reduction techniques and practices these at all times.
- Most modern digital fluoroscopy units use "pulsed fluoroscopy," in which the x-ray beam is only active for approximately one-tenth of the time that the image is showing.
  - This markedly reduces radiation exposure.
  - Particularly important in pediatric fluoroscopy.

HOW ARE IMAGES ACQUIRED?

> **NO STARGAZING!**
> It's tempting to keep watching with fluoroscopy– don't! The dose adds up quickly.
> **Take your foot off the pedal and look at the static image.**

See chapter 1, Radiology Essentials, p. 25, for more information on radiation risk and for techniques to reduce patient dose during fluoroscopy.

Contrast choices

Fluoroscopy studies are dependent on intra-luminal opacification with contrast. This can be radiodense (barium, iodinated contrast) or radiolucent (air, carbon dioxide).

See chapter 1, Radiology Essentials, p. 18 for additional information.

Barium

A naturally occurring element, barium sulfate is insoluble in water, passes through the GI tract and is eliminated completely. It is available in thick and thin consistencies, each of which has a different use.

<u>Indications:</u>
- Use to show anatomy and mucosal detail in the GI tract.
- Use in small bowel obstruction to show site and cause.

Thick consistency: "coats" mucosal surfaces, used in double contrast studies with air or CO2.
Thin consistency: Contains more fluid and is used for single contrast studies where it fills the lumen. Bowel can be compressed, and you can "see through" the thin barium.

<u>Contraindications:</u>
- Known or suspected bowel or esophageal perforation—barium won't be reabsorbed and so will require surgical washout.
- Do not use above the site of known or suspected **colonic obstruction** —the water will be absorbed but not the barium and will form concretions.

Water soluble contrast

Water soluble contrast is reabsorbed if extravasated into tissues, unlike barium. See "Contrast" in chapter 1, p. 18 for more details.

<u>Indications:</u>
- Known or suspected perforation of GI tract.
- Confirmation of position of tubes or catheters.
- Biliary tree injections (cholangiography, ERCP).
- GU tract studies (e.g., hysterosalpingography, urethrography, cystography, nephrostograms, pyelography).
- Neonatal GI studies especially on premature infants.
- Other—sialography, ductography (breast), myelography.
- HOCM agents also stimulate peristalsis and may be therapeutic in the setting of ileus, for example, Ogilvie syndrome.
  - Gastrograffin™ often used for this because it contains a soap; may be helpful especially if constipated.

Contraindications:
See "Contrast" in chapter 1, p. 20.

Types of contrast examinations of the GI tract
Single contrast
Single contrast technique means that the lumen is filled with contrast alone. The density of the contrast is tailored to the clinical question. In general, it should be lucent enough to not completely obscure a filling defect. For example, if the contrast is too dense in a T-tube cholangiogram, a small stone might be obscured.
- Patients are positioned to optimize visualization of area of concern.
- Compression is used to displace overlapping bowel loops and get better images of specific areas.
- Compression also used to oppose bowel walls in order to see the surfaces better.

Double contrast
With double contrast technique, the mucosal surface is coated with thick barium, and the lumen distended with something that is radiolucent (e.g., air, gas from effervescent tablets or methylcellulose).
- Patient is positioned to maximize visualization of all surfaces, for example, upright to view the air distended colonic flexures during a barium enema.
- This technique requires a lot of patient movements, rotations, and cooperation.

Fluoroscopy versus endoscopy of the GI tract
These two methods of studying the bowel provide different information, and have different risk profiles.

Endoscopy
- Allows direct visualization of the bowel mucosa and biopsy of lesions.
- Does not assess motion.
- Cannot visualize bowel wall or adjacent tissues unless endoscopic ultrasound is used.
- May be limited in patients with redundant colons.
- Entire jejunum and ileum cannot be endoscoped and may require specialized "pill cameras," and such.
- Requires conscious sedation, nursing assistance, and recovery time.
- Is more expensive than fluoroscopy.

Fluoroscopy
- Provides information on the lumen and mucosa of the bowel.
- Assesses bowel function (peristalsis) in real time.
- Allows the examiner to challenge the GI tract with different kinds of contrast and different techniques.
- Gives information about the effect of adjacent structures on the bowel.
- Biopsy cannot be performed, and follow-up endoscopy may be necessary.
- Exposure to ionizing radiation.

Of note, neither of these studies gives the level of information about adjacent structures (e.g., pancreas, liver) that computed tomography provides.

Patterns of disease

Lesion Localization

Diseases "intrinsic" to lumen

Contrast fills and defines the lumens of structures. Masses arising from the mucosa (e.g., polyps) will show as filling defects in the column of contrast. Mucosal defects such as ulcers will show as irregularities in the edge of the contrast.

Determining how a lesion abuts the lumen wall is important, so an appropriate differential diagnosis can be made. It is easier to make this distinction with larger lesions.

- The angle the lesion makes with the wall helps to determine the origin of the lesion.
- The location within the gut or GU tract guides the differential diagnosis.

Mucosal abnormalities

- Lesion makes acute angle with bowel wall.
- Loss of normal smooth mucosal pattern.
  - Generally appear as irregularities in the otherwise smooth contour of the wall of the lumen.

Can be very subtle (e.g., herpes ulcers in the esophagus), or very obvious, (e.g., the "apple-core" lesions of colon adenocarcinoma). Small bowel polyps, including hamartomas, adenomas, and adenocarcinomas are all examples of neoplasia originating in the mucosa.

Diseases "extrinsic" to lumen

Extrinsic disease may be within the wall of the structure (<u>submucosal</u>), or outside of it entirely (<u>extrinsic</u>). These both cause "mass effect," that is, displacement of the contrast-opacified lumen.

- Is it a luminal narrowing (a stricture) or is there a mass encircling the lumen? This can be difficult to determine (see Figure 7.1).

Submucosal masses

Lesions originating in the submucosa include GI stromal tumors (GIST), lipomas, metastases (melanoma, breast, lung), and carcinoid tumors.

- Lesion makes obtuse angle with bowel wall (see Figure 7.2).
- Preservation of smooth mucosal pattern unless they ulcerate through.

Extrinsic masses

Extrinsic masses include serosal metastases, endometriosis, and mass effect from focal or diffuse disease in adjacent structures (e.g., pancreatic pseudocysts, abcesses, adenopathy).

- Lesion makes obtuse angle with bowel wall (see Figure 7.2).
- Preservation of smooth mucosal pattern.

CHAPTER 7 **Fluoroscopy**

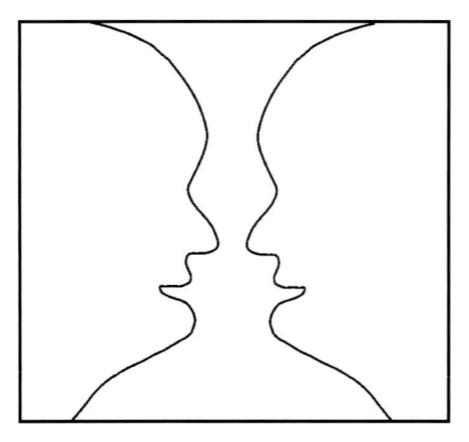

Figure 7.1 Two faces or a goblet? The drawing might be two faces or might be a goblet and is a good analogy for images in fluoroscopy.

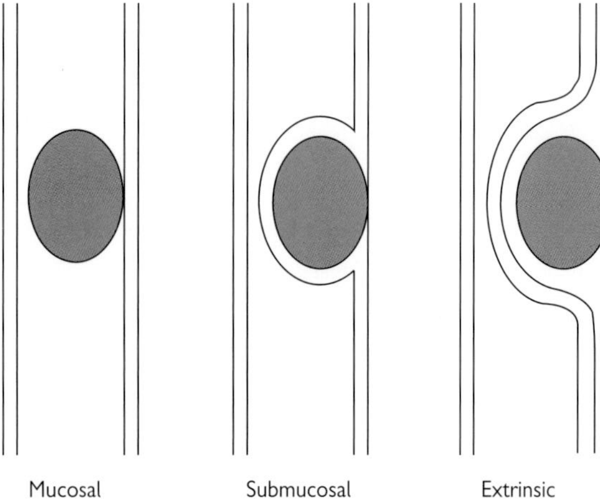

Mucosal Submucosal Extrinsic

Figure 7.2 Localization of lesions within the bowel wall.

> Despite the preceding descriptive criteria, mucosal, submucosal, serosal, and extrinsic lesions can be challenging to distinguish on fluoroscopy.

Filling defects
Filling defects appear as lucent areas outlined by contrast. We need to decide if they are free within the lumen or fixed to the wall by palpating the area under fluoroscopy.

Filling defects on fluoroscopy

Free/Mobile
- Air bubbles
- Ingested material
- Bezoars
- Stones
- Blood clot

Fixed
- Benign or malignant mass
- Thickened fold or edema
- Foreign body
- Ectopic pancreas
- Heterotopic gastric mucosa
- Brunner gland hyperplasia (duodenum)
- Intramural diverticulum (duodenum)
- Post-operative change

Strictures and obstructions

Strictures
Narrowing of the column of contrast reflects the narrowing of the lumen. Because the gastrointestinal tract is very dynamic, fluoroscopy is necessary to determine whether the narrowing is a temporary phenomenon, like peristalsis or spasm, or whether it persists. Strictures can be caused by:
- Cancer.
- Inflammatory disease.
- Extrinsic masses.
- Congenital narrowings.

> Differentiation of benign versus malignant strictures is not always possible with fluoroscopy; endoscopy is often required.

Obstruction
Obstruction is caused when the lumen becomes too tight to allow passage of the contrast (and normal luminal contents). This can be due to an intrinsic or extrinsic lesion.

<u>Imaging findings:</u>
- Abnormal dilatation above the obstruction.
- Decompression (collapse) of lumen below the obstruction.
- +/− abnormal motility (increased or decreased depending on chronicity).

> Etiologies:
>
> Volvulus
> Primary or metastatic cancer
> Hernias
> Stones
> Adhesions
> Inflammatory disease
> Congenital abnormalities
> Foreign bodies

Leaks
Fluoroscopic studies are frequently ordered to "rule out leak":
- In suspected perforation.
- For post-operative evaluation of a new gastrointestinal or ureteral anastomosis.

Patterns of GI perforations
- Free spill of luminal contents into the peritoneal space (air and fluid).
- Spill/leak into a contained, walled off space (e.g., peri-diverticular abscess).
- Communication to another structure as a fistula.
- Spill/leak into the retroperitoneum.
  - Retroperitoneal gas and fluid.

Patterns of GU perforations
- Leaks generally will not result in free air.
- Most leaks are retroperitoneal, except bladder perforation which can be intra- or extra-peritoneal.
- A fistulous communication to bowel will result in air in the GU tract.

Motility disorders
Fluoroscopy is an excellent way to evaluate the motility of any part of the GI tract, with or without contrast. When contrast is administered it is possible to observe the time it takes for the contrast to pass through the area of interest, as well as observing the quality of the peristaltic contractions.

Esophagus
Motility is evaluated in the prone oblique position to eliminate gravity and to isolate peristalsis.
- A primary stripping wave is stimulated by swallowing.
- Secondary waves are triggered by any remaining material.
- Tertiary waves are non-propulsive. They increase with age and are considered to be a sign of dysmotility.

Some disorders that affect esophageal motility can be distinguished by their characteristic appearance or by the portion of the esophagus affected.
- Scleroderma.
- Achalasia and Chagas Disease (mimics achalasia).
- Nutcracker esophagus.
- Reflux esophagitis.
- Primary (idiopathic).

Stomach

Gastric motility can be evaluated qualitatively with fluoroscopy; however, quantitative evaluation requires a nuclear medicine gastric-emptying scan. (See chapter 9, Nuclear Medicine, p. 442). In gastroparesis, the stomach is often enlarged.

Common causes of gastroparesis (delayed emptying):
- Vagotomy and gastric surgery.
- Diabetes mellitus.
- Gastroesophageal reflux.
- Medications (narcotics, anticholinergics, some antidepressants).
- Infection.

Small bowel

Loss of peristalsis occurs in adynamic ileus. In ileus, the entire small bowel will be dilated with diminished peristalsis.

> **Common causes of illeus**
> - Post operative
> - Ischemia
> - Pain
> - Shock
> - Radiation
> - Malabsorption disorders
> - Medications (e.g., opiates)
> - Metabolic disease (diabetes, hypothyroidism)
> - Infection/inflammation
> - Connective tissue disorders

Fold thickening

Fold thickening is a frequent finding in studies of the GI tract. There is a long differential diagnosis, so it is important to identify the location and extent of the abnormality, the pattern of fold thickening, and any accompanying abnormalities.

Characterizing fold thickening
- Straight and uniform—"regular" fold thickening.
- Nodular and irregular thickening.
- Is there accompanying bowel dilatation?

> **Fold thickening—differential diagnosis**
>
> Regular fold thickening:
> - Ischemia: ASCVD, vasculitis.
> - Hypoproteinemia: nephrotic syndrome, cirrhosis.
> - Hemorrhage: coagulopathy, ischemia, vasculitiis.
> - Rare conditions eg. lymphangiectasia, amyloid.
>
> Irregular or nodular fold thickening:
> - Lymphoma.
> - Inflammation: Crohn disease, eosinophilic gastroenteritis, mastocytosis.
> - Infection: giardia, Whipple disease, amyloid, tuberculosis, histoplasmosis.
> - Varices: esophageal and gastric.

Upper GI tract fluoroscopy

Studies are performed by administering contrast into the patient's gastrointestinal tract; either they drink the barium, or it may be administered via an enteric tube if they have one in place.
- Standard studies performed on out-patients are done with various consistencies of barium and may include administration of air or gas (from effervescent tablets).
- When studies are done for specific indications on sick patients, the exam is modified.

Patient preparation

For most studies of the upper GI tract, the patient will fast overnight. This is modified for age (e.g., babies), and critical medications may be permitted with a small amount of water.

> It is preferable to schedule GI exams early in the morning to make fasting easier for patients.

What examination should I order and how is it performed?

Although there is a standard approach to each of the following fluoroscopic examinations, it must be adjusted based on the clinical question, the patient's needs and abilities, and the specific potential risks and benefits of the exam in that patient. It is best to discuss the case with the radiologist so they can tailor the exam as needed.

> Tell the radiologist all the pertinent past medical history. The surgical history is particularly critical to obtaining an accurate study and answering the clinical question.

Modified barium swallow

A modified barium swallow is performed with a speech pathologist in attendance. The study is dynamic, and is saved on a DVD for review and analysis by the radiologist and the speech pathologist.
- Patient is studied upright: standing or sitting in lateral and frontal projections.
- Speech pathologist administers various consistencies of barium, from thin to a solid, such as a barium-coated marshmallow or cookie.
- Patient is imaged chewing and swallowing.
- The effect of different swallowing strategies may be evaluated.
- Patient can bring in foods that they have problems with.

"Combined swallow"

When the modified swallow is done in conjunction with a barium swallow/esophagram, it is called a "combined swallow." In this case, the barium swallow/esophagram portion is done first, since the solid material ingested for the modified swallow can cause artifacts on images of the esophagus.

UPPER GI TRACT FLUOROSCOPY

Barium swallow/esophagram

The barium swallow, or esophagram (more correct terminology) studies the mouth (including pharynx) to the fundus of the stomach, using both single- and double contrast techniques.

Double contrast

- In the standing position, patient is given effervescent granules that create gas bubbles and distend the esophagus and stomach.
- The patient then rapidly drinks thick barium that coats the lumen to evaluate the mucosa of the pharynx and esophagus (see Figure 7.3)..

Single contrast

- In the prone oblique position, thin barium is given to evaluate motility without the effect of gravity.
- The table is lowered and raised several times during the exam, to optimize visualization, and the patient may be instructed to roll to improve coating.
- A barium pill may be given to assess patency of the esophagus if the patient has dysphagia or a stricture.
- Rapid sequence swallows of the pharynx are obtained in frontal and lateral projections.

Patient's symptoms do not accurately localize the site of pathology in dysphagia or "food sticking."
- Lower esophageal problems may have discomfort referred to the neck.
- An esophagram is the most useful study unless there is a history of stroke, aspiration, or head and neck surgery.

Upper GI series

The upper GI series includes a full esophagram, as well as single and double contrast evaluation of the stomach and duodenum. It evaluates from the pharynx to the ligament of Trietz.

Double contrast

- Esophagus is evaluated in double contrast, as described in preceding section.
- Patient is then placed supine and asked to roll several times to coat the gastric lumen with contrast.
- Various patient positions are used to evaluate the stomach and duodenal bulb in double contrast.

Single contrast

- Oblique prone images of the esophagus obtained to evaluate motility.
- Single contrast views with palpation (compression) are obtained of the stomach using either an inflated balloon or a plastic compression device held by the radiologist or attached to the fluoroscopic unit.

NOTE: An upper GI series requires a mobile, cooperative patient as does a double contrast barium enema. Limited single single-contrast studies can be obtained on patients who are immobile or cannot cooperate (via tubes if necessary).

Small-bowel follow-through (SBFT)
The small bowel follow through can be done as a stand-alone examination, evaluating from the duodenal bulb to the terminal ileum or combined with a UGI, in which case it is called an upper GI/small bowel follow through. The isolated SBFT begins with images of the duodenal bulb and c-sweep.
- The patient drinks at least a bottle of thin barium.
- The small bowel is studied with a series of radiographs as well as careful periodic palpation (compression) of the bowel under fluoroscopic observation.
- The study is completed with palpation/compression of the terminal ileum as it enters the colon.

What exam should I order?

Modified swallow
Dysphagia if likely related to stroke or head/neck surgery, suspected aspiration, problems swallowing or eating, suspected neurological disease.

Combined swallow
Dysphagia as above, chest pain, suspected aspiration or stricture, (plus indications for either study alone).

Esophagram
Dysphagia other than earlier description, chest pain, pain with swallowing, globus, suspected reflux, hiatal hernia, stricture, esophagitis, dysmotility, achalasia, cancer, post op.

UGI
Suspected malrotation, ulcer, Crohn disease, gastroparesis, gastric outlet obstruction, s/p nissen (check wrap), weight gain after bariatric surgery.

SBFT
Malabsorption, malrotation, Crohn disease, stricture, obstruction, nausea, vomiting, weight loss, anemia, bloating, pain, rule out mass, cancer, stricture, diverticuli.

Anatomy on upper GI fluoroscopic studies

Esophagus
- 25 cm length muscular tube.
- Upper third consists of striated circular muscle.
- Lower two thirds consists of smooth muscle.
- It has a number of normal extrinsic impressions:
  - Cricopharyngeus muscle in neck.
  - Postcricoid defect (venous plexus).
  - Aortic knob (see Figure 7.3).
  - Left mainstem bronchus.

Stomach
- **Cardia**: the portion of the stomach that begins at the end of the esophagus.

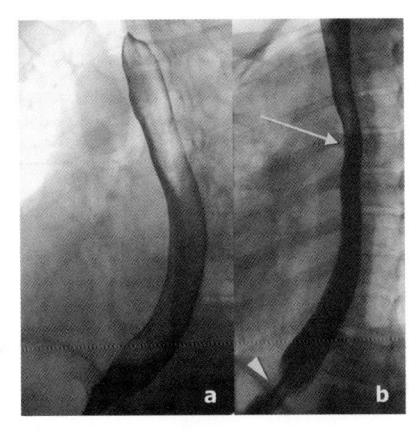

Figure 7.3 (a) Normal double contrast esophagram. Note how mucosal detail is evident. (b) Normal single contrast esophagram. The extrinsic compression of the aortic knob is visible (arrow). Note the normal gastroesophageal junction (arrowhead).

- **Fundus**: the most superior portion of the stomach, above the cardia, and posterior.
- **Body**: the portion of the stomach between the fundus and the antrum.
- **Antrum**: approximately the lower third of the stomach.
- **Pylorus**: connects the stomach and the duodenum, it includes the pyloric antrum, canal, and sphincter.
- **Gastric folds**: = rugae (see Figure 7.4).

Duodenum
Only the first part is intraperitoneal, the rest is retroperitoneal.
- First (bulb).
- Second (descending):
  - Includes ampulla of Vater (hepatopancreatic ampulla).
- Third (horizontal):
  - Crossed by the superior mesenteric artery.
- Fourth (ascending):
  - Ends at ligament of Treitz (suspensory ligament of duodenum).

Jejunum and ileum
- Jejunum starts at the suspensory ligament of duodenum (Treitz).
- Ileum ends with the terminal ileum at the ileocecal valve.
- Attached by mesentery to posterior abdominal wall obliquely, LUQ to RLQ.
- Two borders: mesenteric and antimesenteric.
- Folds are called plicae circulares (also known as valvulae conniventes):
  - Jejunum: closely packed, feathery appearance.
  - Ileum: more widely spaced, less feathery (see Figure 7.5).

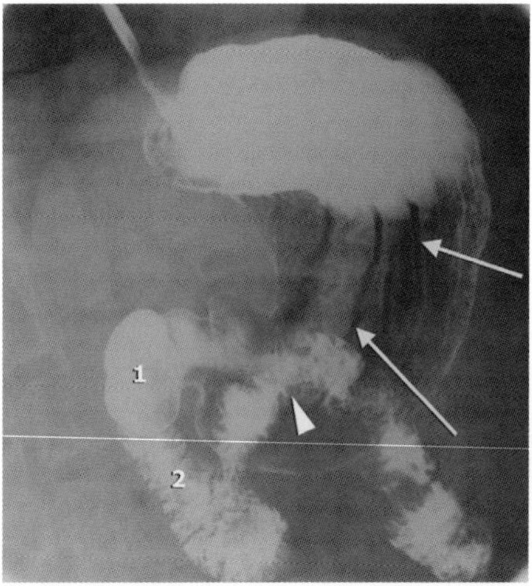

Figure 7.4 Normal stomach on a double contrast UGI (LPO image). Note the normal gastric rugae (arrows). 1st and 2nd parts of duodenum (1 and 2). Duodenal-jejunal flexure = arrowhead.

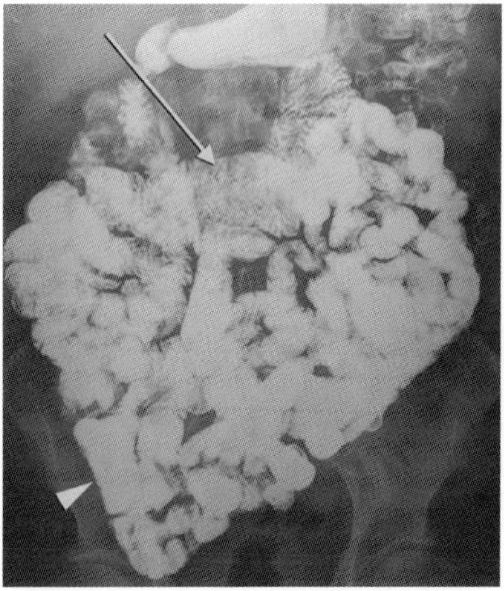

Figure 7.5 SBFT, Normal small bowel follow through. The jejunal folds (arrow) appear feathery and are more closely packed than the ileal folds (arrowhead). Some contrast has passed into the colon.

Post surgical anatomy
Surgeries performed involving the upper GI tract may require a post-op study to evaluate for leak, obstruction or other complications.

> **Include all relevant surgical history on the requisition**
> Knowledge of what surgery has been performed and the typical appearances and complications is important to protocol, correctly perform, and evaluate the study.

Esophagectomy with gastric pull up:
Usually performed for tumor involving the lower esophagus.
- The mid and lower esophagus are resected.
- The stomach is pulled into the chest, with an anastomosis to the upper esophagus.

Fundoplication:
Performed for gastroesophageal reflux (GERD).
- The fundus of the stomach is wrapped around the lower end of the esophagus, reinforcing the lower esophageal sphincter.

Bariatric surgery (gastric bypass or gastric band):
Used to treat obesity.

Gastric bypass
- The stomach is made into a very small pouch, and anastomosed to a loop of jejunum (efferent loop) (see Figures 7.6 and 7.7).
- The unused portion of the stomach (the distal stomach), and the duodenum are drained by a loop of jejunum (afferent loop), which is anastomosed to the efferent jejunal loop.

Gastric banding
- A small gastric pouch is created by encircling the stomach with a band.
- The diameter of the band can be adjusted via tubing connected to a subcutaneous port.
- Less invasive, fewer complications than bypass.
- Slightly less effective.

Pancreaticoduodenectomy (Whipple)
Primarily used to treat tumors, or other significant pathology in the head of the pancreas, but sometimes for disease of the common bile duct or duodenum.
- Excision of the gastric antrum, C-loop of the duodenum, the pancreatic head, common bile duct, and the gallbladder.
- Anastomoses are created to drain the pancreatic body and tail, the biliary tree, and the stomach into small bowel.

CHAPTER 7 Fluoroscopy

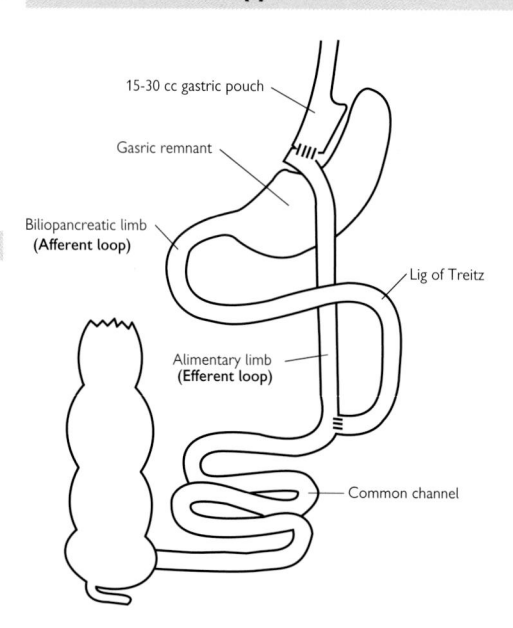

Figure 7.6 Anatomy of gastric bypass surgery.

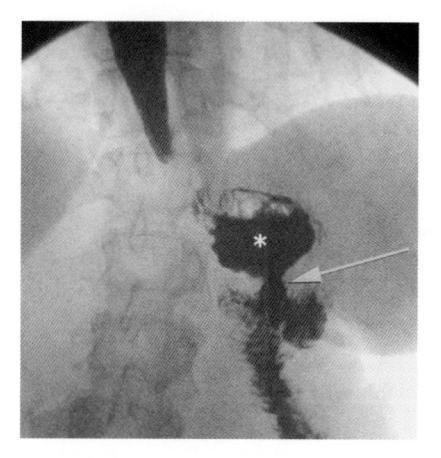

Labels: 15-30 cc gastric pouch; Gastric remnant; Biliopancreatic limb (Afferent loop); Lig of Treitz; Alimentary limb (Efferent loop); Common channel

Figure 7.7 Gastric bypass surgery on single contrast UGI. Note the small size of the gastric pouch (star). The gastro-jejunal anastomosis is patent (arrow).

Common conditions evaluated with UGI/SBFT

Aspiration
Evaluated with a modified barium swallow.
- Aspiration = entry of food, drink, or secretions into the airway below the vocal folds. (Above the vocal folds it is called penetration.)
- This can result in coughing, pneumonia, and lung damage.
- Predisposing conditions include obesity, stroke, prior head and neck surgery, and altered level of consciousness.

Esophageal strictures—benign and malignant
Evaluated with barium swallow/esophagram or UGI.
- A stricture = any narrowing relative to the normal luminal caliber.
- This can be very subtle or very obvious and includes long and short segments.
- Any narrowing requires evaluation, usually with biopsy, because fluoroscopy cannot make a definitive distinction between benign and malignant disease.

Benign causes of esophageal strictures
- Gastroesophageal reflux.
- Barrett esophagus (pre-malignant).
- Caustic ingestion.
- Inflammatory/infection (e.g., Candida).
- Iatrogenic:
  - Post NG tube and post-surgical (anastomoses).
  - Radiation therapy.
- Extrinsic benign disease.

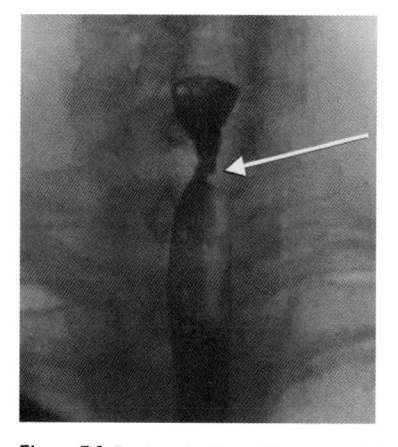

Figure 7.8 Esophageal stricture. The asymmetric, irregular proximal esophageal stricture (arrow), on this image from an esophagram, was a recurrence of esophageal cancer.

Malignant causes of esophageal strictures
- Esophageal carcinoma (squamous and adenocarcinoma) (see Figure 7.8).
- Lymphoma.
- Extrinsic malignant disease.

Esophagitis
- Evaluated with double contrast images from a barium swallow/esophagram/UGI.
- Fold thickening.
- Mucosal irregularity, ulcerations, and nodularity.
- Different types of esophagitis can sometimes be characterized by their double contrast appearance, but generally endoscopy is needed.

Etiologies
Infectious (Candida, herpes, cytomegalovirus [CMV]), reflux, chemical ingestion or drug induced, eosinophilic esophagitis, other inflammatory diseases (e.g., scleroderma or Crohn disease).

Achalasia
Absence of primary esophageal peristalsis and a failure of the lower esophageal spincter to relax and let food into the stomach. The esophagus can become massively dilated, and the distal end can have a characteristic appearance called the "bird's beak" or "rat tail" sign (see Figure 7.9).
- Evaluated with double contrast (barium swallow/esophagram/UGI).
- A timed barium swallow can be performed to assess emptying.
  - The patient quickly drinks a specific amount of barium, and images are obtained at 1, 2, and 5 minutes.
  - The height and width of the remaining column of barium helps quantify emptying.
- Achalasia can be treated with medication (antispasmodics), injected Botulinum toxin, balloon dilatation, or myotomy.

Primary achalasia
- Caused by loss of the ganglion cells in Auerbach's plexus, the esophageal myenteric plexus.

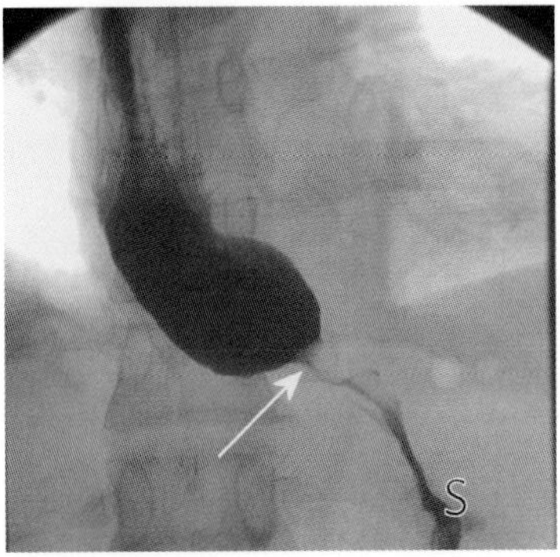

Figure 7.9 Esophogram in a patient with achalasia shows a wide column of barium in the enlarged esophagus leading to a diffusely narrowed gastroesophageal junction (arrow). Some barium has passed into the stomach (S).

Secondary achalasia—causes:
- Malignancy of the distal esophagus.
- Chagas disease (infection from trypanasoma cruzi). The latter is indistinguishable radiographically from primary achalasia.

Hiatal hernias and reflux

Although the radiographic literature distinguishes sliding or axial hiatal hernias and paraesophageal hernias, the surgical literature calls them all hiatal hernias, and divides them into 3 or 4 subtypes, one of which is paraesophageal.

> The key to the fluoroscopic diagnosis of a hiatal hernia is identifying the location of the GE junction.

Sliding/axial hiatal hernia
The gastroesophageal junction is *above* the diaphragm. It is associated with gastroesophageal reflux (see Figure 7.10).

Paraesophageal hernia
- The gastroesophageal junction remains below the diaphragm and the fundus or more of the stomach herniates above the diaphragm, next to the esophagus.
- Occasionally, small bowel, colon, and even liver herniate into the chest.
- Paraesophgeal hernias can be a surgical emergency when obstruction or infarction of the stomach occurs.

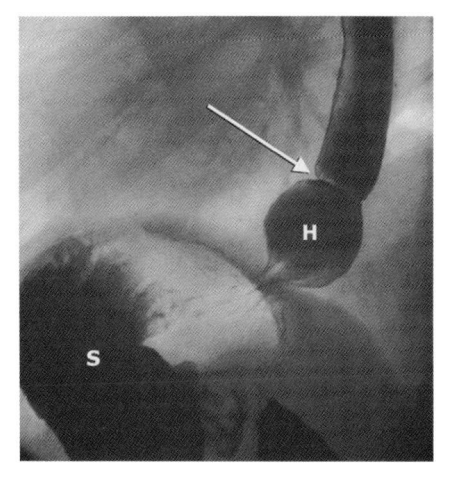

Figure 7.10 Small hiatal hernia, esophagram. The GE junction is located above the diaphragm (arrow), and a portion of the stomach (S) has herniated into the thorax (H).

Gastroesophageal reflux (GERD)
Associated with hiatal hernias, but can occur without a hernia.

Imaging findings
- +/− reflux of barium seen on a Valsalva maneuver or Trendelenburg positioning.
- Thick, irregular folds.
- Ulceration or stricture.
- Barrett's esophagus.
  - Metaplasia of the normal esophageal squamous epithelium to columnar.
  - Conveys an increased risk of adenocarcinoma.
  - Produces a reticular pattern on esophagram.

Gastric volvulus
There are two types of gastric volvulus, a condition where the stomach twists out of its usual orientation.

Organoaxial volvulus
- The stomach rotates along a horizontal axis (the long axis of the stomach, a line drawn from fundus to pylorus).
- Flips upside down; greater curve is cephalad to lesser curve.
- May be asymptomatic.

Mesenteroaxial volvulus
- Gastric rotation is perpendicular to the long axis of the stomach.
- More serious; likely to cause vascular compromise and ischemia.
- This is a surgical condition.

Gastric and duodenal ulcers
Helicobacter pylori (H. pylori), a very common bacterial inhabitant of the stomach, is a major cause of peptic ulcers, causing more than half of peptic ulcers worldwide.
- H. pylori also increases the risk of gastric cancer and a type of gastric lymphoma.

Nonsteroidal anti-inflammatory drugs (NSAIDs), such as aspirin and ibuprofen, are another common cause.

Gastric ulcers
Most gastric ulcers are benign. There are features on the upper GI study that may help distinguish a benign ulcer from a malignant one. A 'malignant' ulcer is actually a tumor that has ulcerated on its mucosal surface.

<u>Benign ulcers:</u>
- Gastric folds radiate gradually up to the ulcer.
- Contrast extends *beyond* the expected margin of the stomach wall, indicating erosion into the submucosa (see Figure 7.11).

<u>Ulcerating malignancy:</u>
- More abrupt and irregular transition of folds at ulcer margin.
- Will appear as a collection of contrast projecting *within* the gastric lumen, because it occurs within a mass that is growing inside of the stomach.

These distinctions are less critical in modern practice because essentially all ulcers will be visualized endoscopically and biopsied.

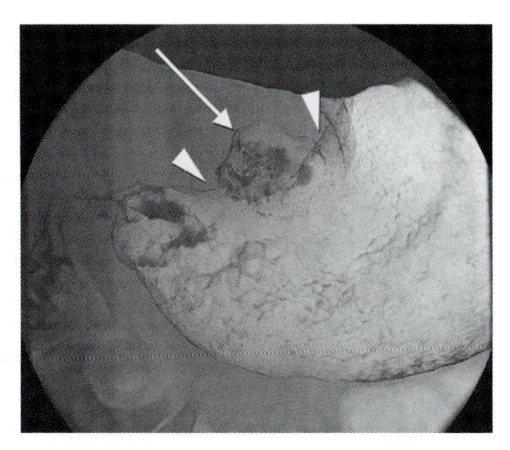

Figure 7.11 Benign gastric ulcer, UGI LPO view. The ulcer crater extends beyond the wall of antrum of the stomach (arrow). An ulcer collar is also seen (arrowheads). These are features of benignity, confirmed at EGD.

Duodenal ulcers

Most commonly seen in the bulb as a manifestation of peptic ulcer disease, and are usually benign in this location. They are more common than gastric ulcers.

Imaging findings (UGI):
- Collection of contrast extending beyond the wall.
- Thickened folds.
- A perforated ulcer of the posterior wall of the duodenum will result in retroperitoneal air.

Gastric outlet obstruction
Results in severe gastric dilatation with retained fluid and food.

Etiologies:
Malignant: gastric cancer, lymphoma, metastatic cancer, gastric invasion from adjacent tumor.
Benign: bezoar, stricture, Crohn disease, and post-operative complications.

Neoplasms of the Upper Gastrointestinal Tract
Gastric adenocarcinoma
Most commonly involves the greater curvature.

Imaging findings
- Superficial mucosal lesion.
- Polypoid lesion.
- Large ulcerated mass.
  - Linitus plastic (see later).

Gastric lymphoma

Most commonly non-Hodgkin lymphoma. It can spread into the duodenum. It can be primary or secondary (much more common).

Imaging findings
- Diffusely thickened wall narrowing the lumen.
- A mass or masses.
- Markedly thickened folds.

Gastric metastatic disease
- Most commonly from melanoma, Kaposi's sarcoma, breast, and lung primaries.
- Often characterized by masses with central ulceration.

Linitis plastica

Primary and metastatic neoplasms of the stomach can infiltrate the wall diffusely, resulting in gastric narrowing, poor distensibility, and poor motility, "linitis plastica." Common etiologies:
- Gastric adenocarcinoma.
- Metastatic disease from breast or lung, lymphoma.
- Corrosive ingestion.
- Some infections such as tuberculosis can give this appearance.

Gastrointestinal stromal tumors (GIST)
- Can occur anywhere in the gastrointestinal tract.
  - 50–70% of GISTs originate in the stomach.
  - 20–30% originate in the small intestine (jejunum and ileum).

<u>Growth patterns:</u>
- Submucosal lesions that most frequently grow endophytically in parallel with the lumen of the affected structure.
- Exophytic extraluminal growths. These tumors have been reported ranging in size from smaller than 1 cm to as large as 40 cm in diameter.
- May have areas of necrosis and cavitation.

Duodenal cancer

The most common type is adenocarcinoma. Other duodenal malignancies include leiomyosarcoma, lymphoma, metastases, and benign lesions that can become malignant, like adenomas. Duodenal cancers can appear as polypoid, annular, or ulcerating lesions.

Crohn Disease

Crohn disease (=regional enteritis, granulomatous ileocolitis) is a form of inflammatory bowel disease. It is an idiopathic, systemic disorder that can affect any part of the GI tract from mouth to anus, but has predilection for the terminal ileum (see Figure 7.12).
- It can affect the eyes, joints, skin, urinary tract, liver, and biliary system.
- Often there are "skip areas"—regions of normal, unaffected bowel between areas of active inflammation.
- Frequently recurs after resection.
- Patients with Crohn disease have an increased risk of colon cancer.

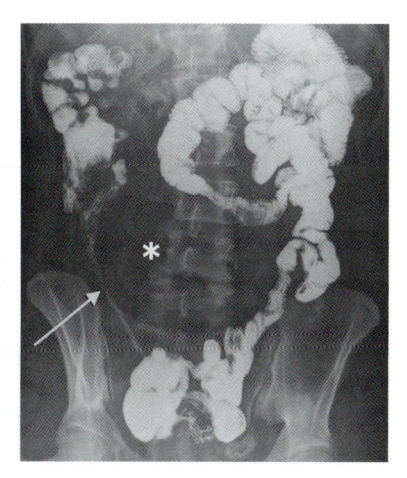

Figure 7.12 Crohn disease of the distal and terminal ileum The terminal ileum is irregularly strictured (string sign—arrow) and ulcerated, and separated from the rest of the loops due to fatty proliferation of the mesentery (*).

Crohn disease is often imaged with fluoroscopy (tailored to the portion of bowel involved), CT, or MRI. MRI is very good for evaluating fistulous disease, and MR enterography is useful to assess the bowel wall.
- Imaging is often done to evaluate a change in symptoms or to assess a change in medication.

Imaging findings
- Apthous ulcers—shallow depressions, seen on double contrast studies.
- Fold and wall thickening.
- Luminal strictures.
- Fistulae.
- Inflammation, fatty proliferation (better seen on CT).
- Filiform polyps.

Complications
Abscess, malnutrition, bowel obstruction.

Lower GI tract fluoroscopy

What examination should I order and how is it performed?
Contrast enema
Benefits of contrast enema over endoscopy include
- Ability to evaluate the colon proximal to a nearly obstructive lesion.
  - Endoscope cannot pass through the obstruction.

- Assessment of fistulas, leaks, and diverticulosis.
- Therapeutic:
  - Water soluble contrast enemas can be performed for the treatment of Ogilvie's syndrome, constipation, or distal intestinal obstruction syndrome, a complication of cystic fibrosis.

Benefits of endoscopy include
- Direct visualization of the mucosa.
- Ability to perform biopsy.
- Ability to remove polyps.

Patient preparation

Adherent stool can both obscure and mimic pathology.
- Study will not exclude polyps or tumor if an adequate bowel prep has not been performed.
- Therapeutic contrast enemas do not require any bowel preparation.

> **Bowel preparation for enemas**
> Although the bowel prep varies in different institutions, it usually involves strong laxatives and dietary limitation, such as clear fluids only. It often takes several days and can be very difficult for old or debilitated patients. Patients with poor fluid intake can become dehydrated.

Contraindications to contrast enemas

Absolute:
- Risk of colonic perforation.
- Toxic megacolon.
- Severe pseudomembranous colitis.
- Suspected perforation.

Relative contraindications:
- Difficult or painful exam.
- Sigmoidoscopy within 24 hours due to excessive gas in colon.
- Recent colonic biopsy (risk of perforation).
- Acute colitis.

Technique

Contrast enemas can be uncomfortable for the patient, causing abdominal pain and cramping, although it is usually tolerated adequately.
- A cooperative, mobile patient is a necessity, since patient rolling and frequent changes in positioning are required to "unwind" the colon and visualize each segment.
- A rectal exam is performed to exclude stricture.
- A catheter tip is then inserted into the rectum and a balloon insufflated with air to help retain it. Air and/or contrast delivered via the tube.

Double contrast enemas
- Thick barium coats the mucosa.
- Air then distends the colon.
- "See through" colon wall.

Indications:
- Colon cancer screening.
- Family history of cancer.
- Evaluation of inflammatory bowel disease.
- Evaluation of diarrhea, mucous, fever, blood in stool.

Single contrast
Thin barium or water soluble contrast is utilized.
- Can't "see through" the wall.
- Palpation and compression is used to oppose walls.
- Profiling abnormalities, that is, position the patient so the lesion is displayed in profile, relative to the wall.

Indications:
- Senile/debilitated patients who cannot tolerate a double contrast study.
- Therapeutic treatment of Ogilvie syndrome and constipation.
- Diagnosis of volvulus.
- Colon obstruction.
- Neonates and infants (see chapter 6, Pediatrics, p. 304).
- Diagnosis and reduction of intussusception (though air enema more common).

What exam should I order?

Single contrast barium enema
Evaluation for site of obstruction, identify fistulas.

Double contrast barium enema
Cancer screening, diagnosis, and assessment of inflammatory bowel disease.

Water soluble enema
Therapeutic for Ogilvie syndrome, distal intestinal obstruction syndrome [DIOS] of cystic fibrosis, rule out colonic leak, identify some fistulae (e.g., to bladder), rule out volvulus.

Tell the radiologist what you are looking for, and they will decide what study is needed!

Colonic anatomy on lower GI fluoroscopic studies
Normal anatomy
- Muscular tube, 5–6 feet long.
- Semilunar folds.
- Outpouching between them = "haustra" (see Figure 7.13).

Post surgical Anatomy
Partial colectomy
Depending on the indication and clinical scenario, the remaining bowel may be joined:
- With an end-to-end primary anastomosis.
- Permanent colostomy and Hartmann pouch.

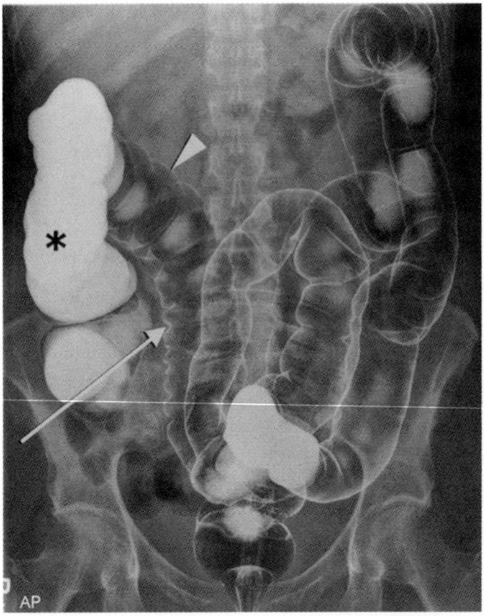

Figure 7.13 Normal double contrast barium enema. Note the accumulation of barium in the ascending colon and hepatic flexure (*), both somewhat posteriorly located, in this supine image. The semilunar folds (arrow) and haustra (arrowhead) are clearly visible. The sigmoid colon forms a large loop in the midline.

- A temporary diverting ileostomy may be created to promote healing:
  - Loop ilestomy—a knuckle of ileum is brought to the skin surface and an opening made to allow efflux of material. This is easier to take down than an end ileostomy.
  - End ileostomy—ileum transected, distal end oversewn, proximal end brought to skin surface.
- Evaluation of the remaining distal colon "Hartmann pouch" may be requested prior to colostomy take down.
  - This is usually done via single contrast enema.

Low anterior resection of the rectum (LAR)
- Indicated for upper rectal cancer or low sigmoid cancers.
- Remaining lower rectum is anastomosed to the colon.
- Sometimes a temporary diverting loop ileostomy is created to allow healing.

Abdominoperineal resection (APR)
- Indicated for low rectal cancers.
- The anus, rectum, and sigmoid colon are excised.
- A permanent sigmoid colostomy is created.

Common conditions evaluated with lower GI tract fluoroscopy

Colon cancer screening
Typically done with endoscopy.
- Double contrast enema typically is reserved for patients who cannot have colonoscopy or for those who have an incomplete colonoscopy (a segment of the colon was not evaluated).
- CT colonography is an alternative, non-invasive method of evaluating the colon that can be used as a screening examination in place of colonoscopy.

Colonic strictures—benign and malignant
Colonic strictures vary in length, cause, and severity. Arriving at a specific diagnosis is often not possible on contrast enema studies.

Malignant
- Adenocarcinoma: produces the characteristic "apple-core" lesion (see Figure 7.14).
- Lymphoma: can cause long segment narrowing.

Benign
- Colitis: all forms will cause narrowing of the colon acutely.
  - Fibrotic stricture may occur after the acute phase.
- Diverticular disease causes a characteristic "saw-tooth" appearance.
- Crohn colitis.
- Ischemia : acute and chronic.

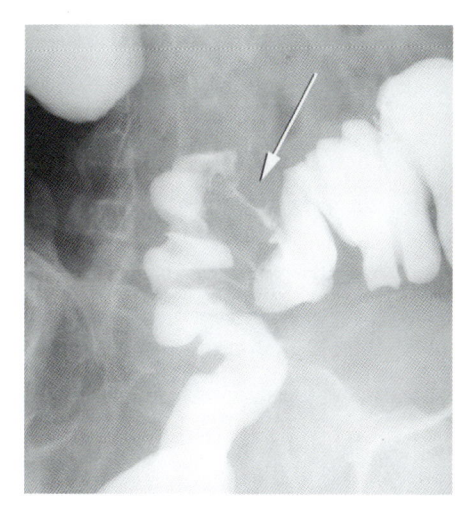

Figure 7.14 Colon cancer. Single contrast barium enema shows an "apple core" lesion (arrow) from an adenocarcinoma of the sigmoid colon.

Colitis
Colitis can be due to ischemia, infection (salmonella, shigella, etc.), inflammatory bowel disease (ulcerative colitis, Crohn and Behçet disease), and radiation.
- Psuedomembranous colitis is seen in the setting of antibiotic use, with resultant overgrowth of *Clostridium difficile*. It can be severe enough to require bowel resection.
  - Most common cause of colitis seen in U.S. hospital setting.

Imaging findings
These are not specific for a causative agent.
- Wall thickening and fold thickening.
- Mucosal ulceration.
- Luminal narrowing.

Diverticular disease
Diverticula are most common in the sigmoid and descending colon; although they can occur anywhere in the colon and less often, the small bowel. Diverticula are very common in the duodenum where they are usually an incidental finding.
- Occur on the anti-mesenteric side of the colon.
- Represent protrusions of the mucosa and submucosa through the muscularis. This occurs where the penetrating vessels pass between the teniae coli.
- Most commonly small; however, they can range from a few millimeters to rare giant sigmoid diverticula.

Diverticulosis
Presence of multiple diverticula. Colonic diverticula become increasingly common with age. When there are many diverticula in a section of bowel, fibrosis can occur, narrowing the bowel lumen, and the patient may complain of constipation or a change in stool caliber.

Imaging findings (see Figure 7.15):
Pouches of variable size that protrude out from the bowel wall.
- When contrast is administered, they often fill with contrast.
- In the absence of contrast, they can sometimes be seen on radiographs or CT as collections of air.

Diverticulitis
Occurs when a diverticulum becomes inflamed or infected. A very small perforation of the diverticulum can occur. This can progress to an abscess, or, less often, to free perforation into the peritoneal cavity.

Imaging findings:
Diverticulitis is usually diagnosed on CT: bowel wall thickening, inflammatory change, and often, a small abscess (see chapter 3, Abdomen, p. 161). Fluoroscopy is not recommended for suspected acute diverticulitis.

Volvulus
Colonic volvulus causes bowel obstruction, edema, and vascular compromise. It is a surgical emergency; if untreated it will result in ischemia and death. Although it is often suspected and sometimes diagnosed on plain

LOWER GI TRACT FLUOROSCOPY

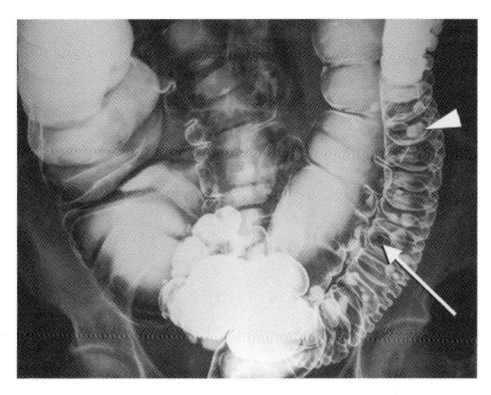

Figure 7.15 Diverticular disease. Air contrast barium enema shows numerous diverticula, predominantly in the descending colon. The dependent ones are contrast filled (arrowhead), and the non-dependent are air filled (arrow).

film or CT, water soluble contrast enema is often confirmatory prior to surgery. (Barium is not used because of the risk of perforation).
- Sigmoid and cecal are the most common types.
- Volvulus can involve other portions of the colon, including the transverse colon.

Imaging findings
Regardless of the site of the volvulus, the column of contrast will end in a tapered twist or "beak." Contrast will not flow beyond this point of twisted bowel.

Cecal volvulus
When the cecum is on a mesentery, it predisposes to volvulus.
- Initially results in cecal distension, then eventually marked upstream dilatation of the small bowel and downstream emptying of the remaining colon.
- It can be diagnosed on radiographs (see Figure 3.19), contrast enema (see Figure 7.16), or CT.

Sigmoid volvulus
When the sigmoid twists, it causes a closed loop obstruction of the sigmoid, which becomes distended, sometimes massively. Upstream dilatation of the entire colon and much of the small bowel can occur.
- It is often diagnosed on radiographs (see Figure 3.18) but contrast enema is sometimes needed (see Figure 7.17). CT can be difficult to interpret due to the mass of gas filled dilated bowel loops.
- Although it is stated that a barium enema can "untwist" the volvulus, in practice this is very rare, but rigid sigmoidoscopy is often therapeutic.

358 CHAPTER 7 **Fluoroscopy**

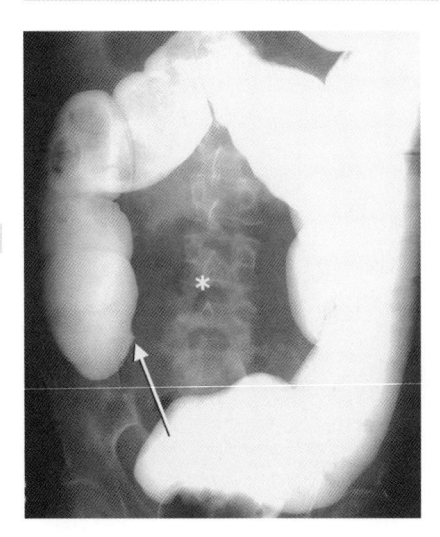

Figure 7.16 Cecal volvulus on barium enema. Large air filled cecum (*) with barium extending to a 'beak' at site of twist. (arrow).

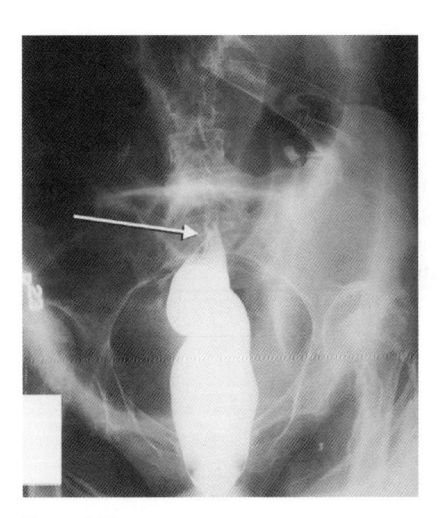

Figure 7.17 Barium enema of a sigmoid volvulus showing barium in the rectum with a "beak" at the site of the twist (arrow).

LOWER GI TRACT FLUOROSCOPY

Polyps
Polypoid lesions in the colon include adenomas, hamartomas, hyperplastic polyps, metastatic lesions and carcinoids. Adenomas have the potential to transform into cancers. There are three forms of adenomas:
- Tubular.
- Villous—highest malignant potential.
- Tubulovillous.

The adenoma-carcinoma sequence is thought to take approximately 10 years, hence the rationale for colonoscopy every 10 years.
- The larger the adenoma, the higher the risk of cancer.

Imaging findings
- Rounded filling defect on a single contrast enema.
- Barium coated lesion protruding into lumen on double contrast enema (see Figure 7.18).
- They are very difficult to see if the colon is not distended or contains stool (which can cause false positive examinations).

Colon Cancer
In 2010, more than 50,000 people died from colorectal cancer in the United States. It occurs most frequently in the rectosigmoid colon. Common complications include bleeding, obstruction, perforation, local recurrence, and metastasis.

Known risk factors for colorectal cancer
- Age>50.
- Colorectal polyps.

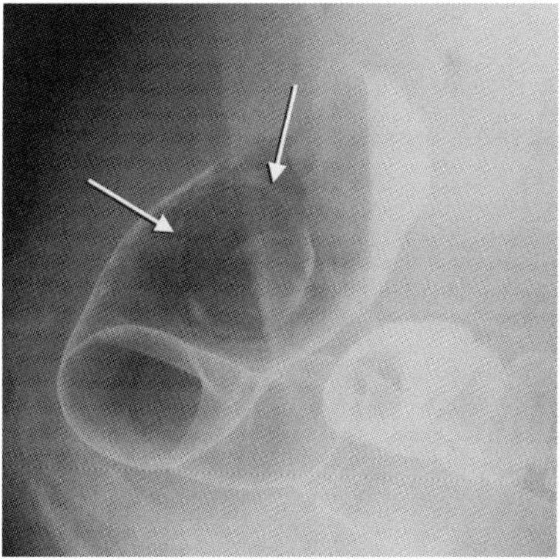

Figure 7.18 Large rectal polyp (arrow) on a double contrast barium enema.

- Family history of colorectal cancer.
- Polyposis syndromes, ulcerative colitis or Crohn disease.
- Personal history of prior colorectal cancer, or women with a history of pelvic or breast cancer.

Imaging findings
There are five radiographic patterns (or a mixture) seen on contrast enemas or CT:
- Polypoid masses.
- Ulcerating plaques.
- Flat plaques.
- Strictures.
- "Apple core lesions" (see Figure 7.14).

GU tract fluoroscopy

What examination should I order and how is it performed?

Voiding cystourethrogram (VCUG)
VCUGs are performed primarily to identify vesicoureteral reflex (VUR) = reflux from the bladder into the ureters/kidneys.
In addition to reflux, this examination can detect:
<u>Bladder</u>: bladder neck dysfunction, bladder diverticuli, tumors.
<u>Ureter</u>: ureterocele, ureteral duplication (if reflux or ureterocele).
<u>Urethra</u>: posterior urethral valves and other pathologies.
(Please refer to the pediatrics chapter for additional information)

Indications
- Infants and young children with first-time urinary tract infection (UTI).
- Because of the high prevalence of familial VUR, asymptomatic siblings are often screened as well.
  - There is considerable ongoing discussion about the best way to image these patients.
  - VCUG is one of many imaging studies that are used.

Technique
- The bladder, after sterile catheterization, is filled to estimated capacity with water soluble contrast via gravity drip.
- The child then voids spontaneously or on request (can be challenging).
  - The voiding phase is key as reflux may only be seen in this phase and it also allows evaluation of the urethra.
- Intermittent fluoroscopy to assess for:
  - Reflux into ureters spontaneously or during voiding.
  - Bladder configuration, capacity, and emptying.

Interpretation
VUR is graded according to the degree of reflux (grade 1–5) and the morphology of the ureters and collecting systems are noted (see Figure 7.21).

Cystogram
A cystogram images only the bladder, not the urethra. Voiding is not performed.

Indications
- To diagnose bladder perforation/leak (trauma or post-surgery). Consider when pelvic fracture/injury with frank hematuria.
- CT cystogram is an alternative (p. 158).

Technique
- After sterile bladder catheterization, the bladder is filled to estimated capacity of tolerance under fluoroscopy via gravity drip.
- AP, oblique, and lateral images are obtained.
- The bladder is emptied and a post-void image taken.

Retrograde urethrogram (RUG)
Indications
- Trauma: including iatrogenic from traumatic catheterization or TURP.
  - Consider in patients with straddle injuries, pubic rami fractures and frank blood at urethral orifice.
- Strictures: post-traumatic or due to infection or tumor.

Technique
- Water soluble contrast is injected into the urethra via a tube placed in the glans of the penis.
- Images are obtained in the oblique/lateral projection to elongate and visualize the entire urethra and to look for strictures, leak, and other pathology.

Anatomy
Divided by the urogenital (UG) diaphragm into 2 segments:
- Posterior: prostatic and membranous, above UG diaphragm.
- Anterior: bulbous and penile, below UG diaphragm.

Imaging findings (see Figure 7.19)

Narrowing—stricture, periurethral hematoma.

Disruption—traumatic rupture.
- Posterior—extravasated contrast in extraperitoneal space, not perineum.
- Anterior—extravasated contrast in perineum.

IVP
An IVP or intravenous pyelogram (sometimes called IVU, intravenous urogram) provides both physiologic and anatomic information about the GU tract. Previously a very commonly performed study, it is now largely replaced by CT urography (see chapter 3, Abdomen/Pelvis, p. 139).
- It remains useful in situations in which specific information is needed, such as the configuration of the ureter.
- Tailoring the exam to the specific indication can reduce radiation dose.

Technique
- Non-contrast tomograms obtained (look for stones).
- IV contrast is injected and a series of images (radiographs and tomograms) are taken, showing phases in the renal metabolism of contrast:
  - Nephrographic phase: uniform renal enhancement.
  - Excretory phase: contrast opacifies the renal collecting sytem, ureters, and bladder.

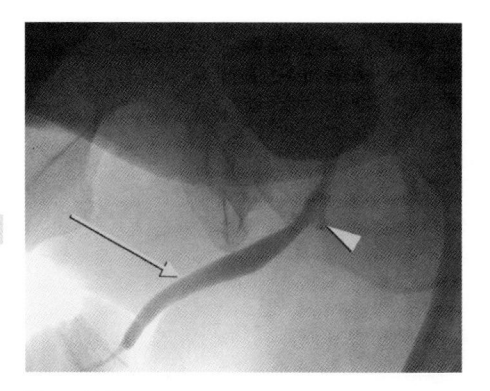

Figure 7.19 Retrograde urethrogram (oblique image) in a patient after a saddle injury. The normal urethra is smooth (arrow). There is extravasation of contrast from the membranous urethra (arrowhead).

Imaging findings

Nephrographic phase:
- Diffuse asymmetric renal enhancement indicates pathology (e.g., obstruction, renal artery stenosis).
- Focal rounded defects: masses (cysts, solid).
- Cortical scars: infection, trauma, surgery.

Excretory phase look for:
- Symmetry of timing of excretion.
- Dilatation of collecting system (calyces, pelvis, ureter)—focal or diffuse.
- Ureteral strictures (tumor, traumatic, inflammatory, iatrogenic).
- Intraluminal filling defects (stones, tumors).
- Extraluminal masses (prostate, pelvic, and retroperitoneal masses).
- Mural irregularity of the collecting system or bladder (tumor, infection, inflammation, bladder hypertrophy).

Hysterosalpingogram (HSG)
HSG is performed as part of an infertility work up. Performed with fluoroscopy (see Figure 7.20).

Technique
- Using sterile technique, the cervix is cannulated and water soluble contrast is injected into the uterus and fallopian tubes.
- AP and oblique images are obtained.

Imaging findings
- Look for opacification of the fallopian tubes, and free spill of contrast out of the distal ends of the tubes into the peritoneal cavity (this indicates tubal patency).
- Look for filling defects or irregularities within the endometrial cavity.

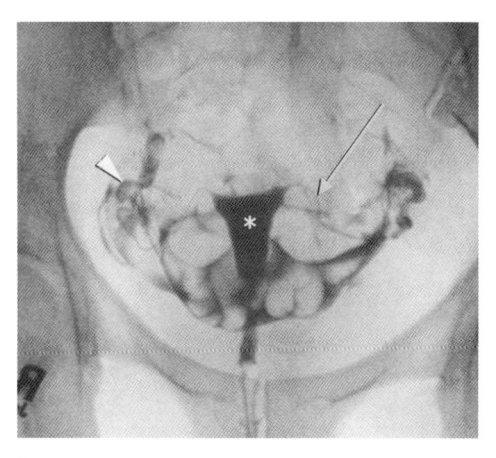

Figure 7.20 Normal HSG. The image shows contrast filling the endometrial cavity (*) and fallopian tubes and spilling into the peritoneal cavity where it surrounds the bowel loops in the pelvis. Note isthmus (arrow) and ampulla (arrow head) of fallopian tubes.

Pathology demonstrable on HSG

<u>Uterus:</u> duplications and other congenital deformity, masses such as fibroids, polyps, synechiae.

<u>Fallopian tubes:</u> obstruction, dilatation, salpingitis isthmica nodosa (Fallopian tube diverticuli, associated with infertility and risk of ectopic pregnancy).

What exam should I order?

VCUG
Urinary tract infection, family history of reflux, prenatal hydronephrosis, evaluation of other known GU anomalies, posterior urethral valves (males).

Cystogram
Pelvic trauma, post op, assess neobladder, leak, fistula.

Retrograde urethrogram
Perineal trauma, infection, disruption/leak, stricture.

IVP
Now uncommonly performed. Indications include hematuria in young patient (less radiation than CT urogram), limited studies in pregnant women usually for stones, trauma, tumor, stricture, stone, obstruction.

Hysterosalpingogram
Infertility, hydrosalpinx, anomalies of the uterus or tubes.

Common conditions evaluated with GU tract fluoroscopy

Renal calculi (stones)
There are several types of renal calculi. Some are radiopaque (visible on radiographs/CT depending on size) whereas others aren't:

Radiopaque:
- Calcium oxalate or calcium phosphate: most common.
- Struvite: Caused by a bacterial infection that alkalinizes urine pH.
  - Most staghorn calculi (calculi that form in the renal pelvis and extend into the calyces) are struvite.

Slightly radiopaque:
- Cystine: cystinuria, an autosomal recessive disease.
  - Results in the formation of cystine stones.

Not radiopaque:
- Uric acid: occur in patients with gout.
- Xanthine: are rare.
  - They can be caused by xanthinuria, a rare autosomal recessive disease, or by treatment for gout with allopurinol.

How to diagnose renal calculi
- <u>Radiography</u>: can demonstrate some radiopaque stones; often stones are too small to be visible.
- <u>CT</u>: easily demonstrable.
- <u>IVP</u>: will be seen on the initial tomographic images, then appear as filling defect on excretory images +/− signs obstruction.

Hydronephrosis
Hydronephrosis or pelvicalyectasis, is dilatation of the renal collecting system due to obstruction. This can be diagnosed on US, CT, MRI, or IVP.
See chapter 3, "Urolithiasis and hydronephrosis," p. 173 for details.

Vesicoureteral reflux (VUR)
Imaging findings on VCUG
- Retrograde flow of contrast up ureters.
  - If small volume, can be obscured by distended bladder on AP view, but visible on oblique views.
- Classification of VUR is based on how high the contrast refluxes and how dilated the system becomes (see Figures 7.21 and 7.22).

Bladder masses
Most bladder tumors are transitional cell carcinomas. A small percentage are squamous cell carcinoma, and rarely adenocarcinoma.
- On IVP or cystogram, bladder cancer will look like a filling defect in the contrast opacified bladder.
- Adjacent pathology can cause mass effect on the bladder, which can be confused for a filling defect.
  - Benign prostatic hypertrophy is a very common cause of extrinsic compression in older men and often causes relative or complete bladder outlet obstruction.

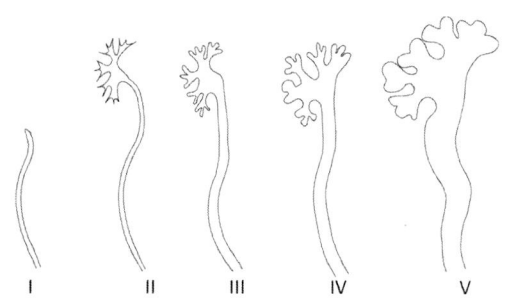

Figure 7.21 Vesicoureteral reflux grading, adapted from the International Classification of Vesicoureteral Reflux.

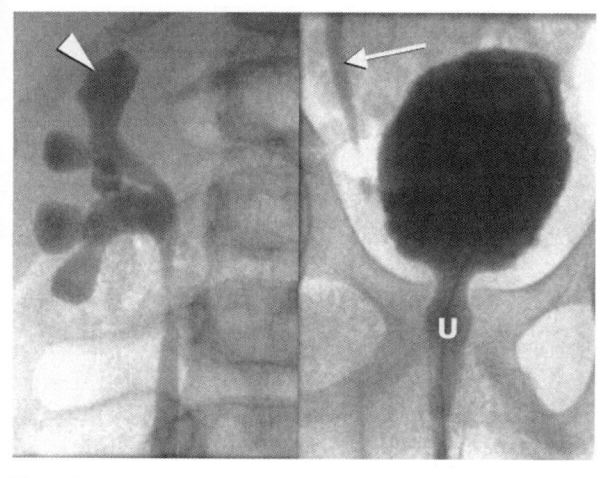

Figure 7.22 Vesicoureteral reflux. VCUG image obtained on voiding shows reflux into lower ureter (arrow). Contrast reaches the calyces, which are blunt without pelvis or ureter dilation making this grade 3 VUR (arrowhead). U = urethra.

> **Bladder Filling Defects: differential diagnosis**
> - Transitional cell carcinoma, other cancers.
> - Stone.
> - Blood clot.
> - Fungus ball.
> - Ureterocele.
> - Prostate cancer or hypertrophy.

Bladder rupture
Bladder rupture occurs in the setting of trauma, including iatrogenic. Diagnosed using a cystogram or CT cystogram.

Extraperitoneal rupture
- Occurs with pelvic fractures.
- Typically involves the base and anterior aspect of the bladder.
- Fluoroscopically, there will be streaky contrast adjacent to the bladder.

Intraperitoneal rupture (see Figure 7.23)
- Usually due to blunt trauma or instrumentation, and is located at the dome of the bladder.
- The contrast will leak into the peritoneum, appearing smooth and surrounding bowel loops.

> What if you cannot differentiate intraperitoneal from extraperitoneal leak? In this situation, limited CT is performed immediately following the cystogram. The extravasated contrast will persist and the compartment can be confidently diagnosed with CT.

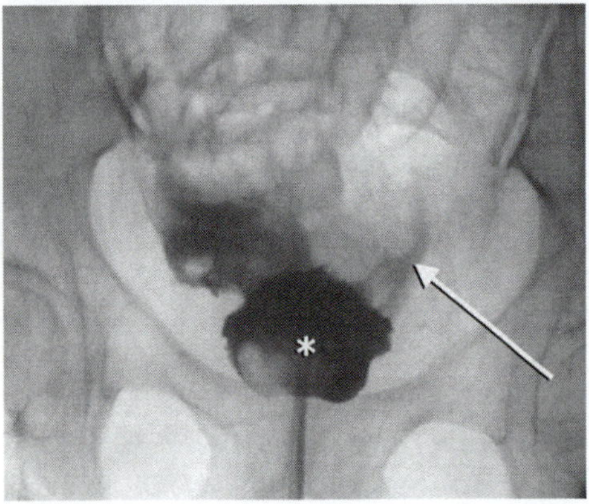

Figure 7.23 Intraperitoneal bladder rupture. Cystogram shows contrast and the foley catheter in the bladder (*). Extravasated contrast surrounds bowel loops (arrow), confirming intraperitoneal rupture.

Tube studies

What examination should I order and how is it performed?
Feeding tubes
Types

<u>Gastric tubes (G tube):</u>
- Placed into the stomach, used for feeding or venting.
- Nasogastric, orogastric, or percutaneous (percutaneous gastrostomy tube, see "Interventional Radiology" section).

<u>Jejunostomy tubes (J tube):</u>
- Placed directly into the jejunum, used for feeding.
- Placed at time of surgery or percutaneously via gastrostomy.

<u>Gastro-jejunostomy tube (GJ tube):</u>
- 2 coaxial catheters, one within the other.
- One lumen is placed into the stomach, and the second component extends into the jejunum.

<u>Dobhoff tube (DHT):</u>
- Fine bore catheter with weighted tip to help it pass into the GI tract.
- Passed through the nose or mouth into the stomach or ideally into the duodenum.
- Used for temporary feeding.

Role of fluoroscopy
- Tube placement under fluoroscopy is done in cases of difficult placement.
- Tube injection studies:
  - Determine location, patency or leakage of percutaneous tubes.
  - Assess adjacent bowel for perforation.
  - Study the GI tract in a patient who cannot drink contrast.
- Lateral view should be obtained to look for contrast reflux along catheter tract.

> **What if you cannot get the feeding tube placed?**
> It can be placed with fluoroscopic guidance, but first try using the right decubitus position; often helps Dobhoff tubes enter the duodenum.
> ALWAYS confirm tube position with a "high" abdominal radiograph (kidneys, ureters, bladder [KUB]) to include lower chest before feeding patients through a tube.

T-tube cholangiogram
During cholecystectomy, a T-tube may be left in the common bile duct for access if there is concern for residual stones.
- After appropriate antibiotics, the tube is injected, under sterile technique, with water soluble contrast.
- The injection is a small quantity, under low pressure to evaluate the intra and extrahepatic biliary tree.

Imaging findings
- Look for filling defects that may indicates stones.
- Assess patency: is there free flow of contrast into the duodenum?
- Look for extravasated contrast, which would indicate a leak.

Drain injections
Any kind of drain can be injected with water soluble contrast.

Indications
- To assess drain patency.
- To determine whether there is communication with bowel.
- To determine if there is any residual abscess cavity prior to drain removal.

References

Eisenber RL, *Gastrointestinal Radiology: A Pattern Approach*, Lippincott Williams & Wilkins, Philadelphia, PA 2003.

Gay SB, Woodcock RJ, *Radiology Recall*, 2nd ed. Lippincott Williams & Wilkins, Philadelphia, PA 2008.

Levine MS, Rubesin SE, Laufer I, Pattern approach for diseases of mesenteric small bowel on barium studies. *Radiology*, 2008; 249: 445–460.

Schueler BA, The AAPM/RSNA physics tutorial for residents general overview of fluoroscopic imaging., *RadioGraphics*, 2000; 20: 1115–1126.

Chapter 8

Neuroimaging

Rihan Khan, MD

Brain
- CT technique *364*
- How do I read a head CT? *365*
- MR technique *366*
- How do I read a head MR? *367*

Patterns of disease *368*
- Normal aging *368*
- Edema *370*
- Mass effect, midline shift, and herniation patterns *371*
- Hydrocephalus and CSF dynamics *375*
- Blood *377*
- Vascular pathology *379*
- Masses *382*
- Meningeal disease *383*

Common conditions *383*
- "Stroke"/Cerebral infarction *383*
- Trauma *385*
- Primary brain tumors *390*
- Cerebral metastases *391*
- Peripheral nerve-sheath tumors *392*
- Infection and inflammation *392*
- Multiple sclerosis *393*
- Seizure disorders *393*

Head and neck *395*
- Sinus disease *395*
- Facial trauma *396*
- Lymphadenopathy *397*
- Infection *397*

Spine *399*
- What imaging test do I order? *399*
- Degenerative disc disease *400*
- Disc herniation *400*
- Masses *401*
- Myelopathy *402*
- Trauma *403*
- Infection *406*

Procedures *408*
Don't miss diagnoses *410*
References *410*

CT

How are images acquired?
Head CT scans can be acquired in one or more planes, and then reconstructed into other planes. The head can be tilted and the gantry can be angled in order to obtain direct coronal plane images (not possible in the chest or abdomen). The reconstructed images may be of lower resolution ('quality') than the primary scanning planes, but do not add additional radiation. When possible, CT scans of the head are acquired at an angle, to avoid irradiating the lens of the eye.

When is IV contrast used?
- CT angiograms (CTA): Carotid arteries, Circle of Willis (COW).
- CT Neck: To differentiate vessels from lymph nodes and other structures. When neoplasm, infection, inflammation are suspected.
- CT Head: When neoplasm, infection, inflammation are suspected.

DO NOT use for trauma—may obscure subarachnoid hemorrhage.

Common CT protocols
Head CT
- Axial images +/− coronal and or sagittal reformats.
- 3–5 mm slice thickness.

Neck CT
- Contrast enhanced axial images with coronal and sagittal reformats routinely performed.
- 3–5 mm slice thickness.

Orbits, face, temporal bones, sinuses
- Helical acquisition with axial and coronal reformats. (Direct axial and direct coronal images obtained at some institutions.)
- Generally, contrast is not indicated unless there is concern for an abscess.
- Thin slices; typically < 3 mm, often 0.6–1.25 for temporal bones.

Spine CT
- Axial images with coronal and sagittal reformats.
- Contrast is rarely indicated.
- Thin slices; typically < 3 mm.

CTA
- Contrast enhanced, with axial, coronal, sagittal, and 3D reformats.
- Slice thickness varies; thin slices to see vessel origins, thicker slices/MIP reformats to evaluate for aneurysm.

Brain perfusion
- A contrast enhanced CT which assesses regional cerebral blood flow and volume, and mean transit time of contrast through a region of brain.
- Most commonly used in tumors to assess for recurrence (post-treatment) and in stroke evaluation, to detect areas of reversible ischemia.

Normal anatomy

A complete review is beyond the scope of this text. See references for sources for study. Selected terms and concepts will be presented.

Compartments
- Intra-axial: includes the brain and spinal cord.
- Extra-axial: everything outside the brain and spinal cord.
- Supratentorial: above the tentorium (the cerebrum, thalamus, and hypothalamus).
- Infratentorial: below the tentorium (the cerebellum and brainstem).

Meninges
- Pia: thin, translucent, innermost layer, firmly attached to the brain and spinal cord.
- Arachnoid: thin membrane adherent to the dura and connected to the pia by cobweb-like strands.
- Dura: firm fibrous, consists of outer layer (the periosteum of the skull) and an inner layer. Dural partitions project inward to incompletely separate parts of the brain (e.g., falx cerebri, tentorium).

Dural venous sinuses
The two layers of the dura split in certain locations to form the venous sinuses. Cortical and deep veins drain into these, which drain primarily via the internal jugular veins.

Spaces
- Subarachnoid: between arachnoid and pia, filled with CSF. Arteries reside here.
- Subdural: potential space between the dura and the arachnoid mater.
- Epidural: potential space bounded by the outer layer of dura mater and the inner table of the calvarium.

Cisterns
Regional enlargements of the subarachnoid space. Contain CSF and blood vessels. Cisterns commonly discussed clinically:
- Suprasellar: above the sella, star shaped. Contains the optic chiasm, arteries, pituitary stalk.
- Peri-mesencephalic: around the midbrain.
  - ambient and interpeduncular (anterior).
  - quadrigeminal (posterior).
- Cisterna magna: around junction of the cord, medulla, and cerebellum.

How do I read a head CT?

There are many methods to read a head CT; the most important point is to be consistent and complete! Develop a search pattern and use it consistently.

Search strategies
Appropriate image windowing should be used; these are listed in parenthesis. See p. 7

Parenchyma (brain)
- Evaluate gray/white matter differentiation: Is it distinct?
  - The internal capsules should be distinct from the thalamus and globus pallidus.

- Look for the normal thin "ribbon" of cortical gray matter.
- Look for symmetry of attenuation, focal areas of abnormal attenuation; either high (blood, enhancement) or low.

Look for mass effect (brain)
- Displacement of falx and appearance and symmetry of ventricles.
- Effacement of sulci.
- Displacement of cortex.

Extra-axial space, ventricles (brain, blood)
- Cerebrospinal fluid should be uniformly low attenuation.
- Lateral ventricles should be symmetric in size and shape.
- CSF cisterns should be patent and symmetric.
- Blood windows improve visualization of small areas of hemorrhage against the inner table of the skull.

Sinuses and mastoid air cells (bone)
- Should be well aerated without mucosal thickening or fluid levels
- Bony margins should be well defined and smooth.

Orbits (soft tissue)
- Orbital fat should be uniformly low attenuation.
- Muscles should be symmetric and well defined.

Bones (bone)
- Follow the contours of osseous structures.
  - Look for fractures, lesions in medullary spaces.

MRI

How are images acquired?
Each MRI exam is comprised of multiple pulse sequences, selected to aid in visualization of pertinent structures and detection of pathology.

Pulse sequences commonly used in neuroimaging

T1: Good for anatomy. CSF dark.

T2: Good for pathology. CSF bright.

FLAIR: Excellent for pathology. Free fluid (i.e., CSF) dark, pathologic fluid (i.e., edema) bright.

Diffusion: Assesses freedom of movement (diffusion) of water molecules. Regions of restricted diffusion of water, (such as in infarcted tissue) are high signal intensity. Other pathologies that are T2 bright may also be bright on diffusion ("T2 shine through").

Apparent diffusion coefficient maps (ADC maps): Are generated from the diffusion images. Translates diffusion information into a quantitative measure of water movement (mm/sec). The contrast on these images relies entirely on differences of diffusion. They are used primarily to differentiate true restricted diffusion from "T2 shine through."

Short T1 inversion recovery (STIR): Has inherent fat saturation. Commonly used in spine imaging to augment detection of bone marrow and paraspinal edema (very useful in trauma).

Gradient recalled echo (GRE): Paramagnetic and ferromagnetic substances (i.e., metal, calcification, most blood products except hyperacute blood) cause loss of signal locally on this sequence, which blooms, making it easier to identify them.

Common MRI/MRA protocols
Brain
- T2, T1, FLAIR, and diffusion sequences. (GRE sometimes obtained).
- Use of contrast depends on indication.
- Additional sequences are obtained for multiple sclerosis, epilepsy, and congenital abnormalities.

Neck
- Contrast is almost always needed.
- Fat saturation is important to increase the conspicuity of pathologic enhancement.

Spine
- No contrast if indication is disc disease/pathology or trauma.
- Contrast required for primary cord tumors and metastatic disease.

Temporal bones and orbits/face
- MRI is usually done with contrast to look for masses, infection, and occasionally perineural spread of tumor.
- Not done specifically to evaluate the bones; CT is superior.

MRA head and neck
- Brain: Contrast not required, 3D time-of-flight (TOF) performed.
- Carotid:
  - Non-contrast techniques are limited due to slow acquisition, large area that needs to be covered, and artifacts.
  - Contrast enhanced (gadolinium) MRA is superior to noncontrast MRA in the neck. Images are reformatted in MIP and 3D.

When is IV contrast used?
- MR angiography (MRA) of the neck.
- MR of soft tissues of neck.
- MR brain, spine, and orbits: for neoplasm, infection, and inflammatory processes.

How do I read a head MR?
With the multiple MRI sequences performed with each study, the approach is somewhat different than CT. Again, a consistent and complete search pattern is essential.

Search strategies
Parenchyma
- Evaluate gray/white matter differentiation—is it distinct?
- Look for symmetry of or alteration in signal intensity
  - Often best seen on T2; many pathologies are T2 bright.
- Look for structural deviations/alterations in normal anatomy.
  - Best appreciated on T1 or any sequence where the signal intensity of gray versus white matter is very different.

- Look for restricted diffusion: Bright signal on diffusion images.
  - May be dark on ADC map (e.g., infarct).
  - May be bright on ADC map (other etiologies)

> **All that is bright on diffusion does not represent infarct**
> - Acute infarcts are bright on DWI and dark on the ADC map.
> - Some T2 bright lesions will show up as bright on diffusion; these will be bright on the ADC map as well.
>   - This is called "T2 shine through" and does not represent truly restricted diffusion.

Blood and calcifications
Often best seen on gradient echo images (GRE).
- Both appear dark and produce artifact.
- Note: hyperacute blood will not look dark.

Mass effect
See CT p. 372

Extra-axial spaces and structures
- CSF should be uniform in signal intensity.
- Lateral ventricles should be symmetric in size and shape.
- CSF cisterns should be patent and symmetric.
- Arteries will look black on T2 images (called a "flow void"). Make sure normal flow voids are present.

Conventional angiography

See chapter 10, "Interventional Radiology," for more details on angiography technique p. 456.
  See "Procedures" section, later in this chapter, p. 414.

Patterns of disease

Normal aging
As we develop and age, there are expected changes in brain that are important to recognize.

Infant and young child
At birth, the majority of the white matter is not yet myelinated and the white matter regions have a high water content.
- CT: White matter is diffusely hypodense.
- MRI: White matter looks T1 dark/T2 bright (opposite of adult pattern).
- In general, as a child develops, myelination occurs from caudal to cephalad and from dorsal to ventral.

How to assess myelination
At certain ages, either T1 or T2 is better for assessing myelination:
- Birth to 6 months: T1 images (see Figure 8.1).

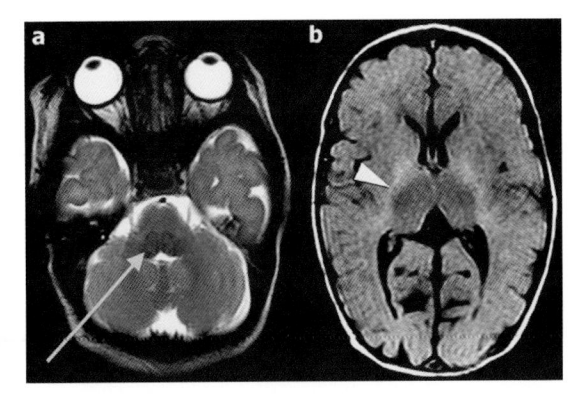

Figure 8.1 Myelination in a 3-day-old infant. (a) T2-weighted axial MRI image shows the myelinated dorsal pons (arrow) to be dark. (b) T1-weighted axial MRI image shows the myelinated posterior limb of the internal capsule (arrowhead) to be bright.

- > 6 months: T2 images.
- > 2 years old: adult myelination pattern present.

Adolescent and adult
Adult pattern of myelination achieved by 2 years of age.
This pattern persists until either normal changes of aging occur, or pathological conditions ensue.

Older adult and elderly
Brain volume loss
A certain degree of parenchymal volume loss occurs with aging, which is deemed age appropriate and not considered pathologic. Gauging what is within normal limits for age comes with experience!
Etiology:
In many cases, loss of brain volume is related to chronic small vessel ischemic disease.
Imaging findings (see Figure 8.2)
- As parenchyma is lost, CSF fills in the space.
- Diffuse enlargement of the subarachnoid spaces.
- Enlargement of the ventricular system ("ex vacuo" dilatation).

Calcifications
Normal senescent calcifications occur at characteristic locations:
- Globus pallidus, typically bilateral and often symmetric.
- Pineal gland.
- Choroid plexus: Can be seen in any portion of the choroid, often seen in the lateral ventricles, and in the foramen of Luschka (lateral apertures).
- Dural calcifications: Usually smooth, may be anywhere along the dura, including the falx and the tentorium.

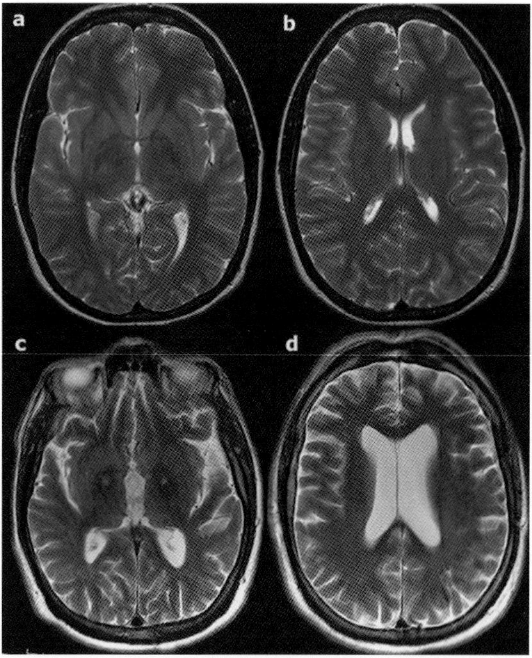

Figure 8.2 (a,b) Normal adult brain volume. (c,d) Cerebral/parenchymal volume loss with aging. Note the enlargement of the third and lateral ventricles with concordant enlargement of the sulcal spaces.

Edema

Edema is nonspecific and can be caused by a variety of conditions including tumor, infection, inflammation,etc.. In the brain, edema is categorized into one of two types and each has different causes.

Vasogenic edema
- Due to leaky capillaries causing fluid to leak into the interstitium.
- Limited to the white matter, as the gray matter is more tightly packed with little room to accommodate fluid.
- Occurs secondary to another process, i.e., peri-tumoral edema, abscess, cerebritis, posterior reversible encephalopathy syndrome (PRES),etc.

<u>Imaging findings</u> (see Figure 8.3):
- CT: Abnormal low attenuation within the white matter, which respects the gray-white matter boundary, sparing the gray matter.
- MRI: High T2 signal in the white matter, again respecting the gray-white junction.

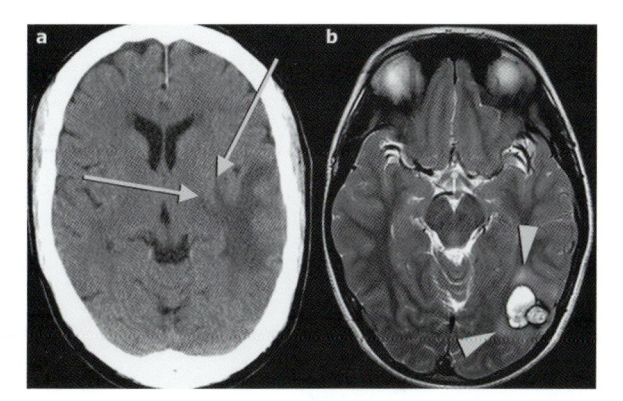

Figure 8.3 Vasogenic edema in two patients. (a) Unenhanced CT shows low attenuation limited to the white matter, sparing the gray matter. The edema involves the internal and external capsules (arrows). The causative mass is not shown. (b) T2-weighted MRI of a cavernous malformation (hypointense rim called a hemosiderin ring) shows more subtle vasogenic edema as increased T2 signal, also respecting the gray-white junction (arrowheads).

Cytotoxic edema
Due to cell dysfunction and ultimately death, (e.g., ischemia, hypoxia).
- Caused by loss of function of normal cell membrane pumps, resulting in accumulation of fluid within the cells.
- Represents cellular edema (not the interstitium as in vasogenic).
- Cortex *and* subcortical white matter involved.

<u>Imaging findings (see Figure 8.4):</u>
- CT: Abnormal low attenuation and swelling in gray and white matter
- MRI: High signal intensity of gray and white matter on T2-weighted images.
- Both: Blurring of the gray-white junction.

> **Keys to categorizing edema**
> **Vasogenic**: Involves the white matter and spares the cortex and other gray matter. Looks like finger-like projections when it involves subcortical white matter.
> **Cytotoxic**: Involves the cortex and/or deep gray matter. Cortex looks thicker, swollen. May efface adjacent sulci.

Mass effect, midline shift, and herniation patterns
Identifying mass effect is critical to patient survival. Identify the primary pathology (i.e., mass, bleed, cytotoxic edema) and then look for the associated mass effect.

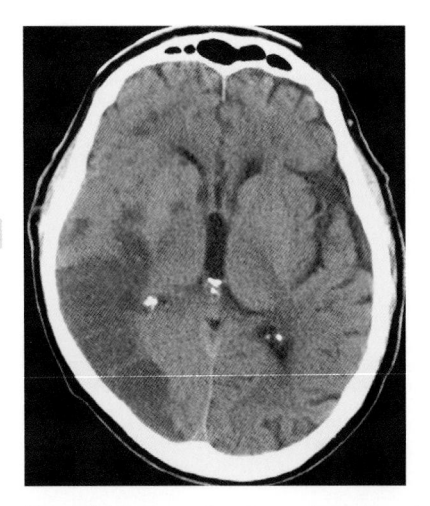

Figure 8.4 Cytotoxic edema from a right middle cerebral artery infarct. Low attenuation involves both gray and white matter throughout a portion of the right middle cerebral artery territory. The adjacent sulci are effaced from mass effect.

Local mass effect
Caused by direct compression (e.g., mass, bleed), or by edematous expansion of the brain (e.g., small infarct).

Imaging findings (see Figures 8.4 and 8.5)
- Effacement of sulci.
- Effacement of adjacent ventricle.

Midline shift and subfalcine herniation
With increased unilateral hemispheric pressure, midline structures (including the falx cerebri) are displaced into the contralateral hemisphere (midline shift). Herniation of the cerebral parenchyma underneath the falx cerebri can occur (subfalcine herniation).

Imaging findings (see Figures 8.5 and 8.6)
Falx cerebri, septum pellucidum or third ventricle deviated from midline position.
- Ipsilateral ventricular effacement.
- Coronal images may show cingulate gyrus herniating under the falx.
- The contralateral ventricle may be dilated due to obstruction of the foramen of Monroe (interventricular foramen).

Along with the brain, the anterior cerebral arteries can also herniate under the falx to the contralateral side. This may lead to ACA compression resulting in an anterior cerebral artery infarct.

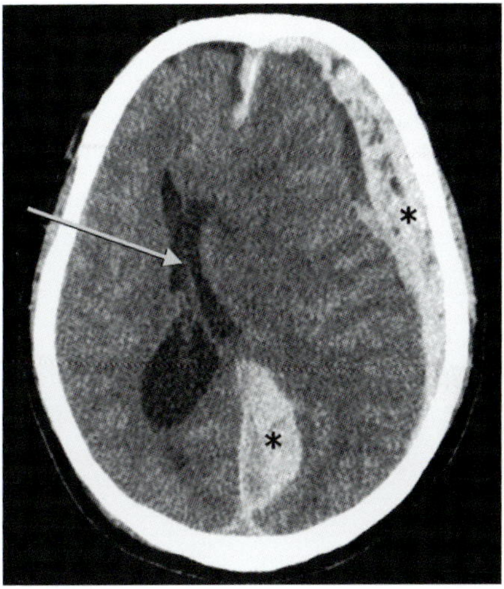

Figure 8.5 Subfalcine herniation. Large left subdural hematoma (*) extends along the anterior and posterior falx and causes local mass effect (sulcal effacement), midline shift and subfalcine herniation. Note the significant rightward displacement of the septum pellucidum from midline (arrow).

Transtentorial herniation

Ascending/upward herniation
Rare. Occurs with infratentorial mass effect (e.g., posterior fossa bleed, tumor, infarct).

<u>Imaging findings</u>
- Cerebellar vermis herniates superiorly through the tentorial incisura.
- Crowding of the quadrigeminal cisterns, displacement of midbrain.
- Effacement of the fourth ventricle.

Descending/downward herniation
Occurs with supratentorial mass effect. Can be unilateral (uncal herniation) or bilateral.

<u>Imaging findings</u> (see Figure 8.7)
- Crowding/loss of the suprasellar cistern and subarachnoid spaces around the midbrain.
- Check for patent CSF spaces under the tentorium.

Uncal herniation
With mass effect in one of the cerebral hemispheres, the ipsilateral uncus (mesial temporal lobe) is displaced medially.
- Can shift over the edge of the tentorial incisura, compressing the midbrain and ipsilateral third cranial nerve (transtentorial herniation).

Imaging findings (Figure 8.6)
- Uncus and medial temporal lobe medially displaced, contact/deform the midbrain.
- Narrowing of ipsilateral suprasellar cistern.
- Narrowing of the contralateral prepontine cistern, and widening of the ipsilateral cistern (as the cerebrum shifts, it pushes the brainstem with it, causing ipsilateral widening and contralateral narrowing).

> Downward transtentorial herniation can cause the posterior cerebral arteries to stretch downward along with the herniating midbrain.
> - May cause PCA compression with resultant PCA infarct

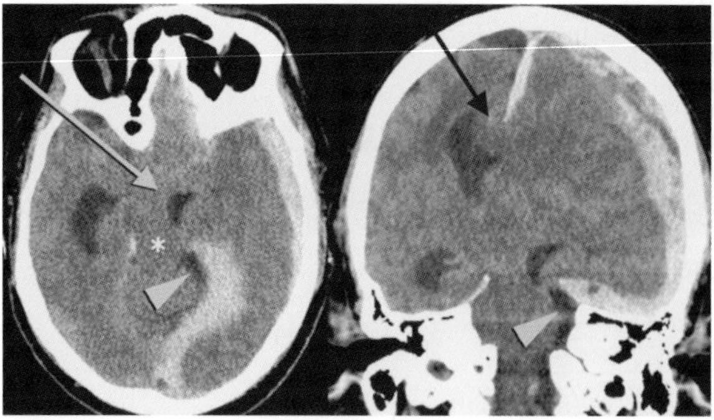

Figure 8.6 Uncal herniation from left subdural hematoma. The left uncus is deviated medially (white arrow), compresses the midbrain (*) and shifts it to the right. Note the widening of the ipsilateral prepontine cistern (arrowheads). The left ventricle is compressed, and the right is dilated (trapped). Coronal image also shows the subfalcine herniation (black arrow).

Tonsillar herniation
Downward herniation of posterior fossa structures.
- Occurs with posterior fossa mass effect (e.g., bleed, tumor, infarct, extension of downward transtentorial herniation).
- Very poor prognosis.

Imaging findings (see Figure 8.8)
- Cerebellar tonsils descend through the foramen magnum and compress the medulla.
- Loss of the CSF space at the foramen magnum (cisterna magna).

> Don't confuse tonsillar herniation with a Chiari malformation (a congenital abnormality)! In a Chiari malformation, the tonsils extend below the level of the foramen magnum, but there is no associated mass effect!

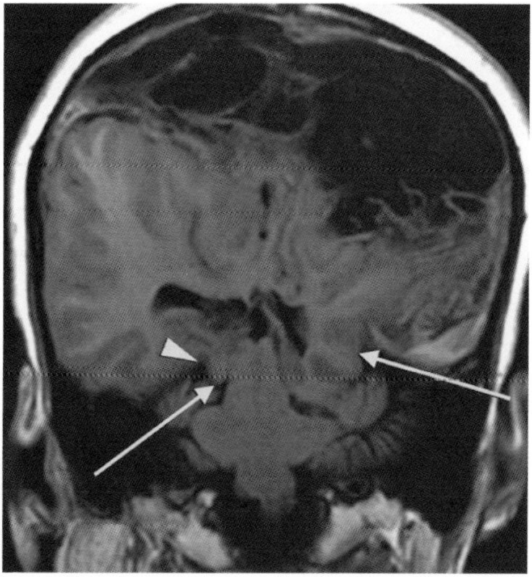

PATTERNS OF DISEASE

Figure 8.7 Large epidural hematoma causing downward transtentorial herniation. Portions of the left occipital and temporal lobes (arrows) are herniating downward through the tentorial incisura; note that these portions of the cerebrum are seen adjacent to the midbrain. Note the contour abnormality of the right parahippocampal gyrus (arrowhead) due to extrinsic compression/impingement from the tentorial free edge.

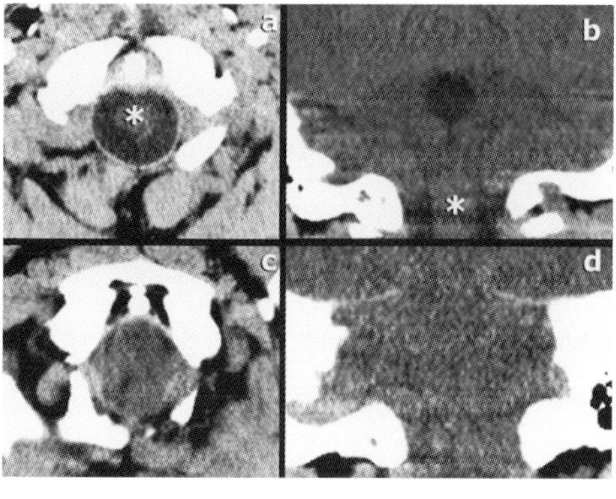

Figure 8.8 Tonsillar herniation. (a,b) On this normal exam, low density CSF surrounds the cervico-medullary junction (*). (c, d) Notice fullness and loss of CSF cisterns at the foramen magnum on both axial and coronal images due to downward herniation of the cerebellar tonsils.

Hydrocephalus and CSF dynamics

CSF is produced by the choroid plexus within the lateral, third and fourth ventricles. It flows out of the ventricular system through the lateral and median apertures (foramina of Luschka and Magendie) in the fourth ventricle, and flows around the spinal cord and brain. It is reabsorbed over the convexity through the arachnoid granulations.

Hydrocephalus

A condition with abnormal dilatation of the ventricles. May be due to overproduction of CSF, obstruction of CSF flow, or lack of resorption.

Overproduction of CSF

Tumors of the choroid plexus overproduce CSF.
- Choroid plexus papilloma and choroid plexus carcinoma.
- Look for intraventricular mass.

Obstructive hydrocephalus

<u>Communicating obstructive hydrocephalus:</u>
Obstruction of CSF resorption at the level of the arachnoid granulations.
- Etiologies: blood products, infectious debris, and tumor such as leptomeningeal carcinomatosis.
- All ventricles should be uniformly dilated.

<u>Noncommunicating obstructive hydrocephalus (see Figure 8.9):</u>
Obstruction of CSF outflow from the ventricular system.
- Etiologies: tumor, cyst, blood clot, mass effect from adjacent parenchymal process, and congenital aqueductal stenosis.
- Continued CSF production by the choroid plexus produces ventricular dilatation upstream from the obstruction.
  - Pattern of dilatation depends on the location of obstruction.

Imaging findings in hydrocephalus
- Ventricular enlargement without sulcal enlargement.
  - Look for temporal horn enlargement, an early sign.
  - Frontal horns of the lateral ventricles appear rounded.
- The sulci become effaced.
- Transependymal edema may be present.
  - As ventricular pressure increases, fluid is forced through the ependymal lining into the peri-ventricular white matter.
  - Hypodensity/increased T2 or FLAIR signal around ventricles.

PATTERNS OF DISEASE

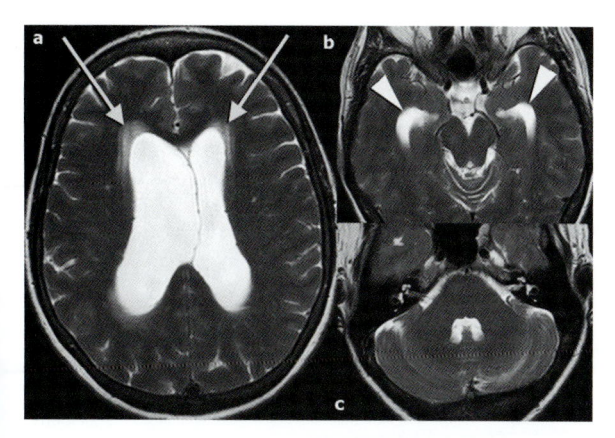

Figure 8.9 Noncommunicating obstructive hydrocephalus. (a) The lateral ventricles are enlarged, with rounded frontal horns, and there is transependymal edema (arrows). (b) Notice the temporal horn tip enlargement (arrowheads). (c) The fourth ventricle is normal in caliber, as was the third ventricle (not shown); obstruction was from a colloid cyst in the anterior third ventricle obstructing the interventricular foramina.

Not all that is dilated is hydrocephalus!
When there is parenchymal volume loss, there is compensatory increased ventricular size. This is called "ex-vacuo" dilatation. (see "Normal aging," p. 375).

Normal pressure hydrocephalus (NPH)
Clinical syndrome with three main findings: incontinence, gait disturbance, and cognitive decline. Imaging findings that have been described are nonspecific but include:
- Enlarged ventricular system out of proportion to the size of the subarachnoid spaces.
- Rim of periventricular T2 hyperintesity.
- Hyperdynamic CSF flow in the cerebral aqueduct, which may be seen as a flow void on conventional MRI imaging.

Blood
Intracranial hemorrhage can result from trauma or occur spontaneously (related to hypertension, infarct, or aneurysm rupture).
Intracranial blood must first be identified and then characterized for acuity (age). Blood varies in appearance on both CT and MRI, depending on its age. There is a natural progression in the density and signal intensity changes over time (see Figure 8.10).

CHAPTER 8 Neuroimaging

CT blood density changes with time

Hyperacute	High attenuation with areas of low attenuation (non-clotted blood).
Acute	High attenuation.
Subacute	Attenuation decreases.
Chronic	Low attenuation, like CSF.

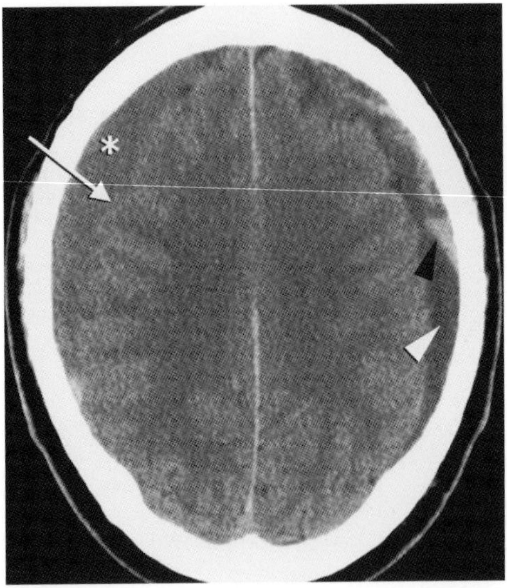

Figure 8.10 Varying age of subdural hematoma. Noncontrast CT image shows a subacute right subdural hematoma (SDH) (*), nearly isodense to brain. The inward displacement of the cortex is evident (white arrow). Mixed acute (black arrowhead) and chronic (white arrowhead) left SDH is also present.

MRI signal intensity changes with time
The signal intensity of blood on both T1 and T2 weighted MR images is based on the oxygenation state of hemoglobin at the time of imaging.

	T1	T2
Hyperacute	**I**sointense	**B**right
Acute (1–2 days)	**I**sointense to Bright	**D**ark
Subacute, early (2–7 days)	**B**right	**D**ark
Subacute, late (7–28 days)	**B**right	**B**right
Chronic (>14–28 days)	**D**ark	**D**ark

PATTERNS OF DISEASE

What do I order for suspected intracranial hemorrhage?
In the non-acute situation, either CT or MRI may be used.
CT: accurate for diagnosis of acute intracranial hemorrhage.
- Fast to obtain, widely available, unstable patients can be scanned.
- Preferred initial imaging test in acute setting.

MRI: can also accurately depict intracranial hemorrhage.
- Remote hemorrhage is easier to see.
- Time consuming to perform (20–30min), undesirable in an unstable patient.

Vascular pathology
Multiple pathologies can affect the intracranial vasculature; the two most important are arteriovenous malformations (AVMs) and cerebral aneurysms.

Vascular malformations
There are several types, some are prone to spontaneous hemorrhage and some are not.

Venous angioma (aka developmental venous anomaly)
- May co-exist with cavernous angiomas.
- Imaging: small radially oriented veins converging into single larger vein. Best seen on postcontrast MRI.

Cavernous angioma (aka cavernous malformation)
- Comprised of vascular sinusoids, and contains slow-flowing or thrombosed blood.
- At risk for bleeding, and it grows when it hemorrhages.
- Imaging: may be calcified. Enhancement is variable. Often have hemosiderin ring on T2 MRI (see Figure 8.3b).

Capillary telangiectasia
- Collection of dilated capillaries, typically are clinically silent.
- Imaging: may see enhancement on MRI. GRE images may show low signal from blood products.

Arterio-venous malformations (AVM)
- Abnormal tangle of blood vessels ("nidus"), between a feeding artery(s) and draining vein(s).
- Prone to hemorrhage. Can cause seizures and other neurological signs.
- Imaging: serpiginous enhancement, +/− hemorrhage and calcifications (see Figures 8.11 and 8.12).

Intracranial aneurysm
A dilated segment of a blood vessel. The morphology may be saccular or fusiform.

Saccular (berry) (see Figure 8.13)
- Focal outpouching of the arterial wall; occur at vascular bifurcations.
- 20% multiple.
- Most commonly involve the circle of Willis.
  - Anterior communicating artery, 35%.
- Posterior communicating artery origin, 30–35%.
- Middle cerebral artery bifurcation, 30%.
- Tip of the basilar artery, 5–10%.

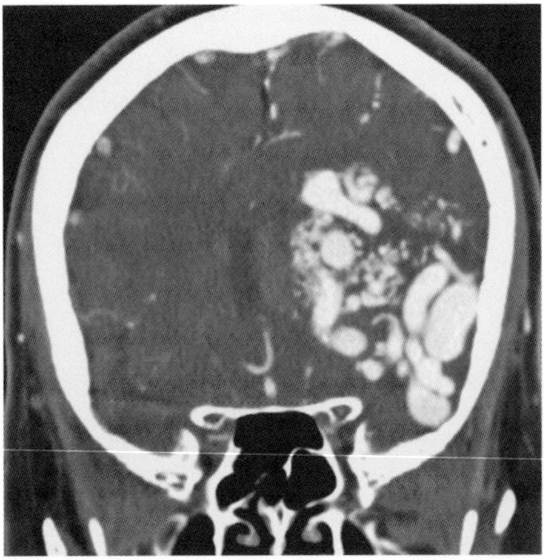

Figure 8.11 Arteriovenous malformation. CTA shows a large tangle of variably sized blood vessels in the left hemisphere. The largest vessels seen are enlarged draining veins.

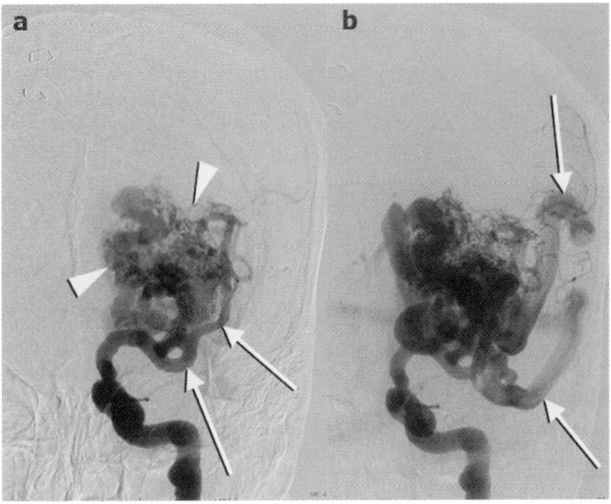

Figure 8.12 Arteriovenous malformation. Conventional left internal carotid angiogram shows the feeding arteries (arrows, a) and the nidus (arrowheads) filling in the arterial phase. (b) Enlarged, early filling draining veins are visible on a more delayed image (arrows).

PATTERNS OF DISEASE

Fusiform
- Circumferential enlargement of a portion of an artery; may occur along any arterial segment, not just at bifurcations.

Risk of rupture
Ruptured aneurysms, resulting in subarachnoid hemorrhage, incur a significant degree of both morbidity and mortality.
- Risk of rupture is related to size: aneurysms greater than 7–10mm more prone to rupture.
- Depending on location, shape, and vascular anatomy, treatment options include surgical aneurysm clipping, percutaneous coiling, or even surgical bypass.

Risk factors for development
Factors that cause degenerative vascular injury such as hypertension and smoking. Less commonly related to connective tissue disorders, trauma, infection, drug use, tumors, high-flow states related to arteriovenous malformations (AVMs).

Diagnosis
CT angiography (CTA):
- Good spatial resolution for identifying small aneurysms.
- Fast and accurate; initial study to order in the acute setting.

MR angiography (MRA):
- Limited for evaluation of small aneurysms beyond the second-order branches of the anterior, middle, and posterior cerebral arteries.
- Not typically done in the acute setting.

Conventional angiography:
- Most often used when CTA does not show an aneurysm in the setting of acute nontraumatic subarachnoid hemorrhage.
- Best spatial resolution, so still considered the "gold standard" when in doubt.

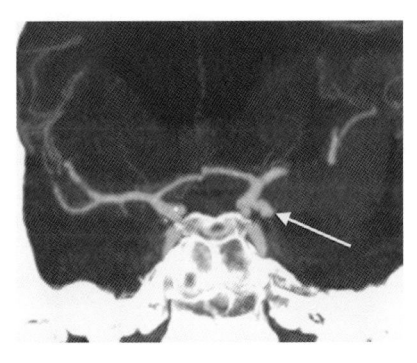

Figure 8.13 Left posterior communicating artery (PCOM) aneurysm. Coronal MIP image from a CTA shows focal saccular outpouching of the PCOM (arrow).

Masses

Intracranial masses are categorized as intra-axial or extra-axial in location; each has a different differential diagnosis.

Intra-axial mass
- Center of the mass is within the substance of the brain.
- If mass is peripheral, may see a rim of parenchyma wrapping around the lesion.

Extra-axial mass
- Center of the mass is outside the brain.
- Adjacent brain cortex and cortical vessels will be displaced, and buckle inwards.
- May see a thin rim of CSF between the mass and the underlying brain.
- CSF space adjacent to the lesion will expand as the mass pushes the underlying brain away from it (see Figure 8.14).

Other characteristics that may narrow the differential diagnosis:
- Size of mass, shape, and margins (sharp, fuzzy, etc.).
- Density on CT or the signal intensity on MRI.
- Presence of calcification, fat, or blood within the lesion.
- Cystic, solid, or mixed.
- Region of the brain (i.e., pineal, cerebellum, corpus callosum).
  - Each has a predilection for certain tumor types.
- Age of the patient.

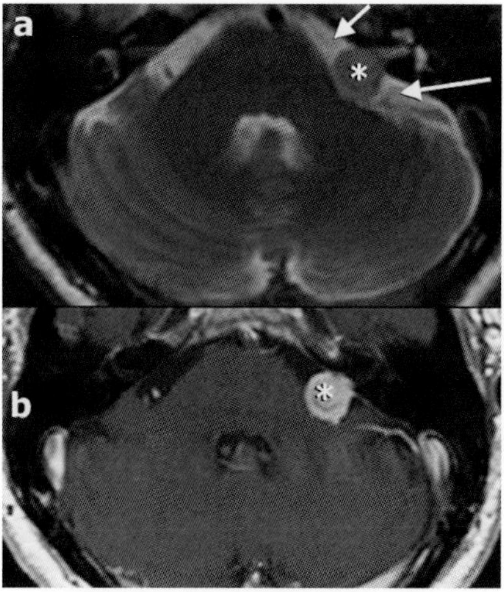

Figure 8.14 Extra-axial mass: acoustic schwannoma. T2 (a) and contrast enhanced T1 (b) MRI demonstrate a mass (*) displacing the adjacent brain, with widening of the adjacent subarachnoid space (arrows). The mass is centered in the cerebello-pontine angle, and enhances homogeneously.

Meningeal disease
Different pathologies arise from/affect each layer of the meninges.

Pachymeninges
- Processes affecting the dura will occur along the skull, falx, and tentorium and will not extend into sulcal spaces.
- Primary tumors, metastasis, hemorrhages, infection.

Leptomeninges
- Processes affecting leptomeninges occur along the surface of the brain, and interdigitate into the sulcal spaces.
- Tumor metastasis, infection, inflammation.

Common conditions

"Stroke" / cerebral infarction (cerebrovascular accidents, CVA)
Stroke is a clinical diagnosis. May be ischemic or hemorrhagic. Both have similar symptoms and physical examination findings. For suspected acute stroke, a CT scan should be performed to evaluate for intracranial hemorrhage and exclude other pathologies.

Ischemic infarct
Ischemic infarction may be caused by arterial thromboembolism or in-situ thrombosis. This causes parenchymal ischemia, which, if prolonged, results in infarction.

- Rapid diagnosis of stroke is critical if thrombolysis therapy is considered.
- Intracranial hemorrhage must be excluded, which is a contraindication to thrombolysis. Always look carefully for hemorrhage.

CT findings
Dependent on the duration since the onset of clinical symptoms.

<u>Acute (0–6 hours):</u>
- CT scan may look *completely* normal.
- Look for subtle signs of cytotoxic edema.

<u>Acute (> 6 hours):</u>
- Cytotoxic edema develops (see "Patterns of Disease," "Edema," p. 377):
  - Loss of the insular ribbon sign: edema will decrease the density of the insular cortex. Look for asymmetry in the R/L insula.
  - Obscuration of the basal ganglia: edema will decrease the density and render them inconspicuous.
- Dense MCA or basilar artery sign: Focal hyperdensity in the artery due to acute thrombus/embolus

> **Caution!** Hyperdensity of intracranial vessels can be seen with any form of hemo-concentration such as dehydration and polycythemia. In these settings the hyperdensity is diffuse, and the patient would not have stroke-like symptoms.

<u>Subacute:</u>
- Mass effect develops.
  - Typically seen from day 1 to 7, peaking around days 3–4.
- Enhancement may be seen 1–8 weeks after the initial event.

<u>Chronic:</u>
- Parenchymal volume loss with adjacent sulcal enlargement, and ex-vacuo dilatation of the adjacent ventricle.

MRI findings

<u>Acute:</u>
- High-signal intensity on diffusion weighted images.
- Low-signal intensity on the apparent diffusion coefficient images (ADC map) (see Figure 8.15).

> **Beware!** All that is bright on DWI is not ischemia/infarction. Regions of truly restricted diffusion (infarction) appear dark on the ADC map, whereas nearly all other causes of bright signal on DWI (T2 shine through) appear bright.

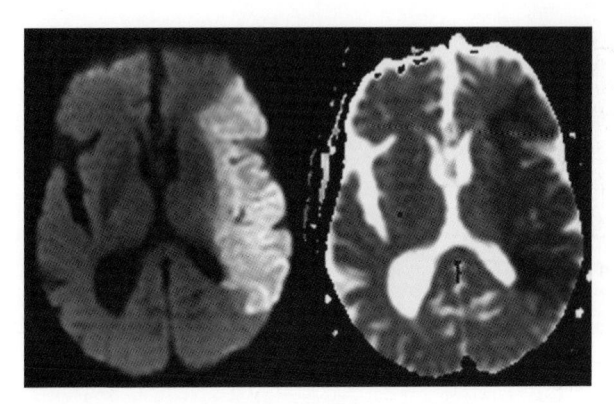

Figure 8.15 MRI Ischemic infarct. (a) DWI image shows bright signal in the left MCA territory, involving both gray and white matter. (b) ADC map shows corresponding low-signal intensity in this region, confirming the diagnosis of acute infarct.

Hemorrhagic infarct
Etiologies
- Hypertensive bleed.
- Tumor hemorrhage.
- Ruptured arteriovenous malformations (AVMs).
- Trauma with cerebral contusions and/or shear injury.
- Ischemic infarcts may also undergo hemorrhagic transformation.

CT findings
- High-attenuation blood.
- May be homogeneous or heterogeneous.
- Assess for associated mass effect (see Figure 8.16).

MRI findings
(See p. 384 for appearance of blood on MRI.)
- Look for intraparenchymal signal abnormalities.
  - acutely: isointense on T1 and hyperintense on T2.
- Assess for associated mass effect.

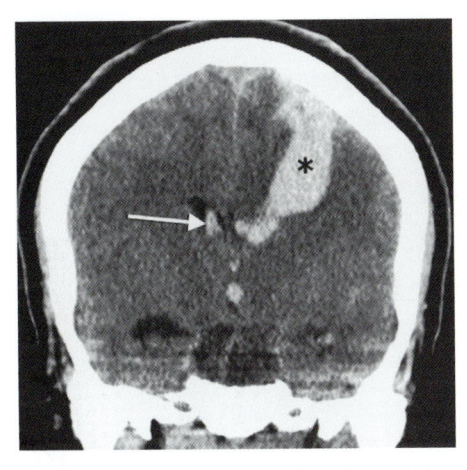

Figure 8.16 Intraparenchymal hemorrhage. 33-year-old hypertensive female with diagnosis of stroke found to have a large parenchymal bleed (*) with both subarachnoid (not shown) and intraventricular (arrow) extension. Patient was a known methamphetamine user.

Head trauma
Trauma is a common cause of intracranial hemorrhage, and imaging is used to diagnose it and to localize it to the proper compartment.
- Blood can involve more than one compartment.
- Blood can extend from one compartment to the next (e.g., subarachnoid blood may reflux into the ventricles).

Extraaxial hemorrhage
Epidural hematoma (EDH)
- The epidural space is a potential space bounded by the dura mater and the inner table of the calvarium.
  - The dura is firmly adherent to suture lines, which limits the epidural space.
- Epidural hematoma is usually caused by arterial bleeding.
  - Classically from a temporal bone fracture lacerating the adjacent middle meningeal artery.
- Arterial bleeding dissects the dura away from the calvarium, causing the classic "biconvex" or "lentiform" appearance on imaging (see Figure 8.17).

Epidural hematoma key imaging findings
- Lentiform/biconvex shape.
- Does not cross suture lines.
- May cross the midline.
- Look for overlying fracture.

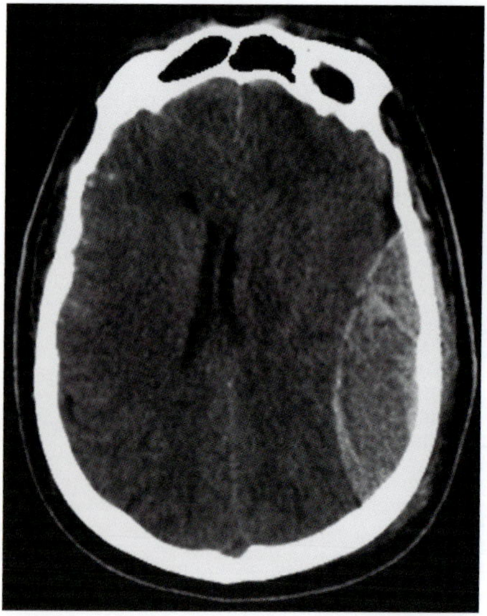

Figure 8.17 Epidural hematoma. Noncontrast CT demonstrates the high-attenuation, bi-convex hematoma that extends anteriorly to the coronal suture and posteriorly to the lambdoid suture. Note the associated mass effect.

Subdural hematoma (SDH)

Subdural hematomas are typically venous bleeds caused by tearing of veins that extend from the cortex to the dural sinuses, "bridging veins."
- More common in the eldery, because the veins are stretched and more taught due to cerebral atrophy.
- Classically "cresentic" shaped.
- They can cross suture lines; however, they cannot cross the midline.
  - Falx is an extension of the dura, and SDH will track back along one side of the falx (see Figures 8.10 and 8.18).

Subdural hematoma key imaging findings
- Crescentic shape.
- May cross suture lines.
- Cannot cross the midline.

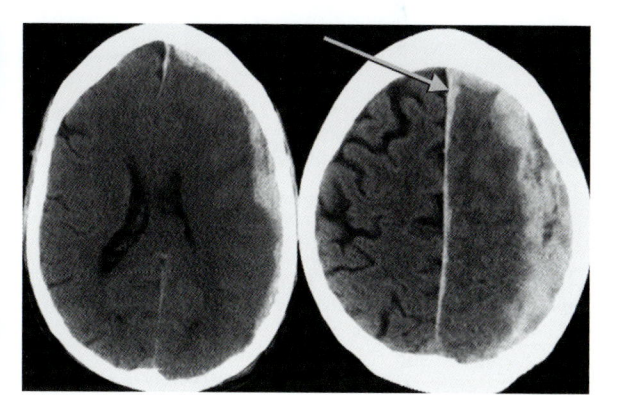

Figure 8.18 Acute subdural hematoma. Noncontrast CT shows a classic, crescent shaped SDH. It does not cross midline, and tracks back along the falx cerebri (arrow).

Subarachnoid hemorrhage (SAH)
- SAH can be limited to the cortical sulci, CSF cisterns, or occur in both.
- Most common causes are trauma and ruptured aneurysm (see Figure 8.19).

Subarachnoid hemorrhage key imaging findings
- High-attenuation filling the normally low-attenuation CSF spaces.
- Lack of visualization of CSF cisterns.
- When in the cortical sulci, appears as linear high-attenuation.
- Can reflux into the ventricles.

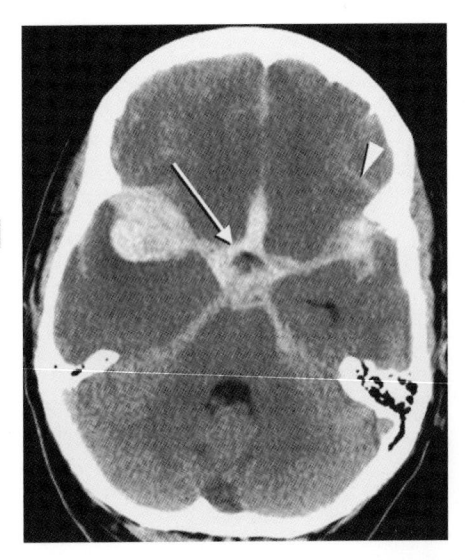

Figure 8.19 Subarachnoid hemorrhage due to ruptured right MCA aneurysm. Noncontrast CT shows high-attenuation acute blood filling the suprasellar cistern (arrow), filling both Sylvian fissures, and extending into sulci (arrowhead).

Intraparenchymal hemorrhage and traumatic brain injury
Two common patterns of brain injuries

Coup-contracoup pattern:
- The site of direct impact is the coup injury (direct injury to stationary brain).
- The contracoup site is directly opposite the site of impact (impact of moving brain on the skull).
- Look for blood and fractures specifically at these sites.

Deceleration pattern (e.g., head in an MVA):
- The skull hits an object (window, dashboard) and the brain is stopped by the skull.
- The head/brain decelerates in a forward flexion motion, causing contusions to the inferior frontal lobes and the anterior temporal lobes.

Types of brain injuries

Contusions:
Think of contusions as brain bruises that occur when the brain impacts the inner table of the skull.
- May be hemorrhagic or nonhemorrhagic.

- Typically involve the cortex.
- Hemorrhagic contusions are often within the anterior-inferior frontal lobes and anterior tip of temporal lobes related to deceleration injury.

<u>Shear injury:</u>
Shear injury (aka. diffuse axonal injury) occurs when structures of different density or rigidity slide past each other during deceleration (i.e., gray nuclei and white matter).
- Shear injuries produce small hemorrhages at gray/white junctions or small foci of edema.
- Common locations include junction of cortex-subcortical white matter, basal ganglia/thalamic region, brainstem, splenium and genu of corpus callosum.
- Can be occult on CT but are well-demonstrated on MRI.

Temporal bone fractures

Temporal bone fractures can have significant clinical consequences due to the potential for injury to the seventh and eighth cranial nerves, the vestibulocochlear apparatus, and middle-ear ossicles.

Classically, two types have been described, although many fractures are a combination of the two.
- **Longitudinal**: fracture through the long axis of the petrous temporal bone. More common, though lower incidence of hearing loss. (May be associated with ossicular chain disruption and conductive hearing loss).
- **Transverse**: fracture through the short axis of the petrous temporal bone. Less common, but much higher incidence of hearing loss. Tends to traverse the cochlea (see Figure 8.20).
- Additional sequelae of both include meningitis and CSF leak if the fracture extends into the cranial vault.

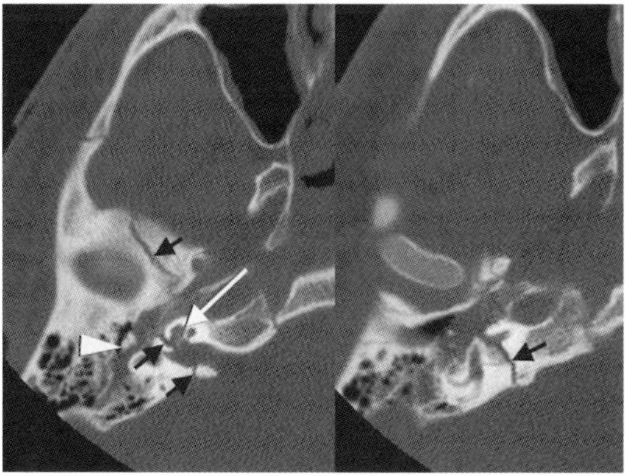

Figure 8.20 Transverse temporal bone fracture (small black arrows) that extends through the cochlea (white arrow) and resulted in disruption of the malleus and incus (arrowhead).

Primary brain tumors

A complete review of brain tumors is beyond the scope of this text; the most common brain tumors are discussed.

Parenchymal

Astrocytic tumors are the most common type of primary brain tumors. There are four main subtypes (WHO grading):
- Pilocytic Astrocytoma (grade 1)
  - Benign. More common in children. Circumscribed and may present as a cyst with an enhancing mural nodule or may be entirely solid and enhancing.
- Diffuse astrocytoma (grade 2).
- Anaplastic astrocytoma (grade 3).
- Glioblastoma multiforme (grade 4).

Grades 2–4 are infiltrative tumors that represent progressively more severe disease, with increasing enhancement, edema, heterogeneity, and ultimately central necrosis on imaging.

Adults

<u>Supratentorial:</u> More common than infratentorial.
- Most common supratentorial primary brain tumor is the glioblastoma multiforme (see Figure 8.21).
  - Infiltrative, heterogenous on imaging.
  - Irregular enhancement, may have central necrosis.

<u>Infratentorial:</u> Most common infratentorial brain tumor is a metastasis.

Children

Incidence of supratentorial and infratentorial tumors is equal. Low-grade astrocytic tumors and primitive neuroectodermal tumors (e.g, medulloblastoma) are the most common primary brain tumors.

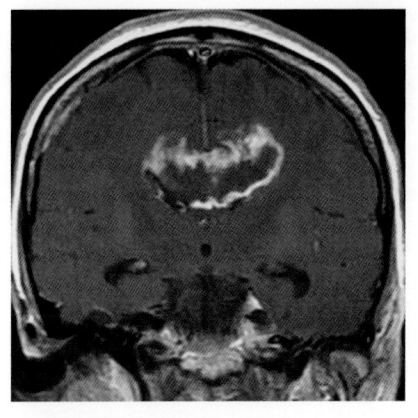

Figure 8.21 Glioblastoma multiforme. Postcontrast T1 MRI image shows a large, irregular, rim-enhancing, centrally necrotic mass centered in the corpus callosum with extension into both hemispheres.

<u>Supratentorial</u>: DDx is based on both age of the child and location (i.e., parenchymal, pineal region, sellar/suprasellar region, intraventricular).

<u>Infratentorial</u>:
- Medulloblastoma: Most common infratentorial tumor in children.
  - Usually midline in the vermis.
- Other tumors:
  - Juvenile pilocytic astrocytoma.
  - Ependymoma.
  - Brainstem glioma.

Meningeal
Meningioma
The most common meningeal tumor. Most are benign but rarely may be atypical and even malignant. ~20% are multiple, particularly in patients with neurofibromatosis type 2.

<u>Imaging findings</u>
- Isointense to brain on T1 and T2.
- Enhances homogeneously and avidly.
- Broad base of contact with dura; may have "dural tail"-extension of tumor along dura.

Other primary meningeal tumors
Rare. Types include hemangiopericytoma, melanocytoma/diffuse melanocytosis, and mesenchymal non-meningothelial tumors.

Cerebral metastases
Metastases may be parenchymal, dural, calvarial, or spread throughout the subarachnoid spaces (leptomeningeal spread).

Parenchymal
- Solitary or multiple lesions with predilection for the gray/white junction.
- Typically with surrounding vasogenic edema, especially as they get larger (due to breakdown of the blood-brain barrier) (see Figure 8.22).
- May be solid and/or cystic, or have central necrosis.
- Lesions enhance: T1W gadolinium-enhanced sequence is the most sensitive for detection.

Dural metastases
- May look just like a meningioma; may even have a dural tail.

Leptomeningeal "drop" metastasis
Metastases that spread from intracranial tumors into the subarachnoid space and "drop" into the spinal canal. More common in children.
- Metastases stud the leptomeninges as "sugar coating" (linear enhancement) and "gum drops" (nodular enhancement).
- Typically multiple/multifocal, and are located in the subarachnoid spaces.
- Gadolinium is required for diagnosis.
- Tumors known to cause drop metastastes:
  - Medulloblastoma.
  - Ependymoma.
  - Glioblastoma multiforme (GBM)
  - Metastatic lymphoma and breast cancer.

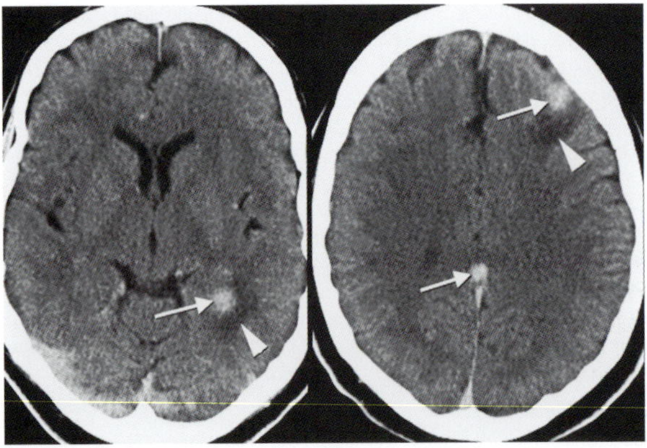

Figure 8.22 Cerebral metastasis. Contrast-enhanced head CT shows vasogenic edema (arrowheads) surrounding the small enhancing metastases (arrows). Note that these are all located at the gray/white junction.

Peripheral nerve-sheath tumors

Most common tumors are schwannomas and neurofibromas.
- May occur along any peripheral nerve (including the cranial nerves).
- Many occur in isolation:
  - Vestibular schwannoma in the cerebellopontine angle
  - Spinal nerve-root tumor within the canal or along the exiting nerve root.
- May occur as part of a syndrome:
  - Neurofibromatosis-1: Multiple neurofibromas.
  - Neurofibromatosis-2: Multiple intracranial schwannomas, classically including bilateral cerebello-pontine angle schwannomas (in addition to meningiomas and ependymomas).

Imaging findings
- Commonly isointense on T1.
- Very hyperintense on T2, though with central areas of lower signal.
- May show central necrosis if they outgrow their blood supply.
- Enhance avidly and homogeneously postcontrast (see Figure 8.14).

Infection and inflammation

Meningitis
Bacterial, viral, and granulomatous processes can affect the meninges (meningitis).
- Certain conditions have a predilection for pachymeninges versus leptomeninges.
- Certain conditions have a predilection for the posterior fossa (e.g., sarcoidosis, tuberculosis).

Imaging findings
Meningitis is most commonly occult on imaging.
- Meninges may or may not enhance following IV contrast.
- Secondary signs of meningitis and possible source of meningitis:
  - Epidural abscess.
  - Cerebritis—focal edematous cortex.
  - Hydrocephalus (from loculations/adhesions).
  - Mastoiditis or paranasal sinusitis.

Cerebritis
Cerebritis is the earliest manifestation of bacterial or other nonviral infection in the brain (encephalitis is typically used to imply viral infection).

Imaging findings
- MRI: cerebral edema and restricted diffusion (bright DWI signal).
- Contrast enhancement may be absent and, if present, is usually streaky.

Abscess
Abscess is the later manifestation of cerebritis, in which necrotic tissue becomes more organized centrally, and a peripheral capsule forms.

Imaging findings
- CT and MRI:
  - smooth ring-enhancement of the capsule.
  - surrounding edema.
- MRI: also look for restricted diffusion centrally, which is a reflection of cellularity and viscosity typical of pus in bacterial abscesses.

Multiple sclerosis
Most common demyelinating disorder. The white matter changes are occult on CT; MRI is required for diagnosis and follow-up.

Imaging findings
- FLAIR sequences are the most sensitive for MS plaques in the brain.
  - They appear as high signal and are commonly ovoid or linear.
- Frequent plaque locations include:
  - Periventricular white matter (those perpendicular to the lateral ventricular surface are known as "Dawson's fingers") (see Figure 8.23).
  - Corpus callosum.
  - Internal capsule.
  - Pons and middle cerebellar peduncle.
- Plaques enhance postcontrast if there is *active* demyelination.
- Lesions may wax and wane or remain stable over time.
- Progressive volume loss occurs over time.

Seizure disorders
MRI is the preferred imaging modality for seizure disorders, and it is helpful in excluding structural causes and identifying surgical candidates. Imaging is often normal in seizure disorders.
- Special sequences with excellent contrast between gray and white matter are performed.

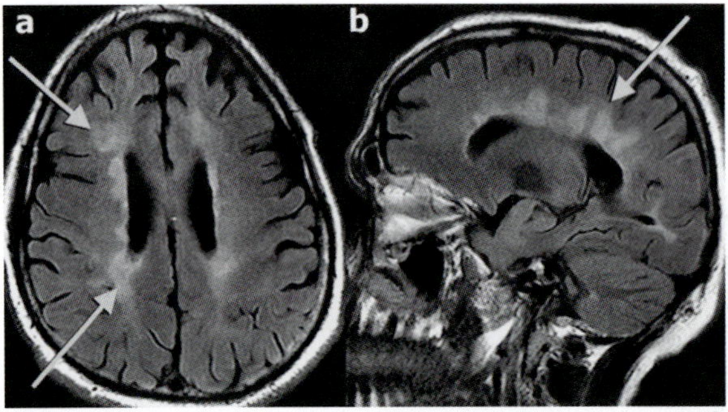

Figure 8.23 Multiple sclerosis. (a) Axial FLAIR MRI shows numerous high-signal lesions in the periventricular white matter. (b) Coronal images demonstrate that these are oriented perpendicular to the lateral ventricles (called "Dawson's fingers," highly suggestive of MS).

- Thin sections are obtained to look carefully at anatomic detail.
- Images oriented perpendicular to the long axis of the hippocampus are often used to evaluate for mesial temporal sclerosis.

Children
Consider congenital causes:
- <u>Cortical dysplasia</u>: focal area of dysplastic cortex.
- <u>Lissencephaly</u>: a neuronal migration anomaly resulting in "smooth brain," thickened cortex related to arrest of neuronal migration.
- <u>Schizencephaly</u>: cleft in the brain lined by dyplastic gray matter.
- <u>Heterotopic gray matter</u>: focus of gray matter in an abnormal location.

Adults
Consider processes that irritate the gray matter:
- <u>Mesial temporal sclerosis (MTS)</u>: temporal lobe seizures due to abnormal hippocampus. Look for hippocampal T2 bright signal and atrophy (see Figure 8.24).
- <u>Brain tumors.</u>
- <u>Vascular malformations</u> (i.e., AVM, cavernous malformation).
- <u>Trauma</u>: with resultant encephalomalacia, gliosis (brain scarring), and/or bleeding.
- <u>Infection</u> (i.e., herpes encephalitis, bacterial meningitis).

Common imaging pitfalls for head CT and MRI
- Small isodense subdural hematomas—easy to miss. Look for displacement of cortex from calvarium, or "thick" looking cortex (see Figure 8.10, p. 384).
- Atrophy versus hydrocephalus.
  - Volume loss causes ex-vacuo dilatation of the ventricles, *and* widening of the sulci and cisterns. If not, consider hydrocephalus.
- Bilaterally symmetric diseases may be overlooked.

- Tunnel vision: looking at the brain and missing a soft-tissue or osseous lesion.
- Places where lesions are commonly missed: dural sinuses, cavernous sinuses, trigeminal (Meckel's) cave, brainstem, skull base, para-pharyngeal tissues.

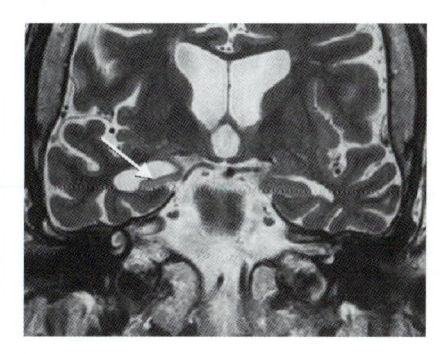

Figure 8.24 Mesial temporal sclerosis. Coronal T2 image perpendicular to the hippocampi shows volume loss and increased signal in the right hippocampus (arrow) relative to the normal left side.

Head and neck

Head and neck radiology is challenging because of the small size of structures, similar densities, and the fact that many appear round or ovoid on axial images. CT and MRI are the modalities of choice in head and neck imaging, and contrast is often used to help differentiate normal structures from pathology.

A review of head and neck anatomy is beyond the scope of this text. See references for suggested resources.

Common conditions

Sinus disease

Sinusitis can be acute, chronic, or acute on chronic. Noncontrast CT has supplanted radiography. Both axial and coronal images are utilized. Coronal images better demonstrates the osteomeatal complexes draining the sinuses.

Imaging findings
Acute sinusitis:
- Air-fluid levels, bubbly secretions, and sometimes complete opacification of the sinus.
- The imaging findings may suggest acute sinusitis in the appropriate clinical setting because it is a clinical diagnosis.

Chronic sinusitis:
- Osseous thickening of the sinus walls, mucosal thickening, often lobular.
- Multiple polyps.

Bone destruction does not occur with typical sinusitis, and that suggests a more aggressive pathogen such as invasive fungal infection (i.e., mucormycosis, aspergillus), or an alternative process such as malignancy.

Facial trauma
- Facial trauma is evaluated with noncontrast facial CT (axial and coronal images, sometimes 3D reformats are generated).
- Nasal bone fractures are the most common facial fracture.
- Facial fractures may be isolated or occur in typical combinations.

Common patterns of facial fractures:

Orbital floor fractures
- Best evaluated on coronal images.
- May be nondisplaced or displaced and depressed.
- If depressed, you must assess the position of the inferior rectus muscle.
  - If it is displaced down into the fracture site, it may become trapped. Alert the clinician!

Medial orbital wall fractures
- Best evaluated on coronal images.
- May be nondisplaced, displaced, or deviated.
- When the medial wall is displaced medially into the ethmoid sinuses, you must assess the position of the medial rectus muscle.
  - If it enters the defect, the muscle may become trapped. Alert the clinician! (see Figure 8.25).

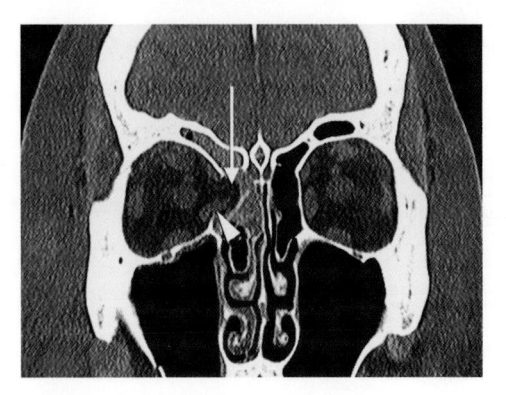

Figure 8.25 Medial orbital wall blowout fracture. Coronal CT demonstrates a displaced fracture of the medial orbital wall. The orbital fat (arrow) and the medial rectus muscle (arrowhead) have herniated through the osseous defect. There is fluid/hemorrhage in the adjacent ethmoid air cells.

Zygomaticomaxillary complex fracture (ZMC)
- Second most common facial fracture.
- Occurs when a patient gets hit in the zygomatic bone. (Note: not the zygomatic arch.)
- The zygoma is displaced inward, which causes fracture of the adjacent bones: lateral orbital wall, orbital floor, anterior and lateral maxillary sinus walls, and the zygomatic arch.

Lymphadenopathy

Identification of lymph nodes in the neck is greatly enhanced by using IV contrast to help distinguish the numerous neck vessels from lymph nodes. Evaluation without IV contrast is fairly limited.

Imaging findings
- Lymph nodes are ovoid with a smooth border.
- Normal nodes often have fat in the hilum, and look like kidney beans.
- Abnormal lymph nodes first enlarge in the short axis and become "fatter" and rounder. The fatty hilum is replaced with tumor.

Classification
A head-and-neck lymph-node-classification system has been developed, which divides the neck into seven regions. This allows for accurate communication of information between physicians.
Lymphatic drainage occurs in a fairly predictable manner (e.g., the palatine tonsil will typically drain via the level II and retropharyngeal nodes).
- In cases of known cancer, look for lymphadenopathy in the expected drainage bed of the tumor.
- The pattern of lymphadenopathy may lead you to identify the primary tumor.
- In lymphoma and viral infections, enlarged lymph nodes may be seen diffusely throughout the neck.

Infection

The location and types of infections in the head and neck is extensive, and beyond the scope of this text. The following are fairly common infections for which CT or MRI is required for diagnosis.

Orbital cellulitis
Categorized as preseptal or postseptal, difficult to distinguish clinically, yet easily distinguishable on CT or MRI.
- Preseptal orbital cellulitis is located anterior to the orbital septum (outside the bony orbit).
- Postseptal orbital cellulitis involves the structures posterior to the orbital septum (within the bony orbit, includes orbital fat and muscles) and may result in vision loss.
  - Most commonly related to ethmoid sinusitis. Infection passes through the thin sinus wall (lamina papyracea) into the orbit.

Imaging findings
- Edema and enhancement in either the pre-septal or post-septal space.
- Enhancing collection adjacent to the ethmoid sinus confined by the periosteum indicates subperiosteal phlegmon/abscess.
- Rim-enhancing collection within the orbit not confined by the periosteum indicates orbital abscess.

CHAPTER 8 Neuroimaging

Tonsillar/peritonsillar abscess
A complication of tonsillitis/pharyngitis.

Imaging findings
- A rim-enhancing fluid collection in or adjacent to the tonsil (see Figure 8.26).
- If there is abnormal enhancement but no defined fluid collection, it is called a phlegmon.

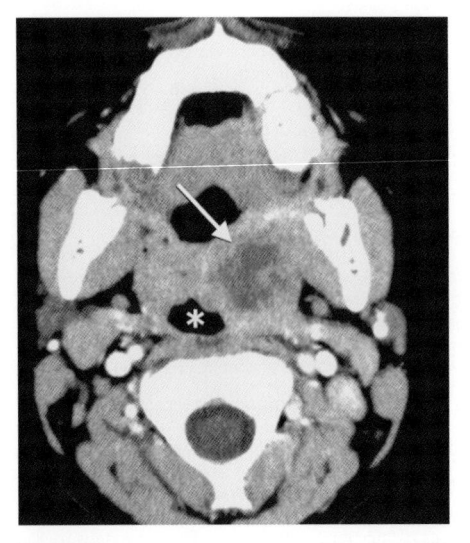

Figure 8.26 Tonsillar abscess. Axial contrast-enhanced CT shows a large left tonsillar abscess with central necrosis and thick rim-enhancement (arrow). This causes mild narrowing and mass effect on the oropharynx (*).

Retropharyngeal abscess
The infection may originate from a pharyngitis, infected retropharyngeal lymph node, or may extend from tonsillitis.

Imaging findings
- Rim-enhancing fluid collection in the retropharyngeal space.
- Potential for airway compromise from edema, and inferior extension into the mediastinum.

Floor of mouth infection/abscess
Usually odontogenic in origin. Particularly problematic because of the potential for soft tissue edema to extend into the retropharyngeal space, thus encircling the airway and pushing the tongue back into the airway.
- This clinical condition is known as Ludwig's angina and may be life threatening.

Imaging findings
- Edema, generalized enhancement (phlegmon), and a rim-enhancing fluid collection (abscess).
- Identify extent of infection and look for mass effect on the airway.
- Identify source:
  - If odontogenic origin, look for dental peri-apical lucency and overlying mandibular cortical erosion where the infection broke through into the soft tissues. Best seen on bone windows.

Spine

The spine is routinely evaluated for both traumatic and nontraumatic conditions with radiography, CT and MRI. It is important to understand the normal spinal anatomy in order to develop a good search pattern and to be able to describe lesions in their appropriate locations.

Anatomy on CT and MRI

What anatomy is seen on CT?
- Vertebral bodies: cortical margins, density, height, shape, and alignment.
- Posterior elements: pedicles, lamina, spinous and transverse processes, facet joints.
- Intervertebral discs (not seen well, but are visible).
- Neural foramina.

What anatomy is seen on MRI?
- Vertebral bodies and posterior elements
  - Cortex: fine-bone detail not as well seen on MRI as on CT.
- Bone marrow: is seen well.
- Intervertebral discs: annulus fibrosis and nucleus pulposis distinguishable.
- Ligaments: posterior and anterior longitudinal, interspinous, ligamentum flavum.
- Neural foramina and nerve roots.
- Spinal cord: signal and morphology can be assessed.
- Subarachnoid and epidural spaces.

What imaging test do I order?

Radiography
Conventional x-rays are good for evaluating the osseous spine, the prevertebral soft tissues, and the width of the spinal canal and neural foramina. Strengths: may be done rapidly and portably, with much less radiation exposure than CT.

Indications:
- Chronic neck or back pain.
- Radiculopathy.
- Low-speed motor vehicle accident with neck pain.

CT
In general, CT is better for evaluating bone than MRI.

Indications:
Acute disease when a rapid diagnosis is needed.
- Trauma.
- Cervical spine vascular dissection or occlusion (CTA).
- Characterizing osseous neoplasm.
- Degenerative disc and joint disease (primarily the osseous effects).
  - Calcified discs, paravertebral ossifications/osteophytes, endplate sclerosis, subchondral cystic changes, facet arthropathy.

MRI
MRI is better for evaluating all soft tissue elements of the spine. MRI can show abnormalities of bone marrow (i.e., infiltrative processes, edema) but does not demonstrate cortical osseous detail like CT.

Indications:
Secondary assessment of trauma/acute disease.
- Trauma: spinal cord injury (edema, hemorrhage), ligamentous injury, epidural hematoma.
- Discitis/osteomyelitis.
- Discs
  - Degenerative disc disease (soft-tissue components).
  - Disc herniations/protrusions
- Spinal metastatic disease: paraspinal and epidural spread, spinal cord compression, pathological fractures.

Common conditions

Degenerative disc disease
Axial loading stresses the intervertebral discs, which act as shock absorbers, and over time the discs may degenerate.

Imaging findings
- Proliferative bone formation (osteophytes) of the endplates
- Disc dessication (lose water content).
  - This causes loss of their T2 bright signal (see Figure 8.27).
- Decreased disc height.
- Vertebral body endplate changes occur as the discs are less effective at absorbing force. There is progressive edema, then fat, then sclerosis, and the signal intensity on MRI varies with the stage of degeneration (e.g., edema will be bright on T2 and dark on T1). These changes are commonly referred to as "Modic" endplate changes.

Disc herniation
Disc herniation may be a result of chronic disc degeneration or an acute disc injury.

Definitions of common terms:
Disc "herniation" / "protrusion"
Defined as a localized displacement of disc material beyond the normal posterior limit of the disc space (see Figure 8.27).

Disc extrusion
A herniated disc fragment that is no longer connected to the parent disc.

Disc bulge
Broad extension of disc beyond the posterior margin of the vertebral body (50–100% of the circumference of the disc).

Imaging findings
MRI is required for diagnosis.
- Disc material posterior to the normal disc margin/posterior margin of the vertebral body.
- May extend cranially or caudally, if extruded.
- Assess for cord compression—flattening, displacement, or effacement of subarachnoid space.
- Assess for nerve-root compression (flattening, displacement).

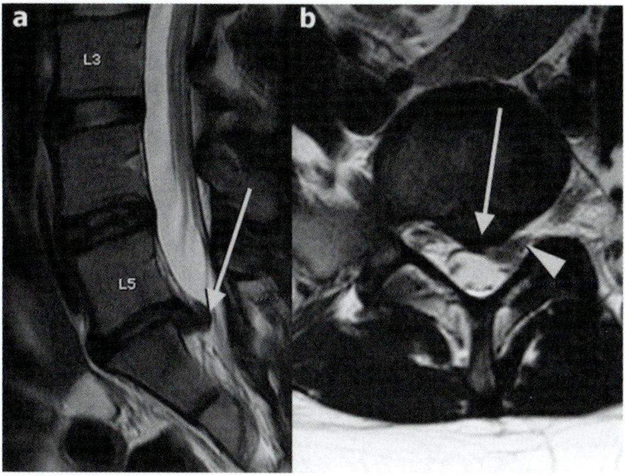

Figure 8.27 Disc herniation (extrusion). (a) Sagittal and (b) axial T2-weighted images show a large disc extrusion that migrates inferiorly (arrows) and compresses the left S1 nerve root within the lateral recess of the canal (arrowhead). There is L5–S1 disc narrowing and dessication from degenerative disc disease.

Masses
Suspected spinal masses, other than osseous metastasis, should be evaluated with MRI. Appropriate differential diagnoses is generated based on identification of the compartment the mass is in. Compartments are shown in Figure 8.28. and explained in the text that follows.

Intramedullary (A)
- Within the substance of the spinal cord. Therefore, it expands the cord.
- Narrows the CSF space around the expanded part of the cord.
- DDx includes: astrocytoma, ependymoma, hemangioblastoma.

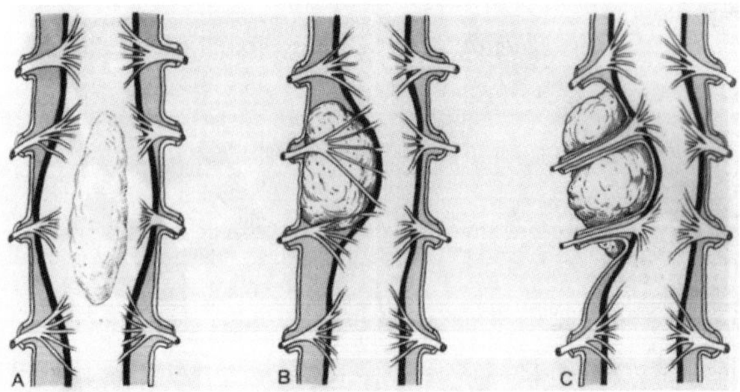

Figure 8.28 Spinal masses; compartments.

Intradural but extramedullary (B)
- Within the thecal (dural) sac but outside the cord.
- Large lesions have mass effect on the cord and displace it. Also widen the CSF space between the cord and dura.
- DDx includes: nerve-sheath tumors (schwannoma, neurofibroma), meningioma, drop metastases.

Extradural (C)
- Lesions outside the thecal sac, cause mass effect on thecal sac.
- "Ball under a rug" appearance—CSF space narrows in the region of the lesion since the adjacent dura is pushed against the cord.
- DDx includes: disc herniation, vertebral metastases, epidural hematoma, abscess.

Myelopathy
Defined as spinal cord damage or disease. This may be acute or chronic, and related to lesions intrinsic or extrinsic to the spinal cord. Myelopathy requires MRI for evaluation.

Imaging findings
↑ T2 signal in cord, solitary or multifocal.
- In conjuction with decreased cord caliber, indicates myelomalacia (chronic volume loss).
- In conjunction with cord expansion, indicates edema or an underlying lesion.

<u>Intrinsic cord lesions:</u>
- Cord tumors: abnormal T2 signal +/− enhancement, +/− blood.
- Demyelination: ↑ T2 signal +/− enhancement (if active demyelination).
- Cord contusion (hemorrhagic or edematous).

<u>Extrinsic cord lesions:</u>
- Masses: intradural or extradural (see Figure 8.28).
- Spinal stenosis resulting in cord compression, look for:
  - Disc herniation (narrows from the front) (see Figure 8.27).
  - Facet overgrowth (arthropathy) and ligamentous hypertrophy (narrow from the back).

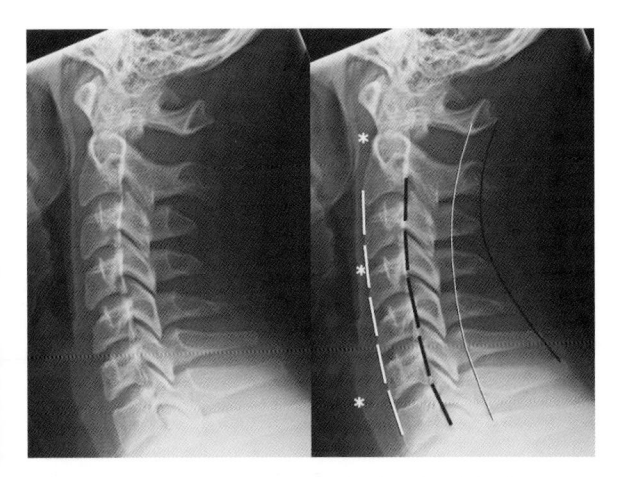

1	Prevertebral soft tissues (PVST) (*)	• Except for the adenoidal soft tissue (occiput/C1 level), should be thin in upper half of cervical spine, and get thicker at ~C4 where the esophagus begins. • Increased in hematoma from spine injury.
2	Anterior spinal line (dashed white)	• Anterior margins of vertebral bodies should be aligned. • Stabilized by anterior longitudinal ligament.
3	Posterior spinal line (dashed black)	• Posterior margins of vertebral bodies should be aligned. • Stabilized by posterior longitudinal ligament.
4	Spinolaminar line (thin white)	• Line formed at the back of the spinal canal where the lamina meet the base of the spinous processes.

Figure 8.29

Trauma

Cervical spine fracture and dislocation
Cervical spine fractures are dangerous because of their potential to cause quadriplegia or death when occurring in the upper cervical spine.

Radiography
Should be performed for suspected spine fractures in patients with mild trauma. C1–T1 must be well visualized in order to exclude fracture.

Views:
- *AP*: to assess vertebral height, uncovertebral joints, lateral masses.
- *Lateral*: to assess vertebral alignment, vertebral height, facet alignment.
- *Odontoid*: AP coned view of C2 (with open mouth). Make sure the interval between C1 and the dens is symmetric bilaterally.
- *Lateral flexion/extension*: performed if there is a concern for ligamentous injury. Usually not obtained acutely.
- *Swimmer's view* (view of cervico-thoracic junction, done with one arm up and one down) if C7/T1 inadequately visualized on lateral.

Four lines to look for on the lateral study:
The four "lines" shown on Figure 8.29 should all be continuous. Any interruption or malalignment should raise a concern for fracture, subluxation, and/or ligamentous injury.

CT
Highly sensitive for fracture, but not for ligamentous or soft tissue injury.
- *Sagittal*: useful for alignment of vertebral bodies and facet joints. Look at the same four lines as described for radiography.
- *Coronal*: useful for evaluating the uncovertebral joints, lateral masses.

Common or well-described cervical spine fractures

Jefferson's fracture:
Axial loading causes fracture of the C1 ring. This results in widening and asymmetry of the C1-dens interval on the odontoid view, and extension of the lateral masses of C1 more lateral than those of C2 (see Figure 8.30).

Hangman's fracture:
Hyperextension injury with fracture of the C2 pedicles bilaterally. Causes anterior subluxation of C2 on C3 (disruption of anterior and posterior spinal lines), avulsion of anterior inferior margin of C2 (avulsion of anterior longitudinal ligament).

Atlanto-axial dislocation:
The occipital condyles are separated from the C1 lateral masses. High morbidity.

Teardrop fracture:
Hyperextension or hyperflexion injury. Avulsion of the anterior/inferior vertebral body by the anterior longitudinal ligament. Unstable. Disruption of the anterior spinal line.

Jumped facets:
Hyperflexion/rotation injury. May be bilateral or unilateral. The inferior facet of the upper vertebral body comes to rest anterior to the superior facet of the lower vertebral body. The facet tips may touch each other instead, termed "perched" facet (see Figure 8.30). Unstable when bilateral.

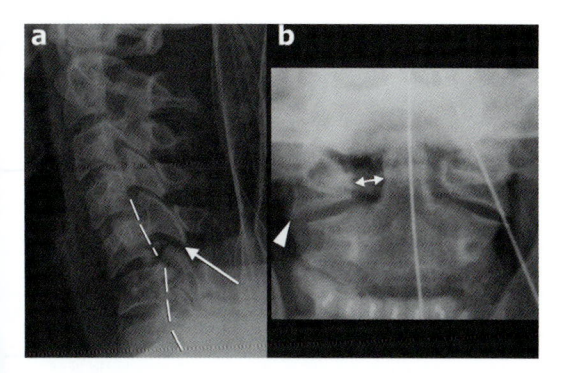

Figure 8.30 (a) (nearly) perched facets. There is widening and subluxation of the C5/6 facet joints (arrow). Note the disruption of the posterior spinal line (dashed line). (b) Jefferson fracture. The interval between the dens and the right lateral mass of C1 (double arrow) is widened, and the lateral mass does not line up with that of C2 (arrowhead). Compare to the normal findings on the left.

<u>Dens fracture:</u>
Divided into types, I, II, and III, describing where the fracture is located (tip versus base). Best seen on odontoid view.

Thoracic and lumbar spine fractures
Radiography should be performed initially for mild trauma. For severe trauma, CT is usually performed in conjunction with CT scans of the head, chest, abdomen, and pelvis.

Compression fracture
This is a compression deformity from a flexion injury.
- Vertebral body typically becomes wedge shaped.
- The posterior vertebral cortex may be intact or it may be displaced posteriorly (retropulsion).
- May be traumatic or osteoporotic.

Burst fracture
Axial loading injury causes vertebral body fracture, with fragment displacement in all directions.
- Retropulsion of fragments into the spinal canal can cause varying degrees of canal stenosis and spinal cord or nerve root compression. Best appreciated on lateral radiograph or CT (see Figure 8.31).
- Widening of the pedicles on AP radiograph.

Spinal epidural hematoma
Anytime a fracture is found, look for an associated epidural hematoma.

CT
- Often occult on CT.
- Use narrow soft-tissue windows.
- Look for hyperdense material in the spinal canal.

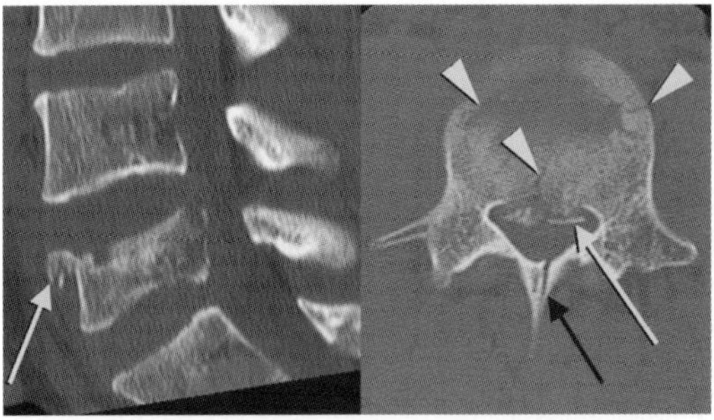

Figure 8.31 L5 Burst fracture; sagittal and axial CT. Multiple vertebral body fracture lines are evident (arrowheads), and there is retro and antero-pulsion of fracture fragments (white arrows). Note the spinous process fracture (black arrow).

MRI
- Fusiform soft tissue in the periphery of the spinal canal.
- Look for abnormal T2 spinal cord signal (to indicate edema or contusion).

Traumatic cord compression
Requires MRI for evaluation. This is a neurosurgical emergency. May result from:
- Retropulsed fracture fragments.
- Large acute herniated disc.
- Foreign body (i.e., bullet fragment).
- Epidural hematoma.

Imaging findings
- Cord flattening, deformity.
- Cord signal abnormality; often T2 hyperintense.
- Effacement of subarachnoid space (see Figure 8.32).

Infection
Infection in the spine usually manifests as discitis/osteomyelitis. Typically, an intervertebral disc is affected as are the adjacent endplates. MRI shows changes earlier than CT.

Imaging findings
Increased T2 disc and endplate signal intensity early on MRI.
- Progresses to endplate destruction.
  - Irregular or mottled appearance of endplates on CT.
  - Loss of black cortical margin on MRI (see Figure 8.33).
- Collapse of the disc space.
- Affected portions of the vertebral bodies will enhance.
- Paraspinal and/or epidural soft tissue phlegmon may be present; this will enhance. Rim-enhancing collections with central areas of nonenhancement represent abscess.

Atypical infections (i.e., tuberculosis, fungal infections) may spare the disc spaces but otherwise appear similar.

COMMON CONDITIONS   413

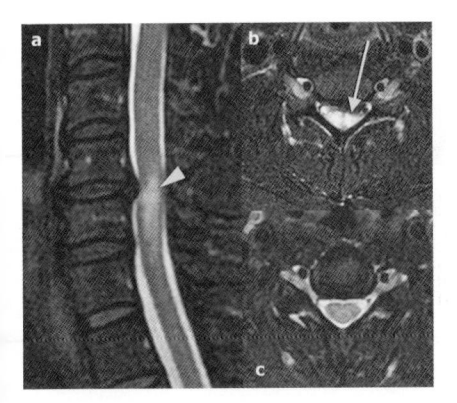

Figure 8.32 Spinal cord compression. Sagittal STIR MRI (a) shows a large disc herniation effacing the subarachnoid space, compressing the cord and causing cord edema (arrowhead). Axial image (b) shows flattening of the ventral cord surface from extrinsic compression (arrow). Compare this to a normal level (c) where the cord morphology and signal are normal.

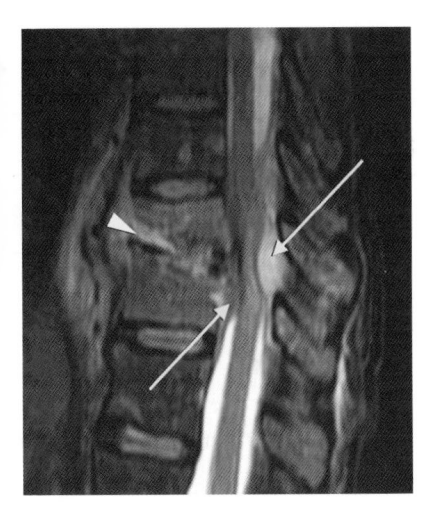

Figure 8.33 Discitis-osteomyelitis. Sagittal T2 weighted MRI shows endplate destruction (loss of the normal dark endplate cortex), hyperintense disc signal (arrowhead), and edema throughout the two involved vertebral bodies (both are brighter than adjacent normal vertebrae). An associated circumferential epidural abscess (arrows) causes cord compression, flattening, and edema.

Procedures

What examination should I order and how is it performed?

Fluoroscopic guided lumbar puncture (LP)

Indications
When cerebral spinal fluid (CSF) needs to be tested, and the procedure cannot be successfully performed without image guidance. e.g., morbid obesity, failed non-guided LP, prior surgery.

Major risks
Rare chance of infection, significant bleeding, nerve-root irritation or injury.

Technique
- Sterile technique and local anesthetic utilized.
- A small gauge spinal needle is advanced into the subarachnoid space.
- Fluoroscopic guidance used to direct needle and avoid osseous structures.

Myelogram

Used much less frequently now that MRI is widely available.

Indications
Usually to assess for cord or nerve-root compression in patients with contraindication to MRI or extensive spinal-fusion hardware, which may distort MR images.

Major risks
- Rare chance of infection, significant bleeding, arachnoiditis.

Technique
- Technique similar to lumbar puncture.
- Small volume of sterile contrast is injected into the thecal sac.
- Patient tilted to get contrast into the thoracic and cervical regions as needed.
- Radiographs and/or CT scan is performed following this.
- Spinal cord and nerve roots appear as filling defects within the contrast-filled subarachnoid space.
  - Contrast may not flow above a stenosis/abnormal level.

Vertebroplasty

Indication
- To stabilize fractures (osteoporotic or pathologic) in order to treat the pain associated with fracture.
- Note: although early studies report 80–90% success rates, recent randomized studies showed no significant difference in pain relief between vertebroplasty and controls.

Major risks
- Epidural cement extravasation with cord compression.
- Cement embolization.

Technique
- Sterile technique imperative. Local anesthesia and conscious sedation used.
- One or two large gauge needles are placed percutaneously into the fractured vertebral body. This is guided with fluoroscopy.
- Cement is injected via the needles, filling the vertebral body.

Carotid and cerebral angiograms
Performed less and less frequently due to availability of CTA and MRA.

Indications
- Diagnosis and treatment of aneurysm, AVMs, AV-fistulas (see Figure 8.12).
- Diagnosis and treatment of vasospasm.
- Small-vessel diseases: atherosclerosis, vasculitis.

Major risks/benefits
- Neurologic injury.
  - 0–5% risk of permanent neurological deficit.
- Reported rate of all major complications of 2%, per ACR practice guidelines. Includes vascular injury, dissection, occlusion, hematoma.
- Advantages include imaging blood flow in real time, excellent evaluation of large and small vessels, and ability to treat certain lesions.

Technique
See Interventional Radiology, chapter 10, "Angiography" for more on techniques.
- A catheter is placed into the carotid and/or vertebral arteries and intravenous contrast is injected.
- Images are obtained in the AP, lateral, and additional supplementary projections.

Therapeutic intracranial procedures
Indications
- Aneurysm coiling.
- AVM embolization.
- Thrombolysis (for acute ischemic stroke).
- Angioplasty (for vasospasm, ASCVD).

Risks/benefits:
- Higher risk procedures with possible death, stroke.
- Benefits
  - Decrease risk of rupture of aneurysm by excluding it from the arterial circulation, avoidance of major surgery (aneurysm clipping).
  - Embolizing AVM may successfully treat it, or decrease its vascularity and operative bleeding risk prior to surgical removal.
  - Reperfusion of brain in setting of acute stroke.
  - Restoration or improvement of blood flow in vasospasm or atherosclerotic stenosis.

Technique
Performed by a neuro-interventionalist. Specific technique varies by procedure. See Interventional Radiology, chapter 10 "General Techniques of Interventions" for further details. p. 456.

Don't miss diagnoses

These critical diagnoses should *not* be missed on imaging because they require urgent treatment. The modality of choice for evaluation and the critical imaging findings to make the diagnosis are listed here:

Cervical spine fracture/subluxation *(Radiography, CT)*
- Discontinuity of bone margins.
- Malalignment.

Spinal cord compression *(MRI)*
- Cord flattening/deformity.
- Cord signal abnormality.
- Effacement of subarachnoid space.

Epidural hematoma, subdural hematoma *(CT)*
- Extra-axial collection, high attenuation when acute.
- Displacement of cortex away from skull.

Cerebral herniation *(CT or MRI)*
- Effacement of CSF cisterns and spaces in specific locations and patterns.

Subarachnoid hemorrhage *(CT)*
- High attenuation in subarachnoid space.

Abscess (cerebral, soft tissues of neck) *(CT or MRI)*
- Peripheral enhancement, central fluid.
- Associated edema.

References

Atlas of the Brain. Structure with functional correlates. (Dartmouth Medical School). (www.dartmouth.edu/~rswenson/atlas/)

ACR–ASNR–SIR–SNIS practice guideline for the performance of diagnostic cervicocerebral angiography in adults. Revised 2005 (Res. 41)*. http://www.acr.org/SecondaryMainMenuCategories/quality_safety/guidelines/iv/cervicocerebral_angio.aspx

Atlas SW. *Magnetic Resonance Imaging of the Brain and Spine.* 4th ed. Philadelphia, PA: Wolters Kluwer/Lippincott Williams & Wilkins; 2009.

Barkovich AJ. *Pediatric Neuroimaging.* 4th ed. Philadelphia, PA: Lippincott Williams & Wilkins; 2000.

Buchbinder R, Osborne RH, Ebeling PR, et al. A randomized trial of vertebroplasty for painful osteoporotic vertebral fractures. *N Engl J Med.* 2009;361(6):557–568.

Capps, E, Kinsella, F, Gupta, M, et al. Emergency imaging assessment of acute, nontraumatic conditions of the head and neck. *RadioGraphics.* 2010; 30:1335–1352.

Enrique M, Elena S, Agustín G, et al. Continuing medical education: CT protocol for acute stroke: Tips and tricks for general radiologists. *Radiographics.* 2008; 28:1673–1687.

Fardon DF, Milette PC. Nomenclature and classification of lumbar disc pathology. Recommendations of the combined task forces of the North American Spine Society, American Society of Spine Radiology, and American Society of Neuroradiology. *Spine.* 2001; 26(5):E93–E113.

Gomori JM, Grossman RI. Mechanisms responsible for the MR appearance and evolution of intracranial hemorrhage. *Radiographics.* 1988; 8(3):427–440.

Hacein-Bey L, Provenzale J Current imaging assessment and treatment of intracranial aneurysms *Am. J. Roentgenol.* 2011; 196:32–44.

Harnsberger R, Osborn A, MacDonald A, et al. *Diagnostic and Surgical Imaging Anatomy Brain Head & Neck Spine.* Philadelphia, PA: Lippincott Williams & Williams; 2009.

Hopper R, Salemy S, Sze R Diagnosis of midface fractures with CT: What the surgeon needs to know *Radiographics.* 2006; 26:783–793.

Kallmes DF, Comstock BA, Heagerty PJ. A randomized trial of vertebroplasty for osteoporotic spinal fractures. *N Engl J Med.* 2009; 361(6):569–79.

Laine FJ, Shedden AI, Dunn MM, et al, Acquired intracranial herniations: MR imaging findings. Pictoral essay AJR. 1995; 165:967–973.

Louis D, Ohgaki H, Wiestler O, et al. *WHO Classification of Tumours of the Central Nervous System.* 4th ed. International Agency for Research on Cancer, 2007.

Som PM, Curtin HD, Mancuso AA. *Am J Roentgenol.* 2000, 174(3):837–844.

SUNY Downstate brain MRI anatomy (http://ect.downstate.edu/courseware/neuro_atlas

University Virginia Evaluation of the Cervical Spine (www.med-ed.virginia.edu/courses/rad/headct/)

University Virginia Intro to Head CT module (www.med-ed.virginia.edu/courses/rad/headct/)

Chapter 9

Nuclear Medicine

Alan Siegel, MD

Principles of physiologic imaging *414*
  Radioisotopes and radiopharmaceuticals *414*
  Diagnosis versus therapy *414*
  How to read nuclear medicine images *414*
Specific radiation precautions related to nuclear medicine *416*
  Nursing mothers *417*
Tumor imaging/PET scans *417*
Bone imaging *420*
  When should I order a nuclear medicine study? *420*
  Radiotracers and protocols *421*
Renal imaging *424*
Endocrine imaging *426*
  When should I order a nuclear medicine study? *426*
  Radiotracers and protocols *426*
  Common conditions *428*
  Therapeutic uses of I-131 *429*
Cardiac imaging *430*
  When should I order a nuclear medicine study? *430*
  Radiotracers and protocols *430*
  Common conditions *433*
GI imaging *435*
  When should I order a nuclear medicine study? *435*
  Radiotracers and protocols *435*
  Common conditions *436*
Lung imaging *438*
  Radiotracers and protocols *439*
  Common conditions *439*
Other nuclear medicine studies *440*
  Central nervous system *441*
  Infection imaging *441*
References *442*

Principles of physiologic imaging

Images created within nuclear medicine are based upon the function or physiology of an organ or structure as opposed to radiography, CT, and MRI, which generally depict anatomy.

Radioisotopes and radiopharmaceuticals
Radioisotope
- A radioactive compound.
- Generally a short-lived isotope (e.g., Tc-99m, I-123).
- For medical imaging radioisotopes are used that emit photons from the nucleus (gamma rays).
- Photons then detected (counted) by a gamma camera, PET scanner, or Geiger counter.

Radiopharmaceutical or radiotracer
- A radioisotope attached (labeled) to a specific compound.
- Administered and taken up by specific target tissues—dictated by the compound selected.
- Compound will be transported or metabolized based on the function of the organ or system being studied.
- For example: hepatobiliary pharmaceuticals are administered intravenously, actively transported into hepatocytes in relation to liver function, and then excreted into and cleared by the biliary tree.
- Route of administration varies with study: intravenously, orally, inhaled, intrathecally, intra-arterially.

Diagnosis versus therapy
Radiotracers can be used for imaging or for therapy. Generally, isotopes that have shorter half-lives and produce gamma rays are used for imaging, whereas those that produce higher energy β-particles are used for therapy.
- Sometimes the same isotope can be used for both (e.g., I-131 which emits both β and gamma), but is given in much higher amounts for therapy.
- Therapeutic radiotracers can be used to treat an overactive thyroid or to treat several different malignancies.
- Therapy may be performed by radiologists, nuclear-medicine physicians, or radiation oncologists.

How are images acquired?
Emission versus transmission scanning
Transmission scanning (radiography, CT, etc.)
- Photons/x-rays produced from a device or source pass through a patient striking a detector or film.

Emission scanning (nuclear medicine)
- Photons are emitted from the patient after the tracer has been administered; the patient is the source of radiation. The gamma/PET camera produces no radiation; it is simply a detector.

PRINCIPLES OF PHYSIOLOGIC IMAGING

Protocols
- Vary depending on the study.

Obtaining images
The time delay from injection to obtaining images varies. An appropriate amount of time must elapse to allow uptake and concentration by the organ or structure of interest. Images may be obtained at one or more times relative to the injection time:
- Immediately (e.g., flow study).
- Minutes (e.g., PET scan).
- Hours (e.g., bone scan).
- Days (e.g., iodine whole body scan).
- Individual image acquisition times are usually 5–45 minutes.

Patient activity level
- Radiotracer administered while patient active (stress): e.g. in cardiac-perfusion scans, the patient is injected during treadmill or pharmacological stress.
- Radiotracer administered at rest: Cerebral-perfusion and PET scans require the patient to be resting during the uptake period.

Postprocessing
Computer analysis enables data to be quantified in multiple ways such as producing uptake and washout curves and comparisons with normal databases. This quantification can be used to display and quantify, for example:
- The differential split function between paired organs (e.g. lungs and kidneys) can be obtained.
- Curves of blood flow into organs (e.g., kidneys).
- Excretion from organs (e.g., kidneys, liver).
- Emptying of structures (e.g., renal pelvis, gallbladder, stomach).
- Graphical representations of radiotracer uptake, e.g., "bulls eye" displays of myocardial perfusion.

Hardware
- Nuclear medicine scanners (gamma or PET cameras) are radiation (photon) detectors.

The standard gamma camera
Camera head has three key components.
- The scintillation crystal converts an absorbed photon into light, which is then detected by an array of photomultiplier (PM) tubes that produce an electric current. This can then be converted into an image or quantitative data.
- Attached to the face of the crystal is the collimator, which markedly improves the spatial resolution of the study.
- Gamma cameras typically have one or more rotating heads that allow "tomographic" reconstruction—images produced as multiplanar slices = SPECT (single photon emission computed tomography).

PET (positron emission tomography) scanners
- Designed to image the photons emitted from isotopes such as F-18 that undergo positron decay.
- These decays result in the simultaneous production of two gamma rays (=annihilation photons) that travel in opposite directions 180° apart.
- Ring of crystals around patient record an event when two photons strike opposite sides of the ring at the same time.
- Tomographic imaging (i.e., images displayed as multiplanar slices) is standard.

Hybrid scanners
- Recently, both gamma cameras and PET scanners have been modified by the addition of CT scanners to their gantries.
- Allows acquisition of SPECT or PET studies with a CT scan (i.e., combined functional and anatomic information).
  - Much improved anatomical localization of abnormalities.
- Allows for correction for attenuation of photons as they pass through different thicknesses of body tissue.
- Data displayed side by side or fused together into one image.

How to read nuclear medicine images

Nuclear medicine images are usually processed and interpreted using specialized software and workstations, although some may be displayed on conventional PACS workstations. Images may be displayed in both grayscale (black on white or white on black) and color scales. Cardiac, brain studies, and "fused" PET or SPECT images are commonly displayed in various vendor-dependent color scales.

- Areas of increased radiotracer uptake are often termed "hot spots," as opposed to areas of decreased uptake, which are termed "cold spots" or "photopenic."
- The physiological nature of nuclear medicine means that images contain areas of normal physiological uptake and excretion as well as pathological e.g., kidneys, bladder, bowel.
- These are specific for a radiotracer, so normal uptake and excretory patterns must be known to interpret images.
- The appearance will vary over time as the tracer is metabolized and excreted.
- These can mask pathological uptake, or be mistaken for it.

Specific radiation precautions related to nuclear medicine

There are differences in the way staff and patients are exposed to radiation in nuclear medicine compared to other areas of radiology, and the radiation precautions that must be undertaken differ as well. As always, the risks of radiation exposure must be weighed against the potential benefit of the study. Extra care must be taken for circumstances in which radiation effects are greater: children and pregnant women.

What is the radiation exposure to the patient dependent on?
- Dose given (mCi/MBq administered).
- Radioisotope used (longer half-life = more radiation exposure).
- Physiological kinetics of the radiotracer compound (which organs it goes to and how long it stays in the body).

What about relatives, staff, and other contacts?
The dose that contacts receive depends on:
- How long they spend near the patient.
- How close to the patient they are (radiation falls off with distance squared).

Instructions may need to be given to patients about how to minimize the radiation dose to others. Therapeutic studies are special circumstances in which particularly high doses of radiation are administered. Post-procedural instructions are mandatory and, in some instances, hospital admission is required.

Nursing mothers
- Need to express and discard milk for a variable period depending on the radioisotope (usually around 4 half-lives).
- If iodine-131 is given, nursing cannot resume.
- Need to avoid close contact with baby for similar period.

Tumor imaging

Radiopharmaceuticals can be targeted toward glucose transporters, tumor-specific antigens, and peptide-binding receptors on tumors.

When is nuclear medicine used to image tumors?
- PET-CT using F-18 FDG is routinely used for the diagnosis, staging and follow-up (evaluation of therapy) of many common tumors.
- Iodine-131 scanning is the standard of care for the evaluation and treatment of patients with differentiated thyroid cancer following thyroidectomy.
- The other commonly used tumor-seeking pharmaceuticals, octreotide, and MIBG are typically used as problem solvers when presence of particular tumors is suspected but not detected by conventional imaging modalities.

Radiotracers and protocols
F-18 FDG (F-18 fluorodeoxyglucose)
Specific features
Used in the vast majority of PET CT scans:
- Analog of glucose.
- Intensely accumulated by most malignancies > than surrounding tissue.
- Most tumors have high levels of glucose transporters.
- F-18 FDG is phosphorylated by hexokinase but then does not undergo further glycolysis. Therefore, it accumulates and remains trapped in the tumor cell.

- F-18 FDG avid tumors include lung cancer (both small-cell and non-small-cell), lymphoma, melanoma, breast, colorectal and esophageal cancer.
- FDG PET tends to be fairly <u>insensitive</u> for prostate and many renal cell cancers and is not routinely used in these conditions.

Patient preparation

In order to reduce the background uptake of radiotracer by muscles, the patients are injected with F-18 FDG while resting quietly and after a 6-hour fast.

- Patients are kept warm and may be pretreated with benzodiazepines to reduce brown fat uptake, which is a common cause of a false positive study (seen in neck, mediastinum, paraspinal, peri-renal regions).

Normal study (see Figure 9.1)

F-18 FDG is taken up by all normal tissues in varying amounts.

<u>High uptake:</u>
- Brain, urine (collecting systems, bladder), heart when not fasting.

<u>Moderate uptake:</u>
- Muscle, liver, spleen, gut (can be high sometimes).

<u>Low uptake:</u>
- Bone, fat, lung.

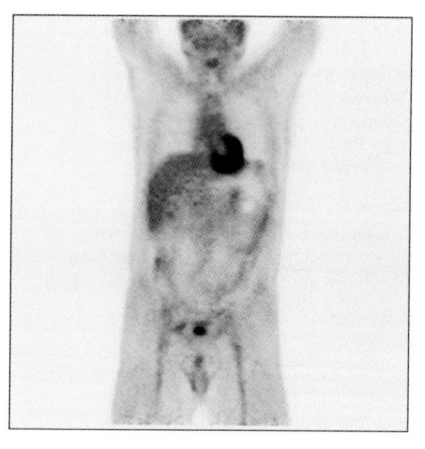

Figure 9.1 Coronal slice of a PET scan demonstrates a normal distribution of FDG. Moderate activity is visible in the soft tissues of the liver and in the blood pool including vascular structures and the mediastinum. There is more intense activity in the myocardium and in urine.

Causes of a false positive FDG study
- Misinterpretation of physiological uptake of F-18 FDG.
- Muscle activity (e.g., working out, talking).
- Gut activity (very variable).
- Infection (granulocytes accumulate F-18 FDG).
- Inflammation (arthritis, surgical sites, radiation pneumonitis).
- Granulomatous disease (e.g., sarcoidosis—has intense uptake).
- Brown fat (especially in neck, mediastinum. Most common in young women during cold weather).

Causes of a false negative FDG study
- Tumors that may not accumulate F-18 FDG (e.g., prostate, renal, some mucinous tumors, extranodal MALT lymphomas, HCC).
- Diabetic patients, especially if serum glucose >200 mg/dl.
- Non-fasting patients.

Applications

<u>Differentiating benign versus malignant masses:</u>
- Malignant tumors usually have increased FDG accumulation whereas benign disease will have minimal to no activity (see Figure 9.2).

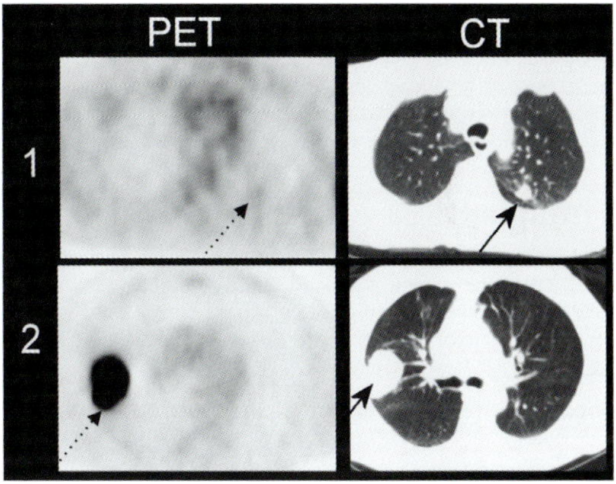

Figure 9.2 Axial PET-CT scans are from two patients who presented with pulmonary nodules. The nodule from patient 1 is a granuloma and has been stable with little FDG uptake (dashed arrow) where the nodule in patient 2 has intense FDG accumulation and subsequently diagnosed as non-small-cell lung cancer.

<u>Staging and response assessment:</u>
- FDG PET also has proven value in assessing response to therapy and restaging of many cancers.

- The intensity of uptake of FDG by many tumors (quantifiable by computer—as the standardized uptake value or SUV) correlates with outcome.
- Tumors with greater FDG activity tend to indicate poorer prognosis with many tumor types.
- Decreasing FDG accumulation early after the initiation of treatment with chemotherapy often implies improved outcomes.
- This "metabolic response" occurs before visible tumor shrinkage.

For other applications of F-18 FDG PET, see cardiac and neuroimaging sections, later in this chapter.

I-131 iodine and I-123 iodine
See p. 432 below, Endocrine section.

In-111 pentetreotide
Indium-111 labeled pentetreotide (Octreoscan®) is an example of a peptide utilized for imaging.

Specific features
- Analog of somatostatin (similar to octreotide), a peptide that binds somatostatin receptors.
- Somatostatin receptors are present on a variety of tumors such as neuroblastoma, carcinoid, pheochromocytoma, meningiomas and neuroendocrine tumors of the pancreas.

Applications
- Diagnosis in patients with clinical suspicion of a neuroendocrine tumor (e.g., carcinoid syndrome) when anatomic studies unhelpful.
- Stage patients when a neuroendocrine tumor has been diagnosed.
- Determine if a known tumor has somatostatin receptors if therapy with octreotide is being considered.

Bone imaging

Bone scanning is one of the most common procedures performed in nuclear medicine. These studies use tracers that distribute within the skeleton in relation to the degree of bone turnover (blood flow is also a determinant). The skeleton attempts to repair itself after injury by laying down new bone.

When should I order a nuclear medicine study?

Metastasis
- Staging and follow-up of malignancy, particularly those that have a predilection for skeletal metastases.

Suspected fracture
- In patients with suspected fractures, bone scans are of value when radiography is negative but the suspicion of injury remains high.

Suspected child abuse
- Due to its excellent sensitivity, bone scanning is often routinely performed in cases of suspected child abuse. (see p. 324, chapter 6, Pediatrics).

Suspected infection
- Particularly in painful prostheses or in children in whom the site of infection may be uncertain or multifocal (e.g., young child with a painful extremity).

Radiotracers and protocols
Tc-99m MDP
Virtually all bone scanning uses Tc-99m methylene diphosphonate (Tc-99m MDP).

Three phase bone scan versus single phase
When a patient is being evaluated for an infectious, traumatic or inflammatory process, a three-phase bone scan should be performed. This provides information on blood flow, blood pool, and bone turnover. Processes that have an infectious, traumatic or inflammatory component will display abnormally increased activity in all three phases of the bone scan.

Single-phase bone scan
The agent is administered intravenously and the scan performed approximately three hours later. About half the administered dose localizes within the skeleton and the remainder clears from the background through the renal system.

Three-phase bone scan
The agent is administered intravenously, and imaging obtained at three time points:
- Initial immediate set of images focused on the area of interest are acquired during the injection of the tracer. This creates an angiographic or "flow" phase.
- Five minutes later, an image focused on the area of interest is again obtained and reflects activity within the extracellular fluid. This is called the "blood pool" phase.
- The third phase is the three-hour delayed bone scan.

Normal Tc-99m MDP bone scan
- A normal bone scan generally displays uniform activity throughout the skeleton, with some exceptions:
- Some areas may appear focally "hot" but are normal: the inferior tips of the scapulas, the medial iliac bones, the superolateral aspects of the orbits and posteriorly in the skull.
- Tc-99m MDP is renally excreted and, therefore, activity is seen in kidneys, renal collecting system, bladder, urinary catheters, etc.
- Soft-tissue activity should be a very low level uniformly throughout the body.

Common conditions
Metastatic cancer
Indications
Staging of malignancy and evaluation of response to therapy are the most common indications for performing bone scans.
- Prostate and breast cancer are the most common indications (high incidence of bone metastases and high sensitivity bone scans in these conditions).

CHAPTER 9 **Nuclear medicine**

- Metastases usually appear as focal areas of increased activity (almost always multiple) in the axial and proximal appendicular skeleton.
- Metastases are uncommon distal to the elbows and knees.

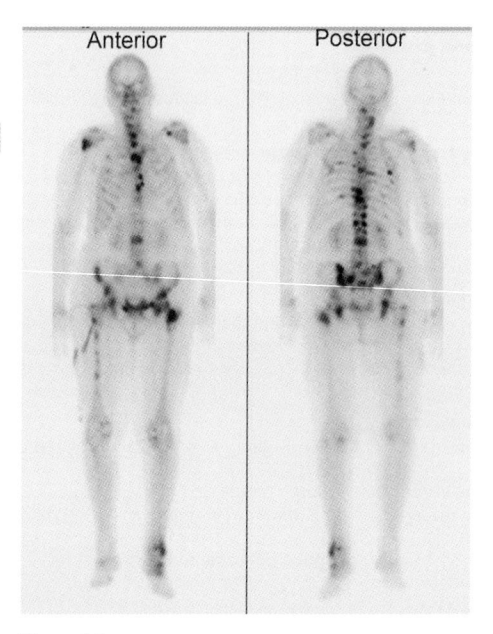

Figure 9.3 Multiple foci of increased activity indicating widespread metastatic disease in a patient with known prostate cancer. Tracer in catheter tubing lies across right thigh.

False negatives
Highly aggressive metastases may produce bone destruction so great that no new bone formation is detected. In these cases, metastases may appear as "cold defects" or they may be invisible.
- Multiple myeloma is a typical example, and bone scanning is not usually indicated for this disease.
- Also common in renal cell cancer, occasionally in small cell lung cancer.

False positives
Bone scanning has a high sensitivity but low specificity. False positives can be caused by:
- Degenerative arthritis or inflammatory arthritis (common), particularly in the spine.
- Trauma (e.g., rib fractures).

- Infection (uncommon).
- Postoperative changes.

It may be necessary to correlate with other studies in order to interpret an examination: plain films, CT scans, and prior bone scans. These are used to confirm a benign cause of uptake, such as a rib fracture, but cannot exclude a metastatic lesion.

Fractures

Bone scanning is an ancillary study in the workup of patients with suspected fractures; radiographs are always first line. Bone scans are highly sensitive shortly after the traumatic event (majority positive within 24 hrs). Typically focal increased activity is seen in all three phases.

Indications

Consider when x-rays are negative and there is continued suspicion of fracture:
- Suspected non-displaced fracture in a patient with osteopenia (for example a proximal femoral fracture or sacral insufficiency fracture).
- Suspected acute stress fracture (see Figure 9.4).
- These show focal, often intense, increased activity often with a completely normal x-ray.

Osteomyelitis

- Bone scans are an excellent means of diagnosing osteomyelitis, because they are highly sensitive (often positive before radiographs).

Typically focally increased activity is seen in all three phases.

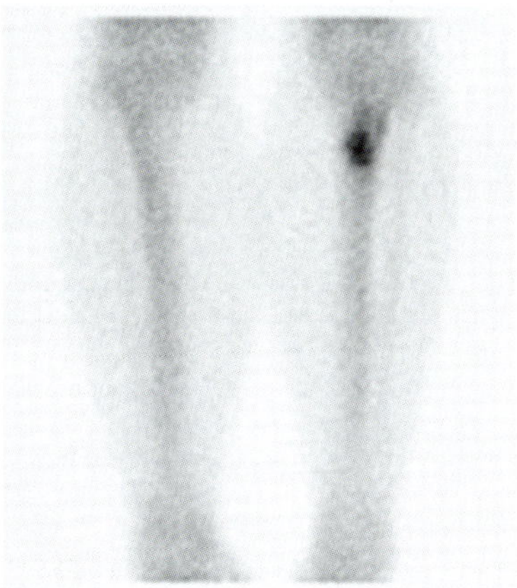

Figure 9.4 Stress fracture. 22-year-old marathon runner with left tibial pain and a normal x-ray. Bone scan demonstrates a focal area of intensely increased activity in the proximal shaft of the left tibia indicating a stress fracture.

Indications
- Excellent study for suspected osteomyelitis when radiograph is normal.
- Especially useful in pediatric patients because the disease can be multifocal and a bone scan imaging the entire skeleton can be performed.
- Scans can be difficult to evaluate when fractures and postoperative changes are also present. MRI or In-111 labeled white cell scan (+/– bone scan) should be considered in these circumstances.
- MRI preferred in chronic osteomyelitis.

Renal imaging

Nuclear medicine examinations enable evaluation of renal perfusion, renal function, and urinary clearance. Nuclear methodology also exists for the detection of vesicoureteral reflux.

When should I order a nuclear medicine study?
Assessment of renal function and clearance
- Suspected renal obstruction (e.g., newborn with prenatally diagnosed hydronephrosis, patients s/p ureteric surgery).
- Renal transplants (vascular compromise, obstruction, ATN).

Assessment of functioning renal parenchyma
- History of febrile urinary tract infections or vesicoureteral reflux to detect cortical scars or atrophy.
- Congenital renal anomalies, to evaluate residual renal function (e.g., polycystic dysplastic kidney).

Detection of vesicoureteral reflux (nuclear cystogram)
- Follow-up of known reflux.
- Screening of siblings.

Radiotracers and protocols
Multiphase renogram: Tc-99m MAG3 or Tc-99m DPTA

These two radiotracers are commonly used to evaluate renal function and clearance. Tc-99m DTPA is exclusively excreted via glomerular filtration whereas Tc-99m MAG3 is principally excreted via tubular secretion with a small proportion via glomerular filtration. Generally, MAG3 is the preferred tracer because higher intra-renal concentrations can be achieved in impaired renal function.

Protocol
- <u>Perfusion phase</u>: rapid imaging for the first minute depicts blood flow to the kidneys.
- <u>Uptake phase:</u> after one minute, the tracer is concentrated in the renal cortex allowing detection of scars, atrophy, and asymmetry of renal function.
- <u>Excretion phase</u>: activity then excreted into the collecting systems and then to the bladder.

Poor clearance of tracer from collecting system can be due to obstruction, but it may also be caused by dehydration, diminished renal function, or a dilated but non-obstructed collecting system. In cases of poor clearance, a fourth phase is added:
- <u>Lasix phase:</u> if clearance is inadequate, the study is supplemented by additional imaging after the administration of furosemide (see Figure 9.5).

Quantification is performed on all phases and provides an estimate of the split renal function and the clearance of tracer from the collecting system (clearance curve):
- Normal collecting systems should show a clearance t½ of <10 mins.
- Borderline obstruction t½ 10–20 mins.
- Obstruction t½ >20 mins.

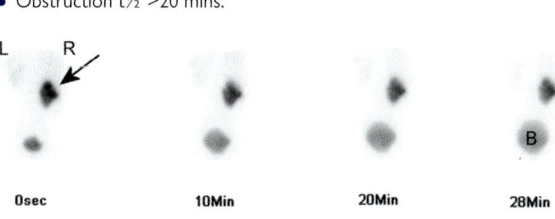

Figure 9.5 Congenital UPJ obstruction. Renal scan performed in a girl with a history of prenatal hydronephrosis. Posterior post-lasix images show that the left collecting system has cleared but there is very slow clearance from the dilated right-sided renal collecting system (arrow). B = bladder.

Tc-99m DMSA
Tc-99m DMSA differs from the DPTA and MAG3 because it has a component that binds to tubular cells and, therefore, it remains within the cortex. It is used for detection of renal cortical scars or atrophy and in the evaluation of relative right- versus left-sided renal function.

Protocol
- Administered intravenously and images obtained two hours later.
- Images in multiple projections or tomographic images obtained.

Nuclear cystogram: Tc-99m sulfur colloid (or DPTA)
- Highly sensitive, low-radiation dose means of evaluating for vesico-ureteral reflux.
- No anatomy so may need VCUG as first examination to exclude ectopic ureters, posterior urethral valves, etc.

Protocol
- A small catheter is placed in the bladder using sterile technique.
- Tc-99m tracer is mixed with saline and infused into the bladder.
- Sequential images are obtained, including both bladder and kidneys, in the posterior projection.
- The bladder is filled to capacity and imaging continued through voiding.

Endocrine imaging

Because the normal thyroid gland actively accumulates iodine to synthesize thyroid hormone, these tracers are examples of the isotope itself acting as the radiopharmaceutical. The two most commonly used isotopes are I-123 and I-131.

When should I order a nuclear medicine study?
Thyroid scans and thyroid uptake
Nuclear thyroid studies include qualitative scans of tracer distribution in the thyroid (thyroid scan) as well as quantitative measurement of iodine concentration by the thyroid (thyroid uptake).

Thyroid nodules
- Assessment of function in palpable nodules.

Hyperthyroidism
- Differentiation of Grave disease, toxic nodular goiter, and subacute thyroiditis.
- Quantification of uptake for planned I-131 therapy.

Hypothyroidism
- Other than in the newborn, where it is occasionally used to identify the cause of hypothyroidism, nuclear medicine has little value in the patient with hypothyroidism.

Neck/substernal masses
- Identification of functioning thyroid tissue in a neck or substernal mass (substernal goiter, ectopic thyroid tissue).

Evaluation for thyroid cancer metastases
- After thyroidectomy to screen for thyroid metastases.
- Routine scanning post-ablation with I-131.
- If serum thyroglobulin rises after surgery/ablation.

Therapy
- Treatment of hyperthyroidism.
- Ablation of thyroid remnants in patients with thyroid cancer s/p thyroidectomy.
- Treatment of metastatic thyroid cancer.

Parathyroid scan
Hyperparathyroidism
- Localization of parathyroid adenomas including ectopic (e.g., mediastinal) adenomas.
- Only performed in patients with diagnosed hyperparathyroidism.
- Localization prior to resection will shorten the intraoperative procedure and limit the extent of the neck dissection/morbidity.

Radiotracers and protocols
Thyroid scans are performed with Tc-99m pertechnetate or iodine isotopes, whereas the uptakes are almost always measured with iodine.

ENDOCRINE IMAGING

I-123 and I-131
Iodine is an essential component of thyroid hormone. Iodine is actively trapped by the thyroid gland and then bound to thyroglobulin ("organification").

Two isotopes of iodine that have been used for thyroid uptake measurements and scanning:

I-123
- Relatively low dose of radiation to the thyroid gland.
- Excellent for thyroid nodule evaluation.
- Scans of thyroid obtained at 24 hours after oral dose.
- Also used for thyroid uptake measurements.
- Uptake measured usually 24 hours after oral dose +/– a 4 to 6 hour measurement.
- More expensive than other thyroid tracers and sometimes difficult to obtain.
- Not used for cancer imaging because the half life of I-123 is too short for the delayed images that are required to allow physiological bowel and bladder activity to clear.

I-131
- Emits energetic beta particles as well as high-energy gamma rays.
  - Results in a fairly high dose of radiation.
- Not used for routine imaging of the thyroid due to radiation dose to thyroid and poor imaging characteristics (due to high energy).
- Used for detection of metastatic thyroid cancer only after a patient has had a thyroidectomy.
- Intense uptake by normal thyroid impairs visualization of tumor elsewhere.
- Enables visualization of tissue deep within the body as the high energy gamma rays can penetrate tissue effectively.
- Whole-body images of patients are obtained usually 8–10 days after an ablative dose of I-131 or 48 hours after a diagnostic dose.
- Iodine is normally only accumulated in the stomach, kidneys and bladder, salivary glands, and bowel.
- Used in tiny doses for uptake measurements.
- Uptake measured at 24 hrs post-oral dose.
- Used for treatment of thyrotoxicosis and thyroid cancer.

Tc-99m pertechnetate
Tc-99m pertechnetate is trapped by the thyroid gland but does not undergo organification. It can be administered in a relatively high dose, providing excellent, rapid images and imparts a low dose of radiation to the patient.
- Both benign and malignant nodules may trap technetium (though it is not common with malignancy).
- Malignant nodules are never hyperfunctioning.
- Patients are scanned 20 minutes following IV injection.

Normal thyroid scan
- Normal thyroid scan (either I-123 or Tc-99m) is homogeneous without hot or cold nodules; the thyroid lobes may be asymmetric in size.
- Normal 24-hour uptake ≈ 10–30%.

Tc-99m sestamibi parathyroid study
Parathyroid scanning is performed with Tc-99m sestamibi (or Tc-99m tetrofosmin). Normal parathyroid glands are not visible on a parathyroid scan; only parathyroid adenomas will be seen.

Protocol
Initial images at ≈10 minutes:
- Sestamibi accumulates in both the parathyroid and thyroid glands.

Delayed images at ≈2 hours:
- Sestamibi is retained by the parathyroid glands but washes out of the thyroid gland. Parathyroid adenomas, if sufficiently large, are seen as foci of increased activity on the delayed studies.
- Thyroid adenomas can retain the tracer as well, so additional thyroid imaging may be needed (I-123/Tc-99m pertechnetate, or ultrasound). With thyroid adenomas, the thyroid scan will show focally increased or decreased uptake concordant to the parathyroid scan.

Normal parathyroid scan
Homogenous uptake and washout of tracer by the thyroid gland with no residual "hot" spots. Little residual tracer on the delayed images.

Common conditions
Grave disease
Grave disease is a common cause of hyperthyroidism. This autoimmune process will result in diffusely increased activity within an enlarged gland with no nodules. The thyroid uptake measurement will be elevated (see Figure 9.6).

Toxic nodular goiter
Toxic nodular goiters can be due to single or multiple hyperfunctioning adenomas.

Solitary toxic nodules
- Single "hot" nodule, with decreased uptake in rest of gland due to suppressed TSH.
- The overall uptake may or may not be increased.

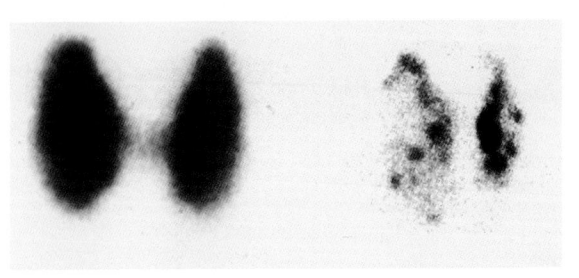

Figure 9.6 Two patients with hyperthyroidism. Grave disease (left) shows diffusely increased uptake compared to multinodular goiter (right), which shows multiple foci of increased and decreased activity.

Toxic multinodular goiters (TMNG) (see Figure 9.6).
- Heterogeneous radiotracer accumulation, also with an elevated uptake. TMNG, in general, have lower uptakes than Grave disease and occur in older populations.
- Note, not all multinodular goiters are "toxic," that is, they do not all have raised thyroid hormone levels.

Thyroid nodule evaluation

Nodules on iodine scans can be "cold" (nodules taking up less iodine than the rest of the gland) or "hot" (nodules taking up more iodine than the rest of the gland).

"Cold" nodules
- Differentiated thyroid cancers (papillary and follicular) concentrate iodine to a lesser degree than the normal thyroid gland, so thyroid cancer usually presents as a solitary cold thyroid nodulenodule (see Figure 9.7).
- 15% of solitary cold nodules are malignant.
- Cysts and adenomas also usually appear as cold defects.

"Hot" nodules
- Indicate that the nodule is a benign, often hyperfunctioning, adenoma.

Therapeutic uses of I-131
The high energy beta particles emitted by I-131 enable this isotope to be used as an effective therapy because both the normal thyroid and thyroid cancer cells will accumulate the tracer and be killed by the radiation.

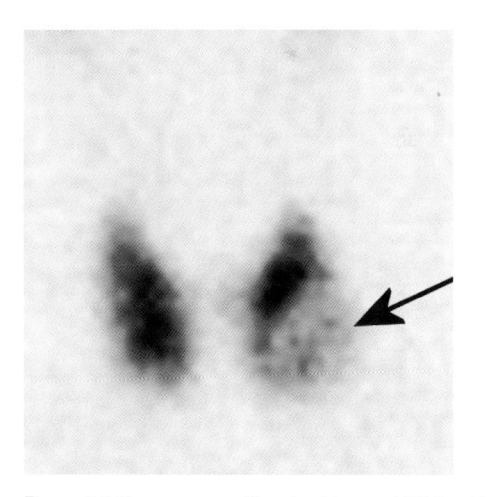

Figure 9.7 Biopsy proven papillary thyroid cancer. I-123 thyroid scan performed in a patient with a lump in the left side of the neck. Thyroid scan shows a cold defect in the left lobe (arrow).

Thyrotoxicosis
- Patients with Grave disease or toxic nodular goiters can have their disease controlled by one or two doses of I-131 (usually 5–30 mCi).
- Few side effects, high success rate.
- Higher doses needed in toxic nodular goiters than Grave disease.
- Eventual outcome is often hypothyroidism necessitating lifelong hormone replacement.

Thyroid cancer
In patients with differentiated thyroid cancer:
- I-131 can ablate residual thyroid tissue following surgery and potentially cures patients with thyroid cancer remaining within the neck (thyroid bed or cervical lymph nodes).
- Extremely effective, though rarely curative, in patients with distant metastases.
- Usually 100–200 mCi I-131 given.
- Total body radiation doses from this treatment are low and side effects are not common.

Cardiac imaging

The two major types of nuclear cardiac imaging are stress myocardial perfusion imaging and gated blood pool scans.

When should I order a nuclear medicine study?

Gated blood pool scans ("MUGA" scans)
MUGA = "multi-gated acquisition," also called gated blood pool scans (GBPS), and equilibrium radionuclide angiocardiography (ERNA).
- Evaluation of wall motion and ejection fraction of the left ventricle.
- Commonly performed in patients receiving cardiotoxic therapies such as adriamycin.

Stress myocardial perfusion imaging
- Detection of coronary artery disease in patients with symptoms or risk factors, particularly intermediate risk levels.
- Assessment of the significance of existing coronary lesions.
- Follow-up of patients being treated for coronary artery disease.

F-18 FDG glucose metabolism PET scan
Used to distinguish viable myocardium versus myocardial infarction in some patients prior to surgery.

Radiotracers and protocols

Gated blood pool scans (Tc-99m labeled RBC MUGA)
- By labeling the red blood cells, MUGAs display the blood pool in the ventricular chamber.
- This study can be used to quantify the size of the LV chamber, motion of the walls, and calculate the LV ejection fraction.
- It does not provide direct information regarding myocardial perfusion.

CARDIAC IMAGING

Perfusion imaging

Stressing patients with suspected coronary artery disease carries a small but definite risk of them having a cardiac event during imaging. The test must be carried out by caregivers familiar with the test and skilled at providing emergency life support.
- A normal scan at an adequate stress level is a powerful indicator of a low likelihood of future adverse cardiac events.

Patient preparation
- Patients should not eat due to the small risk of a cardiac event.
- Patients may be asked to discontinue beta blockers in order to be able to increase heart rate during the exercise test.

Pharmacologic stressors related to adenosine are counteracted by caffeine, so patients are asked to avoid coffee and other caffeinated beverages prior to the exam.

Tc-99m Sestamibi or Tetrofosmin perfusion imaging

These are the two most commonly used tracers for perfusion imaging. Both tracers are accumulated in the heart in relation to blood flow *at the time of the injection*. These two tracers have similar mechanisms of uptake, acquisition protocols, and scan appearances.

Protocol
Following injection, 2 SPECT scans are obtained:
1. During stress (treadmill or pharmacological).
2. During rest.

Thallium-201 chloride perfusion imaging

Tl-201 chloride is an older cardiac tracer that functions differently than sestamibi and tetrofosmin.

Protocol
Tracer is injected during stress, and 2 scans are obtained:
1. During stress.
2. Delayed images: obtained at 3–4 hours.
    - The stress scan is a depiction of blood flow during the stress phase.
    - Over time, thallium will "redistribute" in the myocardium.
        — Areas of normal myocardium wash out tracer faster than ischemic zones.
        — Stress-induced ischemia will appear as a reversible defect.

Thallium images are:
- Lower image quality than the Tc-99m tracers, especially in obese patients.
- Superior to the Tc-99m tracers in detecting hibernating myocardium (viable myocardium with decreased blood flow and function).

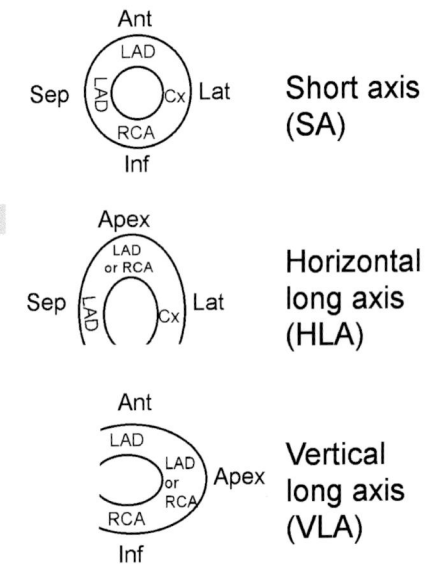

Figure 9.8 Schematic diagram of heart in each of the standard reconstruction planes with wall names and coronary vascular supply. LAD = left anterior descending artery, RCA = right coronary artery, Cx = left circumflex artery.

Methods of stress

Treadmill exercise
- Ideal because it increases myocardial oxygen demand and allows assessment of patient's exercise tolerance.
- Patient exercises to maximal capacity.

Coronary vasodilators
- Given when patients cannot exercise.
- Normal vessels dilate (↑myocardial perfusion 3–5x) but stenotic vessels will not (no change in myocardial perfusion to the supplied territory).
- Resultant scan appearance will be that of a flow defect distal to areas of stenosis.
- The most commonly used pharmacologic vasodilator is adenosine and its analog, regadenoson. Dipyridamole (persantine) was used previously.
- Contraindicated in some patients with reactive airways disease.

Image quantification and display
- Comparison of the two image sets may reveal a stress induced defect not present at rest (inducible ischemia) or defects in both sets (myocardial infarction).
- The data can be compared to normal data sets, usually displayed as a "bulls eye" showing areas of perfusion that are <2SD of normal.
- Images are gated to the cardiac cycle with an ECG, and displayed in cine format, showing wall motion in a 3D format.

Normal perfusion scans
- Uniform activity throughout the myocardium.
- Septum appears shorter in length than the other walls of the LV.
- Slightly less activity in the apex.

F-18 Fluorodeoxyglucose (FDG)
F-18 FDG PET can be used to detect viable myocardium in patients with chronic ischemia to select appropriate candidates for revascularization.
- Ischemic or "hibernating" myocardium preferentially metabolizes glucose, whereas normal myocardium utilizes fatty acids as its substrate.
- Viable myocardium with decreased blood flow (as determined by myocardial perfusion scanning by PET or SPECT) or abnormal wall motion (seen with echocardiography) will accumulate FDG, whereas infarcted segments will not.
- It is more expensive than SPECT with Tc-99m or Tl-201 agents, although more accurate, and may require protocols that need very careful control of patient's blood glucose levels.

> **Hibernating myocardium**
> Hibernating myocardium is myocardium that is so severely ischemic that it does not contract properly or at all (hypo- or akinetic), but is still viable. It can appear as a myocardial infarct (fixed defect) on myocardial perfusion imaging, but will take up F-18 FDG and may take up Tl-201.

Common conditions
Myocardial Ischemia
Best evaluated with stress perfusion imaging.

Imaging findings
- Focal decreased radiotracer uptake on the stress image set that is normal/improved at rest (see Figure 9.9).
- The distribution of ischemia often indicates the coronary artery(s) involved.
- On an F-18 FDG scan, the ischemic areas should accumulate FDG.

Myocardial infarction
Best evaluated with stress perfusion imaging.

Imaging findings
- Decreased blood flow at stress that remains unchanged at rest. Distribution of the defect may indicate the occluded vessel (see Figure 9.10).

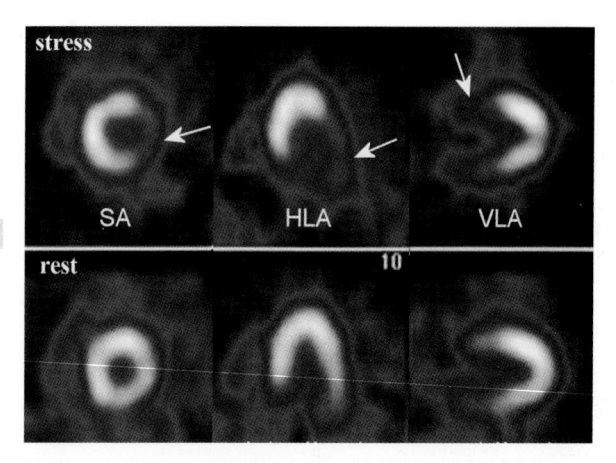

Figure 9.9 Coronary ischemia. Myocardial perfusion scan performed on a patient with chest pain. Decreased blood flow in the lateral wall on stress (arrows) that is normal at rest. Cardiac catheterization confirmed stenosis of the left circumflex coronary artery. See Color Plate 13.

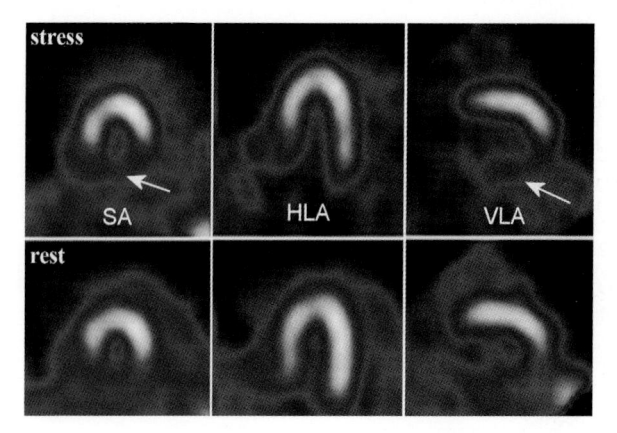

Figure 9.10 Myocardial infarct. Myocardial perfusion scan performed on a patient with a history of MI and dyspnea. Fixed defect in the inferior wall indicating infarction (arrow). No ischemia detected. See Color Plate 14.

- Large areas of infarction may be accompanied by chamber dilatation.
- Wall motion abnormalities are usually present in the area of infarction.
- Thallium is superior to the Tc-99m tracers at distinguishing scar from hibernating myocardium, and F-18 FDG PET better than Tl-201.

Cardiomyopathy

Dysfunction of the cardiac chambers has various causes in addition to coronary artery disease, e.g., viral, toxic, chemotherapeutic agents, alcohol. Wall motion abnormalities may be seen on both MUGA and myocardial perfusion scans as well as echocardiography, but a perfusion scan may be needed to exclude coronary artery disease as a cause.

Imaging findings
- LV chamber may be enlarged.
- Wall motion abnormalities may be focal or diffuse.
- If non-ischemic, no focal perfusion defects seen.

GI imaging

Nuclear imaging of the gastrointestinal tract includes a large variety of studies. This chapter will concentrate on the most commonly performed: hepatobiliary scans, GI bleeding scans and gastric emptying studies.

When should I order a nuclear medicine study?

Hepatobiliary scans
- The most accurate means of diagnosing acute and chronic cholecystitis.
- Detection of bile leaks.
- Diagnosis of biliary obstruction.
- Diagnosis of biliary atresia in neonates.

Bleeding scans
- Patients with active lower GI bleeds, or GI bleeds of uncertain origin.
- Usually performed prior to endoscopy or angiography.

Gastric emptying studies
- Patients with suspicion of gastric motility disorders.
- Assesses function rather than anatomy (in contrast to an UGI study).

Radiotracers and protocols

Tc-99m hepatobiliary scan

Hepatobiliary scans (often called "HIDA" scans after Tc-99m HIDA, a tracer that is no longer used) are a method for evaluating the flow of bile from the liver. Disofenin (DISIDA) and mebrofenin are the most common agents used.

Protocol
- Patients should be fasting for 4–24 hours prior to the study.
- Tracers are injected intravenously, taken up by hepatocytes and then excreted into the bile where they will follow the flow of bile.
- Images are obtained at 1-minute intervals for 60 minutes.

If the gallbladder is not visualized at one hour, either:
- Delayed images are obtained 4 hours later.

- Morphine is administered and imaging continued for 30 minutes (morphine will constrict the sphincter of Oddi).
- Evaluation of the gallbladder's ability to contract can be made by infusing an analog of cholecystokinin (sincalide) after visualization of the gallbladder.
- This procedure may be used to diagnose acalculous chronic cholecystitis (gallbladder dyskinesia).
- Sometimes sincalide is given before the start of a hepatobiliary study if the patient has fasting for a longtime (e.g., ICU patient) to prevent a false positive scan from an overfilled gallbladder.

Normal hepatobiliary scan
- Prompt and uniform concentration of activity by the liver.
- The gallbladder is visualized within the first 60 minutes of the study.
- Small bowel activity is typically seen within the first 60 minutes, but later visualization is not necessarily abnormal.

Tc-99m labeled RBC GI bleeding scan
Bleeding scans are the most sensitive imaging tests for detecting sites of GI bleeds; able to detect bleeding rates of 0.1–1.0ml/min. They typically are the first study ordered in patients with lower GI tract bleeds, and, if positive, angiography with embolization may ensue. Only active bleeding can be evaluated.
- Bleeding scans are less sensitive for upper tract bleeds; endoscopy is usually the first test performed.

Protocol
- The patient's own red blood cells are labeled with Tc-99m pertechnetate and then reinjected.
- Dynamic imaging performed over at least 1 hour.
- Sites of active bleeding seen as foci of activity that appear in the GI tract and move along the course of the bowel on sequential scans.
- Delayed imaging (e.g., if patient rebleeds on floor) rarely helpful for localization due to rapid antegrade and retrograde transit of blood in bowel.

Gastric emptying studies
These studies are performed in patients in whom delayed (or occasionally increased) gastric emptying is suspected, for example, diabetic patients with postprandial bloating and vomiting.

Protocol
- A standardized meal (e.g., egg sandwich) is labeled with Tc-99m sulfur colloid and ingested.
- Images are obtained at 0, 1, 2, and 4 hours and the % emptied calculated and compared to normal database.
- Normally >90% has emptied by 4 hours.

Common conditions
Acute and chronic cholecystitis
Acute cholecystitis
Usually due to obstruction of the cystic duct by a gallstone.

Imaging findings:
- Non-filling of the gallbladder even on delayed imaging or after administration of morphine (see Figure 9.11).
- Acalculous cholecystitis produces the same imaging findings.

Chronic cholecystitis
- Usually manifests as delayed filling of the gallbladder (after one hour), though in some cases, the gall bladder may fill normally.
- The gallbladder will fill by the 4-hour image or during the post-morphine phase.
- The diagnosis also can be made by detecting abnormal emptying of the gallbladder after a sincalide infusion.

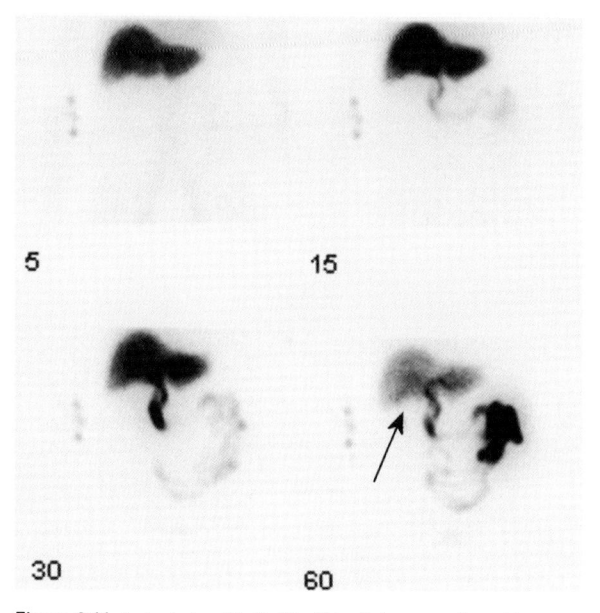

Figure 9.11 Acute cholecystitis. Tc-99m Mebrofenin scan performed in a patient with RUQ pain, fever, and leukocytosis. Images shown were taken 5, 15, 30, and 60 minutes after tracer injection. Activity is present in the liver and small bowel, but there is no filling of the gall bladder (arrow = empty gallbladder fossa).

Common bile duct obstruction
- No visualization of activity in the small bowel or the gall bladder with retained liver activity due to lack of excretion.
- High pressures in the biliary system prevent gallbladder filling.
- The diagnosis of concurrent acute cholecystitis cannot be made in this circumstance.

GI bleeding

Typically used in UGI bleeds when endoscopy is negative, especially if chronic.

May be used as first study in lower GI bleeds or if endoscopy is negative in both acute and chronic bleeds (can direct angiography).

- GI bleeds are characteristically intermittent, so, abnormal foci of tracer may appear at anytime during the study.
- Blood in the bowel can move in both an antegrade and retrograde direction (see Figure 9.12).
- The sensitivity of the study will increase with longer imaging times.
- Bleeding sites within the large bowel may move very slowly along the course of the bowel.
- Small-bowel bleeds move rapidly and, due to dilution by the fluid in the bowel, may appear and disappear during the course of the study.

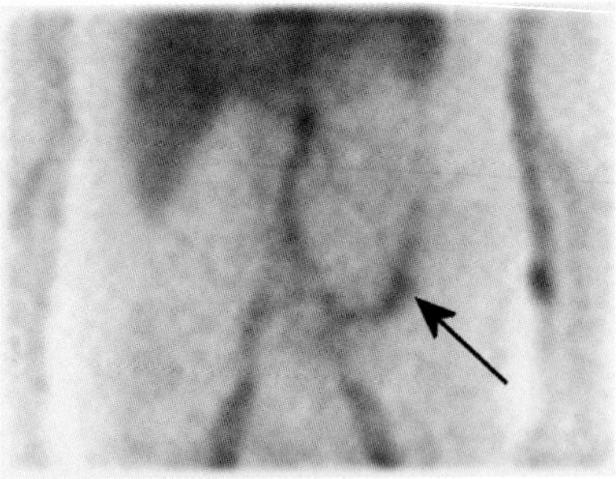

Figure 9.12 Sigmoid colon hemorrhage. Patient presented to the emergency room with bright red blood per rectum. Single image from bleeding scan shows extravasated blood in the sigmoid colon (arrow) with both retrograde and antegrade movement.

Lung imaging

Lung scanning (ventilation–perfusion (VQ) scanning) has generally been replaced by CT pulmonary angiography as the first line test for the diagnosis of pulmonary emboli; however a role remains for this study.

When should I order a VQ scan?

Patients with suspected pulmonary embolism with:
- Renal dysfunction or a history of severe contrast reactions.
- Patients with no history of pulmonary disease and normal chest x-rays and in young women, because of the relatively low-radiation dose to the breast compared to CT.
- Patients with impaired lung function in whom lobectomy/pneumonectomy is considered. A "split lung function" can be obtained with the perfusion scan.
- A current CXR is vital for appropriate interpretation of the VQ scan.

LUNG IMAGING

Radiotracers and protocols
Tc-99m MAA (Perfusion imaging)
- MAA particles are small, slightly larger in size than a capillary.
- When injected intravenously, they will distribute within the lungs according to blood flow.
- The percentage of the pulmonary capillary bed that is obstructed is minimal and carries no significant risk unless severe pulmonary hypertension or a large right to left cardiac shunt is present.

Xe-133 and Tc-99m DTPA aerosol (Ventilation imaging)
Xenon is a gas and DTPA is an aerosolized solution.
- Both are inhaled and will distribute according to airflow.
- Xenon will flow into and then wash out from the lungs, making it difficult to image the lungs in more than one projection.
- Xenon requires special negative-pressure rooms to evacuate the radiotracer from the atmosphere.
- DTPA is fairly static and allows acquisition of multiple views, but it suffers from clumping in the airways, particularly in patients with COPD.
- A normal ventilation scan will show no defects in the radiotracer distribution.

Ventilation and perfusion images may be taken in either order, but, most commonly, ventilation is performed first.

Images are obtained from multiple projections (anterior, posterior, obliques) to increase the accuracy of the study.

Common conditions
Pulmonary emboli (PE)
The hallmark of pulmonary embolism is a mismatch between perfusion and ventilation. The VQ image findings must be correlated with the CXR.

Imaging findings
- Normally, there should be no defects in the radiotracer distribution in the lungs.
- If the perfusion scan is normal, a clinically significant PE is not present, regardless of the appearance of the ventilation scan.
- PE causes occlusion of pulmonary arteries leading to perfusion defects that are segmental or subsegmental, wedge-shaped, and pleural based.
- Because airflow is not obstructed, the perfusion defect is "mismatched," that is, defect on the perfusion scan but not on the ventilation scan (see Figure 9.13).
- Defects due to abnormal airflow are much more common, typically caused by obstructive airways disease.
  - Because airflow abnormalities are accompanied by pulmonary arterial shunting, this may produce matched defects.
- PE can, at times, lead to areas of consolidation visible in chest x-rays. This may be related to pulmonary infarction or atelectasis.
- Once consolidation occurs, the mismatched perfusion defect may become "matched" (seen in both the ventilation and perfusion scans).

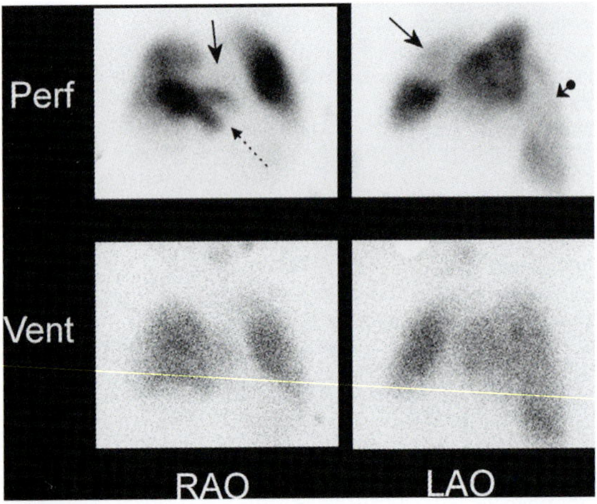

Figure 9.13 Pulmonary emboli. VQ scan from a patient with shortness of breath and tachycardia. Right anterior oblique (RAO) and left anterior oblique (LAO) views are shown. There are wedge-shaped, pleural-based mismatched perfusion defects seen in the RUL (arrow), RML (dotted arrow) and LLL (ball arrow) = high probability of pulmonary emboli.

Prospective Investigation of Pulmonary Embolism Diagnosis (PIOPED) criteria

PIOPED is the standardized interpretation scheme for VQ scans based on a large prospective multicenter trial in which conventional pulmonary angiography was used as the gold standard (the PIOPED study).
- Key findings include the number and size of perfusion defects, regardless of whether they are matched by ventilation defects and the appearance of the chest radiograph.

Probability of PE using PIOPED criteria
- High probability > 80%.
- Intermediate probability 20–80%.
- Low probability < 20%.
- Normal studies < 1%.

It is imperative to modify the results based on the pretest probability of disease.

Other nuclear medicine studies

These exams are not performed as commonly as those discussed earlier, but they may have specific useful indications.

OTHER NUCLEAR MEDICINE STUDIES

Central nervous system
Cerebral perfusion tracers (e.g., Tc-99m ECD)
- Confirmation of brain death.
- Localization of seizure foci in patients with epilepsy (ictal and interictal).
- Diagnosis of dementia/dementia subtypes.

Tracers placed within the subarachnoid space
- Tracer introduced via a lumbar puncture or via a cerebral shunt.
- CSF flow dynamics (e.g., normal pressure hydrocephalus, checking shunt patency).
- Detecting CSF leaks.

Thallium-201
Thallium is not only used for cardiac imaging, but can be used for tumor imaging in the brain.
- Evaluate for brain-tumor recurrence after surgery/radiation therapy due to the low normal background uptake (unlike FDG).

F-18 FDG PET
Early confirmation and subtyping of dementia
The most common forms of dementia have characteristic patterns of decreased glucose metabolism. For example:
- Alzheimer dementia typically produces biparietal, bitemporal hypometabolism.
- Fronto-temporal hypometabolism in Fronto-Temporal Dementia (FTD, Pick disease).

Epilepsy
- Detection of areas of focal hypometabolism at sites of seizure origin on studies performed interictally.

Infection imaging
Gallium-67
- Non-specific infection (and tumor) imaging agent.
- Relatively high radiation dose to patient with low resolution images.
- Mostly supplanted by MRI, FDG, and labeled white cell studies.
- Still a role in chronic osteomyelitis, diagnosis of Pneumocystis jiroveci and other atypical infections.

In-111 or Tc-99m labeled white blood cells
- Both can be used to detect sites of infection or inflammation.
- In-111 gives a higher radiation dose, but allows delayed imaging and can be used in combination with Tc-99m MDP for patients with suspected osteomyelitis, especially if there is underlying chronic bone disease (e.g., neuropathic feet).

F-18 FDG
- Accumulates at sites of infection and has been used for infection imaging (e.g., of aortic grafts).

Bone scintigraphy
- Sensitive method for identifying osteomyelitis.

References

Habibian MZ, Delbeke D, Martin WH, et al. (eds): *Nuclear Medicine Imaging: A Teaching File*. 2nd ed. Lippincott Williams & Wilkins, 2008.

Sandler MP, Coleman RE, Patton JA, et al. *Diagnostic Nuclear Medicine*. 4th ed. Lippincott Williams & Wilkins, 2002.

Ziessman HA, O'Malley JP, Thrall JH: *Nuclear Medicine: The Requisites*. 3rd ed. Mosby, 2005.

Chapter 10

Interventional Radiology

Nancy McNulty

When should I use image guidance? 444
Methods of imaging guidance 444
Patient preparation for interventional radiology 445
Patterns of vascular disease 446
General techniques of interventions 450
Extremity arteriography 453
Venography 456
Angiography of dialysis fistulas 456
Renal/mesenteric angiography 457
GI interventions 460
GU interventions 461
Biliary interventions 462
Aspiration, biopsy and drainage 464
Image guided tumor ablations 466
Vascular access 467
References 468

When should I use image guidance?

Imaging guidance should be used when a procedure cannot safely be performed without it, for example, when accessing masses or fluid collections that are not clinically palpable or visible.

Imaging guidance can also be used to increase the safety of procedures that *can* be performed without imaging, such as using ultrasonography to guide central line placement or thoracentesis, particularly in challenging patients (e.g., obese) or at risk patients (e.g., severe lung disease).

Methods of imaging guidance

Multiple imaging modalities can be used for guiding interventional procedures, each with its own benefits and drawbacks.

Fluoroscopy
Benefits
- "Real time" imaging allows continuous visualization of procedure.
- Used to target structures visible on radiographs (e.g., using the air in stomach to guide a G-tube placement).
- Used to guide placement of catheters/wires/stents and other devices.

Limitations
- Radiation dose: can result in high doses to both patient and operators. (See chapter 1, Radiology Essentials, Radiology Essentials, "Risks of Imaging," "Interventional Procedures and Fluoroscopy," p. 25 for techniques to reduce dose.)
- Structures not clearly defined by x-rays cannot be seen with fluoroscopy (e.g., it cannot be used for targets in the solid abdominal organs).

Indications
Angiography and vascular interventions, central venous catheter (CVC) placement, chest tube placements, tube placements, and interventions in the GI and GU system; tube changes and manipulations.

Ultrasound
Benefits
- No radiation and no known risks.
- Portability: can be used for bedside procedures in the ICU.
- Flexibility of imaging planes: not limited in angling needle, etc.
- Doppler: can differentiate arteries and veins, look for vessels in path of needle that you may want to avoid.

Limitations
- Learning curve to develop the hand-eye coordination required.
- If patient is obese or target too deep, target may not be visible.
- Target conspicuity: not all pathologies are seen on US, and it cannot image structures deep to air or bone (e.g., lung, bone, bowel).

Indications
Vascular access, access of fluid containing structures (ascites, gallbladder, bile ducts, etc.), biopsy of solid organs, masses, lymph nodes, breast.

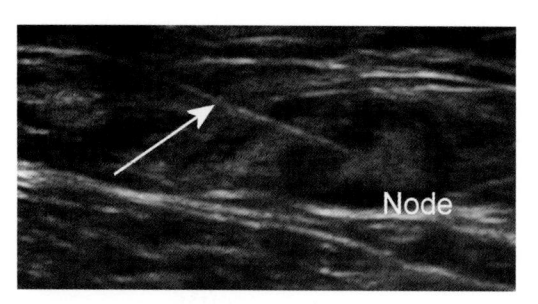

Figure 10.1 US guidance for lymph node biopsy. The needle is echogenic (arrow), and can be watched in real time as it is advanced into the target.

CT

Intermittent low dose CT images are acquired to guide placement of needle to check position. Images are not obtained "real time," that is, not *during* needle adjustments.

Benefits
- Enables visualization of, and access to, many more tissues and tissue types than fluoroscopy or US.

Limitations
- Radiation exposure (though low dose techniques are utilized).
- Needle position somewhat limited to the axial or shallow axial oblique plane that CT provides.

Indications
- Mass and solid organ biopsy, fluid aspiration and drain placement, percutaneous ablations, nerve blocks, joint injections.

MRI

Benefits
- Ability to biopsy/localize abnormalities only visible on MRI (e.g., some breast cancers).
- No ionizing radiation.

Limitations
- Technically challenging (lack of real time imaging, need for non-ferromagnetic instruments).

Patient preparation for interventional radiology

Diet
Many, if not most, interventional procedures are performed with conscious sedation. In preparation of this, patient should be NPO for 6 hours prior to procedure (may need to adjust insulin dose in diabetics).

Pre-procedure considerations
Contrast allergy
- Steroids prophylaxis (see chapter 1, Radiology Essentials, "Contrast Allergies," p. 20).

Renal Insufficiency
- Use carbon dioxide for intravascular contrast when possible.
- Pre and postprocedure IV hydration or prophylactic medications such as N-acetylcysteine (see chapter 1, Radiology Essentials, "Intravenous Iodinated Contrast Agents," p. 16).

Anticoagulation reversal—Is it necessary?
Usually handled on a case-by-case basis, depending on the potential risks and benefits. If anticoagulation needs to be held, these are the general recommendations:
- IV heparin—discontinue 2 hours prior to procedure.
- Lovenox—hold dose morning of procedure.
- Coumadin—discontinue 5 days prior to procedure.
- Aspirin/plavix—discontinue 5 days prior to procedure.

Pre-procedure medications
Many procedures require antibiotic prophylaxis. Some require coverage of skin flora (e.g., port placement), others require broader coverage (e.g., percutaneous transhepatic cholangiography). See individual procedures.

Pre-procedure labs
No standard guidelines exist, and labs required prior to a procedure will vary from institution to institution. Some generalizations can be made:
- Angiography—creatinine, coags, platelets, hemoglobin.
- Biopsy—coags, platelets.
- Gastrointestinal, genitourinary procedures, abscess drain—coags, platelets.
- Vascular access—coags, platelets.
- Hepatobiliary—LFTs, coags, platelets, CBC.

Patterns of vascular disease

Figure 10.2 is a schematic drawing of different types of pathology which affects arteries. Each is discussed in detail in the text following.

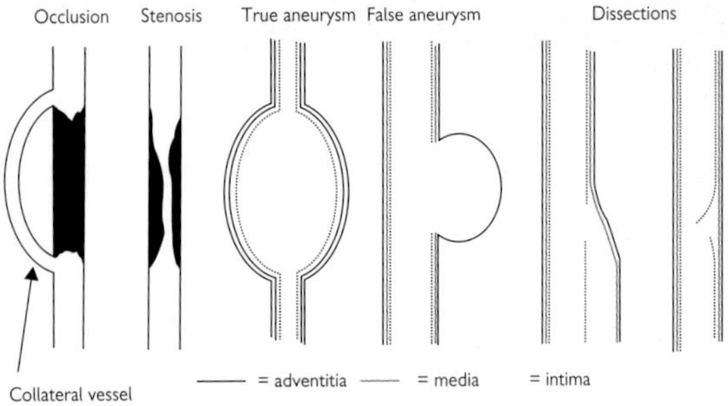

Figure 10.2

PATTERNS OF VASCULAR DISEASE

Occlusion
Segment of vessel without flow. May be short or long segment, acute or chronic. Angiographic findings can help to narrow the differential.

Angiographic findings
Acute: Often embolic or post-traumatic, though can be caused by in-situ thrombosis of a pre-existing stenosis. Abrupt clinical presentation.
- Abrupt vessel cut-off, "reverse meniscus" sign, with contrast in lumen surrounding the proximal edge of the occluding embolus, creating a meniscus (see Figure 10.3).
- May appear as endoluminal filling defect if non-occlusive.
- No significant collaterals.
- Distal vessel may or may not reconstitute.

Chronic: Indolent or slowly progressive clinical presentation.
- Tapered vessel to point of occlusion.
- Numerous collaterals—serpiginous vessels spanning the occlusion to reconstitute the distal vessel (see Figure 10.3).

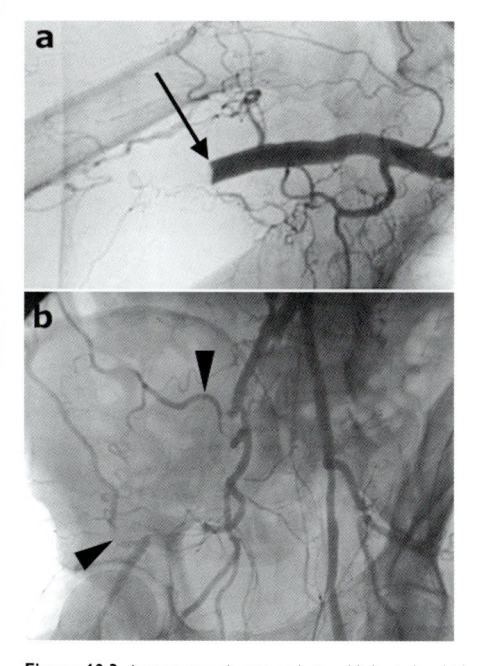

Figure 10.3 Acute versus chronic occlusion. (a) Acute brachial artery embolic occlusion. Abrupt termination of the vessel with "reverse meniscus" sign (arrow) and lack of collaterals. (b) Chronic external iliac occlusion. The vessel tapers at its termination, and large collateral vessels (arrowheads) reconstitute the distal segment.

Stenoses

Vessel narrowing of any length and any severity. Not all are hemodynamically significant; they are typically clinically relevant when there is > 50% decrease in luminal diameter on angiography, or vessels have a pressure gradient > 10 mmHg (systolic).

Etiology
Most commonly due to atherosclerosis, but they may also occur from radiation therapy, chronic dissection, tumor encasement, and rarer entities.

Angiographic findings
- Decreased caliber of vessel—focal or diffuse, regular or irregular morphology, concentric or eccentric (see Figure 10.7).
- If hemodynamically significant, collateral vessels will develop.
- May see post-stenotic dilatation.

Aneurysms and pseudoaneurysms

(See chapter 3, Abdomen/Pelvis Imaging, "Aneurysms and Dissections," p. 163 for more information.)
Enlargement of the normal caliber of an artery.

<u>True aneurysm</u>: dilatation of all three layers of the vessel wall.

<u>False (pseudo) aneurysm</u>: one or more layers of the arterial wall are dilated; blood contained by the adventitia.

Morphology
<u>Fusiform:</u> for example, standard infrarenal aortic aneurysm.
<u>Saccular:</u> focal/irregular outpouching of part of the vessel, possibly related to penetrating ulcer.

Etiologies/types
- Degenerative: atherosclerosis associated.
- Inflammatory: immune mediated reaction to vessel wall.
- Mycotic: infectious, often expand rapidly.
- Post traumatic: usually causes false aneurysm.

Aneurysms may be occult on angiography!
Angiography only displays the lumen of the vessel. If there is significant mural thrombus in an aneurysm, the lumen can look normal on angiography.
- Cross sectional imaging is more accurate, as it displays both the lumen and vessel wall.

Dissection

(See chapter 2, Chest Imaging, "Aortic Dissection," p. 104 for more information.)

Angiographic findings
- Parallel lumens: occurs when both true and false lumens are patent.
- Fusiform narrowing: occurs when the false lumen is thrombosed.
- Intimal flap: intimal tissue projects into the lumen as a linear filling defect (see Figure 10.4).

Etiologies
- Post traumatic (e.g., vertebral artery dissection).
- Iatrogenic: post catheterization/intervention/PTA.
- Spontaneous: often associated with hypertension.

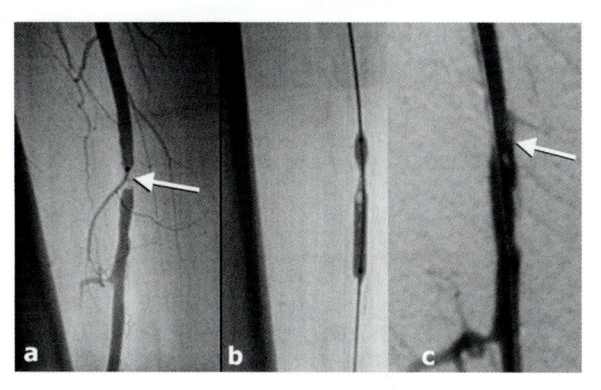

Figure 10.4 Post angioplasty dissection. (a) Focal, short segment right SFA occlusion (arrow) was treated with PTA. (b) The waist on the partially inflated angioplasty balloon is at the level of the occlusion. (c) Magnified view. Non-flow limiting, linear intimal dissection flap is seen post PTA (arrow).

Leak/extravasation

Extravasation of contrast from injured arteries can be seen on angiography if the rate of bleeding is brisk enough (approximately 0.5 ml/min). Active bleeding can be treated with percutaneous embolization.

Angiographic findings
Extraluminal collection of contrast (see Figure 10.5):
- Amorphous configuration.
- Pooling or puddling of contrast.
- Persists after contrast bolus no longer seen in vessel.

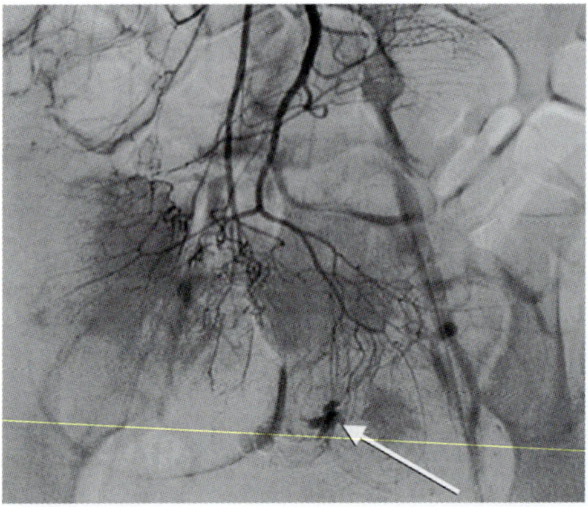

Figure 10.5 GI bleed. Image from a selective superior mesenteric angiogram shows an amorphous collection of extraluminal contrast which has extravasated from a distal SMA branch. Embolization was subsequently performed.

General techniques of interventions

Seldinger technique
Used for gaining vascular access (arterial or venous). Vessel is punctured with a needle, wire advanced through needle into vessel lumen, needle removed and a catheter passed over the wire into the lumen.

Angiography
A general term which includes both arteriography and venography. Arteriography is most commonly performed via common femoral (CFA) or brachial arteries.

Technique
- Seldinger technique is used. Catheter tip is positioned in the vessel of interest.
- Contrast is injected via a power injector.
  - The rate of injection and total volume given depends on the size of the vessel and its vascular distribution.
- An image is obtained prior to the injection, and then multiple rapid sequential images are taken during the injection (range ~ 3–7/second).
- The preimage is subtracted from the contrast opacified images to yield a "subtraction" image (digital subtraction angiography or DSA).
  - This increases the conspicuity of vessels.

> In patients with renal insufficiency, carbon dioxide (CO_2) can be used in the arterial or venous system as a contrast agent. It looks hyperlucent on angiography. This agent must be used with extreme caution to ensure that no contamination with air occurs.
> It is resorbed rapidly in the pulmonary circulation; however, it can cause arterial "blocks" in nondependent vessels, and, therefore, should not be used above the aortic arch.

Benefits over CTA or MRA
- Better quality images of small vessels (hand, foot, intracranial, etc.).
- Enables *therapeutic options* (e.g., PTA, stenting, or thrombolysis).
- Allows dynamic assessment of flow characteristics.
- Contribution of collateral circulation and reconstitution beyond stenosis or occlusion can be assessed.

Complications
- Bleeding at puncture site—focal hematoma (3%), pseudoaneurysm.
- Injury to access or other vessel—occlusion, dissection, distal embolization, AV fistula.

Percutaneous transluminal angioplasty (PTA)
Angioplasty (balloon dilatation) is used to treat stenoses within the vascular system, as well as the biliary and genitourinary systems. In arteries, it works by stretching the media, and cracking or splitting the intimal plaque. In veins and the GU/GI system, it works by stretching the wall.

Balloons
- Come pre-mounted on catheters, in a variety of lengths and diameters.
- Upon inflation, will expand to a pre-set diameter.

Technique
- Select balloon size 10–15% greater than transverse vessel diameter of the normal vessel.
- Inflate to the pressure that fully expands the stenosis and effaces the waist (see Figure 10.3).

Complications
- Dissection, occlusion, rupture, distal emolization (see Figure 10.3).

Percutaneous stent placement
Implanted metal devices that are used to treat stenoses, dissections, occlusions, and injured vessels. Both balloon expandable and self-expanding stents exist, and both covered (polytetrafluoroethylene [PTFE]) and uncovered stents are available. The indications for each type of stent are beyond the scope of this text. Some generalizations are possible:
- Covered stents: used to treat (exclude) aneurysms and to cover damaged segments of arteries (dissection, traumatic injury).
- Precise stent placement is easier to achieve with balloon expandable stents, and these are often used when placement is critical (e.g., in an ostial renal artery stenosis) (see Figure 10.7).

Technique
- Select stent size 10–15% greater than the transverse diameter of the normal vessel.
- Precise placement is critical—use bony landmarks or angiographic images to guide placement.

Complications
- Mal-deployment, vessel injury.

Embolization
- The injection of material into blood vessels to stop flow.

Indications
- Active bleeding—trauma, post intervention/surgery, tumors.
- Devascularization of tumors/organs pre-operatively to reduce blood loss (e.g., pre-splenectomy), or therapeutically to reduce tumor bulk.

Technique
- Catheter tip placed within the vessel to be embolized.
- Administration of embolic agent via catheter.

Embolic agents
- Gelfoam: mechanical blockage, temporary, vessel will recanalize. Used often in trauma. Mix with IV contrast to make radioopaque for delivery.
- Particles: mechanical blockage, permanent, a variety of types and sizes are available. Mix with IV contrast to make radioopaque for delivery.
- Coils: mechanical blockage, permanent, a variety of types and sizes are available. Allows precise occlusion of a vessel.

Complications
- Non-target embolization: occlusion of a vessel not intended. Consequence depends on the organ and vessel occluded.

Thrombolysis
Indicated in acute vascular (arterial or venous) occlusions in patients without immediate danger of limb loss. Thrombolysis removes intravascular thrombus and reestablishes blood flow. Generally performed following diagnostic angiography via a catheter or other device.

Technique
<u>Mechanical</u>: A variety of devices are available that macerate or aspirate the thrombus. For example:
- Balloon maceration.
- Corkscrew wire—rotational aspiration.
- Catheters that allow pulse spray and also aspirate the thrombus.
- <u>Pharmacologic</u>: Fibrinolytic agents that are administered directly into the thrombus, which break down thrombin. Generally given as continuous low dose infusion over hours; patients typically will be monitored in the ICU during the infusion.
  - Fibrinogen levels must be monitored and the dose of thrombolytics decreased or stopped if the levels drop below 150mg/dl and 100mg/dl, respectively.

Contraindications to pharmacologic thrombolysis
- Active hemorrhage, known bleeding diathesis, recent stroke, craniotomy or trauma, intracranial tumors.

Complications
- Hemorrhage: may occur at vascular puncture site, or remote location (e.g., intracranial).
- Distal embolization, limb loss, death.

Drain/pigtail catheter placement
Pigtail catheters are used for a wide variety of indications, including abnormal fluid (e.g., pus, ascites), obstructed structures (e.g., renal collecting system, gallbladder, and for drainage of air (e.g., PTX).

Technique
- Seldinger technique used to pass wire into structure of interest.
- Soft tissues must be dilated to accommodate the diameter of the catheter.
- Pigtail catheter is passed over the wire. A string within the catheter tightens the pigtail; this aims to prevent catheter dislodgement.

Complications
Inadvertent puncture of non-target structures, for example, vessels.
- Bleeding.
- Catheter occlusion/malfunction.

Central vascular access
A catheter is placed into a vein (e.g., basilic, jugular, femoral) to provide a conduit for blood draws or administration of medications. Those placed in interventional radiology are typically for central venous access.

Technique
Sterile precautions are used, and sterile technique employed.
- Pre-procedure antibiotics given for some placements.
- US guidance and Seldinger technique used to access vein of choice.
- Catheter tip positioned in SVC or at cavo-atrial junction (for HD catheters, right atrium).

Extremity arteriography

Technique

Upper extremity
Includes images of the aortic arch to the hand. For vessels distal to the arch, catheter tip typically placed in the subclavian artery, but can be positioned more distally. Performed via CFA access.

Contrast
- Full strength contrast is painful to the digits.
  - Iso-osmolar agents better tolerated.
  - Intra-arterial lidocaine administration (for analgesia prior to contrast injection) has been used with varied success.

Ancillary techniques: to better visualize hand vessels.
- Intra-arterial vasodilators given prior to angiogram.
- Hand warming prior to angiogram (warm towels, water).

Complications (See "Angiography," p. 457 for complications of angiography.)
- Stroke: rare.

Lower extremity
Includes angiography of the aortic bifurcation to the toes. Digital subtraction technique usually employed. Performed via CFA access.
- "Outflow" or "run-off" can be evaluated using a moving angiographic table. As contrast is injected, the table moves and sequential images of the legs are obtained, following the contrast bolus from pelvis to feet.
- As with upper extremity angiography, iso-osmolar contrast is better tolerated.

Anatomy and terminology
Using proper terminology is important to convey accurate information.
A complete review of the anatomy is beyond the scope of this text; please see references for review.

Upper limb arterial system
The brachial artery bifurcates into the radial (lateral) and ulna (medial), both of which continue into the hand to form the palmar arches.
- <u>Superficial arch:</u> formed primarily from ulnar artery, is located more distally. Gives rise to common palmar digital arteries.
- <u>Deep arch:</u> formed primarily from radial artery, is located more proximally. Gives rise to the palmar metacarpal arteries.

Lower limb arterial system
The common femoral artery bifurcates into the:
- <u>Profunda femoris artery</u>: gives many muscular branches in thigh. In cases of external iliac stenosis/occlusion, the internal iliac artery provides collaterals to the leg via anastomoses with the PFA branches.
- <u>Superficial femoral artery</u>: very few branches in thigh, becomes the popliteal artery at the adductor hiatus.

Blood supply to the foot is via:
- <u>Dorsalis pedis</u>: a continuation of the anterior tibial artery.
- <u>Medial and lateral plantar arteries:</u> terminal branches of the posterior tibial artery.

Common conditions
Peripheral vascular occlusive disease (PVOD)
Angiographic findings
Focal, multifocal or diffuse irregular stenoses and/or occlusions.
- In diabetics, both proximal and distal vessels are affected, often with severe distal small vessel calcifications.
- Collateral vessel development parallels the chronicity and severity of the stenosis (see Figure 10.3).

Percutaneous interventions
- PTA and stenting are frequently used to treat stenoses or occlusions (see Figure 10.4).
- Newer techniques are emerging, including catheter embolectomy devices and laser treatments.

Trauma
Mechanism of injury is typically arterial stretch injury, compression, or penetrating trauma. In fractures and dislocations, the proximity of an artery to the bone places it at risk:
- Shoulder and elbow: axillary and brachial artery at risk.
- Knee: popliteal artery at risk.

Angiographic findings
- Transection and occlusion.
- Dissection: usually a stretch injury, often causes intimal flap.
- Pseudoaneurysm: +/− distal embolization (see Figure 10.6).
- Fusiform narrowing: from dissection or intramural hematoma.

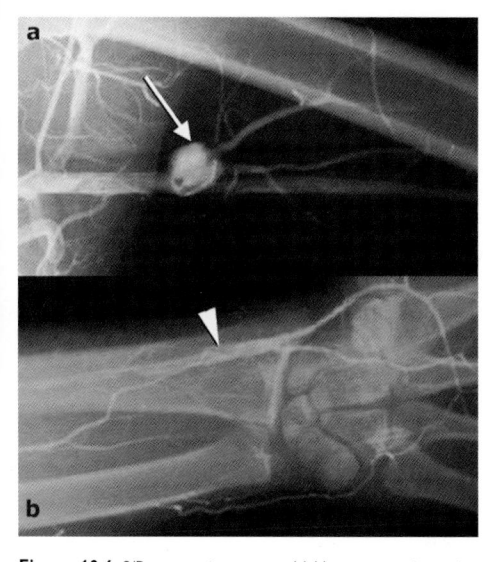

Figure 10.6 S/P penetrating trauma. (a) Upper extremity angiogram demonstrates a pseudoaneurysm of the brachial artery involving the origin of the profunda brachial artery (arrow). (b) Angiogram of the forearm reveals subtle irregular filling defects in the radial artery (arrowhead) and occlusion of the ulnar artery from distal embolization.

Vasospastic disorders of the upper limb
Raynaud's phenomenon
- Intermittent vasoconstriction of small hand arteries, incited by cold and stress, causing reversible ischemia. Usually bilateral, UE > LE.
- Primary Raynauds' phenomenon has unknown etiology and mechanism. Strong female predominance.
- Secondary Raynauds' phenomenon is associated with an underlying condition, for example, scleroderma, systemic lupus erythematosus, rheumatoid arthritis.

Angiographic findings
- Slow blood flow and poor opacification of distal small vessels of hand.
- Improved blood flow and digit perfusion following direct intra-arterial vasodilator administration (this is diagnostic on angiography).

Venography

Indications
- Venous mapping prior to AV fistula creation for dialysis access.
- Assessment of central stenosis pre-pacemaker or central line placement.
- Diagnosis of deep venous thrombosis (largely supplanted by US, however, still used for central veins, which are difficult to evaluate with US).
- Diagnosis of venous insufficiency.

Technique
Position of angiocatheter
- Hand→ pre-operative venous mapping for dialysis fistulas.
- Antecubital fossa→ central venography for stenosis evaluation.
- Foot→ lower extremity assessment of DVT or venous insufficiency.

Contrast
Iodinated contrast or carbon dioxide (CO_2) can be used. CO_2 recommended in patients with renal insufficiency.

Ancillary techniques
Tourniquets can be used to compress superficial veins and thereby maximize deep vein filling.

Angiography of dialysis fistulas

Upper extremity arterio-venous fistulas are created surgically for hemodialysis access. These frequently require intervention to maintain adequate flow and function.

Technique
- Seldinger technique used to access the fistula.

- Venography of outflow veins performed.
- Assessment of arteriovenous anastomosis made by compressing the outflow vein so that injected contrast refluxes back through the arterial anastomosis.

Common conditions

Outflow vein stenosis

Results in prolonged bleeding after hemodialysis, decreased flows, and increased pressures at dialysis. It may also result in upper extremity edema (more common with central venous stenosis than peripheral).

Angiographic findings

- Stenosis anywhere along outflow vein or central veins. Most commonly within several centimeters of the anastomosis.
- Collateral veins bridging the stenosis very common.

Treatment

- PTA. Occasionally, stents are used when PTA fails; however, surgical revision should also be considered in cases refractory to PTA.

Renal/mesenteric angiography

Usually performed for the purpose of an intervention, as CTA and MRA have largely, but not entirely, supplanted diagnostic angiography.

Technique

A variety of shaped catheters are available, which aid in selecting the mesenteric and renal vessels, which often originate from the aorta at a 90 degree or more acute angle.

Mesenteric angiogram: catheter tip is placed just beyond origin of vessel. Continue imaging until veins have opacified to evaluated SMV, IMV, and portal vein patency.

Renal angiogram: catheter placed at origin of vessel. Continue imaging until kidney is fully enhanced to assess the nephrogram.

Anatomy of renal and mesenteric system

Table 10.1

Vessel	Level of origin	Site of origin	Angle of origin
Celiac axis	T12	Anterior aorta	~90 degrees
SMA	L1	Anterior aorta	Down-going
IMA	L3/4	Anterior aorta	Down-going
Renal arteries	L1/2	Lateral aorta	~90 degrees

References for anatomy are provided at the end of the chapter.

Common conditions

Mesenteric ischemia
- The clinical hallmark of ischemia is abdominal pain.

Angiographic findings in acute ischemia
- Emboli to mesenteric vessels (accounts for 40–50% of acute ischemia).
  - Abrupt vessel cut off, usually at branch point.
- In situ thromboses usually superimposed on severe stenosis.
- Mesenteric vasoconstriction: pruned, attenuated vessels.

Angiography enables potential thrombolytic administration or injection of intra-arterial vasodilators (in cases of vasoconstriction).

Angiographic findings in chronic ischemia
- Atherosclerotic stenoses or occlusions—usually ostial/proximal
- Clinical significance of stenoses is uncertain; many asymptomatic patients have significant stenoses, and so clinical context is important.

Angiography enables potential PTA or stent placement.

GI bleed
Angiography can identify GI bleeding if the rate is at least 0.5 ml/min. Angiography is typically performed for the purpose of embolization.

Indications for angiography and embolization
- Known active GI bleeding (e.g., positive tagged red blood cell scan) with ongoing transfusion requirements.
- Failure of endoscopic treatment or inability to perform endoscopy.

Technique
- Selective angiography of the three mesenteric vessels to identify site of active extravasation.
  - Extravasation seen: sub-selective catheterization of bleeding vessel and embolization (gelfoam, coils, occasionally particles all used).
  - No extravasation seen: embolization typically cannot safely be performed. Vasopressin can be infused in lieu of embolization (*beware of risk of cardiac ischemia in the elderly).

Special considerations in intestinal embolization
- There is risk of ischemia to normal intestine. Greatest in the colon.
- GI bleeding tends to be intermittent, and angiography will not detect it if not actively bleeding during imaging.

Renal artery stenosis
Most common causes include atherosclerosis and fibromuscular dysplasia (FMD). Angiography performed for both diagnosis and treatment.

Angiographic findings
<u>Atherosclerotic cardiovascular disease (ASCVD).</u>
- Irregular stenosis, most commonly ostial (see Figure 10.7).
- Post-stenotic dilatation.

<u>FMD</u>
- The classic form of FMD produces alternating arterial stenoses and dilatation, giving a beaded appearance.

- Other less common forms of FMD exist and have a different angiographic appearance (e.g., solitary fusiform stenosis).

Treatment
- Indications to treat: hypertension and/or renal insufficiency.
- FMD: excellent response to PTA alone.
- ASCVD: primary stent placement is the treatment of choice, yielding higher procedural success and lower re-stenosis rates than PTA.

Renal revascularization is not beneficial in the following situations
- Significant renal atrophy.
- Severe renal failure (creatinine >4.0mg/dL).

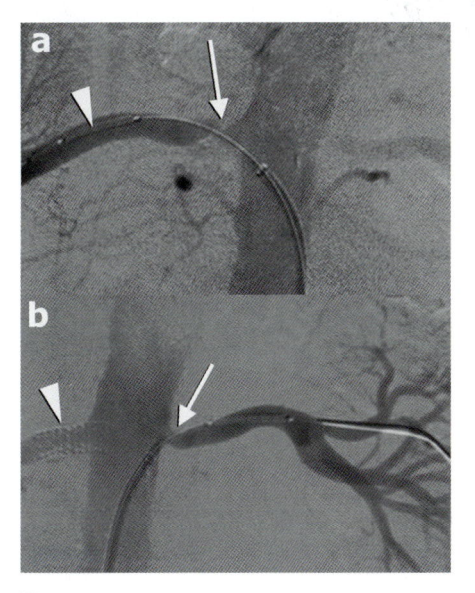

Figure 10.7 Renal artery stenosis. Irregular narrowing of the proximal right renal artery (arrow, a), and smoother narrowing of the proximal left renal artery (arrow, b) from atherosclerosis. (a) Note the undeployed stent on the renal artery wire (arrowhead). (b) The right renal stent has been deployed (arrowhead), and the stenosis has resolved.

GI intervention

Feeding tubes are commonly placed in IR. They will occlude eventually, and so require routine tube changes to maintain patency.

Gastrostomy and gastrojejunostomy tubes
Indications
- Unable to take enough PO to maintain weight.
- Swallowing dysfunction: stroke, neuromuscular disorders.
- Obstruction: for example, esophageal cancer.
- Aspiration.

G-tubes
- Technically easier to place, clog less frequently.
- Function of stomach preserved, any type of diet can be used.

GJ tubes
- Technically more challenging to place, requires more manipulation.
- Types of feedings that can be used are more restricted.
- Smaller caliber tube, becomes clogged more frequently.
- GJ tubes are indicated in patients with aspiration and known gastroesophageal reflux, and in delayed gastric emptying.

Technique and preparation

Review prior cross sectional imaging; anatomy of stomach, and adjacent structures. Ensure patient has not had prior gastric surgery.
- Pre-procedure antibiotics to cover skin flora.
- Glucagon given to decrease gastric peristalsis and emptying.
- Stomach is distended with air via NGT (see Figure 10.8).
- Percutaneous anterior gastric wall puncture under fluoroscopic visualization (make sure colon is not in the path!).
  - Air is aspirated and contrast injected to confirm intra-gastric position.
  - Deployment of stay sutures (anchor anterior gastric wall to anterior abdominal wall).
- The SQ tract is dilated over the wire, and the tube is placed.
- For GJ tubes, the wire and then tube must be advanced to the ligament of Treitz (duodenal suspensory ligament).

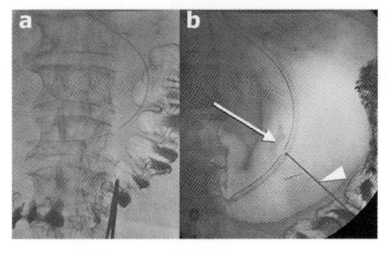

Figure 10.8 G-tube placement. Oral contrast given the night prior to the exam opacifies the colon. Note the stomach (indicated by the NGT) and colon before (a), and after (b) insufflation of the stomach with air. In (b), a needle (arrowhead) has been placed into the stomach, and contrast injected into the lumen to confirm position prior to tube placement (arrow).

GU interventions

Percutaneous nephrostomy (PCN)
A tube placed through the skin of the flank into the renal collecting system.

Indications
- Relief of ureteral obstruction.
- To gain access to collecting system for a variety of interventions, including: stone extraction, antegrade chemotherapy, stricture dilatation, brush biopsy of urothelial tumors.

Techniques and patient preparation
Review prior cross sectional imaging: ensure the spleen, colon and gallbladder are sufficiently away from the kidney.
- Pre-procedure antibiotics to cover urinary flora.
- Imaging guidance options:
  - US: direct visualization of needle entering collecting system.
  - Fluoroscopy: first give IV contrast to opacify collecting system.
- Access a posterior calyx (least vascular area), confirm position with aspiration of urine and contrast injection, and place pigtail catheter. (See "General Techniques of Intervention," p. 459 for details of pigtail catheter placement.)

Follow-up
Routine tube changes are needed every ~ 8–12 weeks to maintain patency; tubes tend to clog with debris or become encrusted.

Ureteral stents
Indications
- Nephroureteral obstruction.
- Ureteral injuries or fistulas.
- Stents also often placed pre-surgically and pre-extracorporeal shock wave lithotripsy (ESWL), but this is more commonly done retrograde with cystoscopy by urology.

Stent types
There are two types of stents (which are actually catheters) that can be placed in IR. If needed chronically, each must be changed routinely to maintain patency.

Nephroureteral
- Percutaneous catheter with an external portion, a proximal pigtail in the renal collecting system, and a distal pigtail in the bladder.
- Advantage is that external access is maintained, allowing for recurrent interventions such as ureteroplasty.
- Disadvantage is the risk of dislodgement.
- Routinely changed in IR.

Double J
- Internal catheter with proximal pigtail in renal pelvis and distal in urinary bladder; external access is not maintained.

- Requires cystoscopy for routine change.
- Advantageous for patients with chronic ureteral strictures, because it is more comfortable and less inconvenient than chronic external catheter.

Techniques and patient preparation
- A PCN should already be in place. Over a wire, this is removed, and the wire is advanced down the ureter into the urinary bladder.
- Nephroureteral stent: placed over the wire. External portion of tube then flushed and capped to allow internal drainage.
- Double J stent: placed over the wire, and wire removed. Placement and positioning is more complicated than a nephroureteral stent.

Biliary interventions

Techniques and patient preparation
Review cross sectional imaging studies:
- Confirm and determine level of biliary stenosis (PTC).
- Assess for focal hepatic masses (these should be avoided).

Antibiotics
Must cover both Gram-positive and Gram-negative organisms. The rate of colonization in malignant biliary obstruction is 25–35%, and even higher in patients with choledocholithiasis.

Cholecystostomy
Placement of pigtail catheter to drain gallbladder externally.

Indications
Acute cholecystitis in non-operative or high risk patient.

Technique
Usually performed with a combination of US and fluoroscopic guidance (see general techniques of drain placement p. 459).

Key points
Cannot be removed for at least 4–6 weeks, until a mature tract has formed to prevent bile spill into peritoneal cavity.

Percutaneous cholangiogram (PTC) and drainage
Indications
- <u>Diagnostic</u>: bile duct inflammatory disorders, identifying site of suspected bile leak.
- <u>Therapeutic</u>: decompression of biliary obstruction, angioplasty of strictures, removal of stones.

Technique
- US or fluoroscopic guided puncture of a peripheral bile duct. Seldinger technique utilized.
- For drainage, a catheter is placed over a wire through the biliary tree, with distal pigtail of catheter positioned in duodenum.
- Multiple side holes in the catheter allow bile to flow from intrahepatic ducts through tube and out into the duodenum.

Risks
Cholangitis, bleeding (could require surgery, embolization or transfusion), bile duct or gallbladder injury, including leak.

Biliary stent
Indications
Metallic stents are nearly universally reserved for the palliation of malignant biliary obstruction (non-operative).

Technique
Placed over a wire via pre-existing PTC access. Stent position depends on the level of the obstruction. PTA is then performed to fully open the stent.

Key points
- Median patency 6–8 months.
  - Patients may require repeat PTC to re-establish patency of stent.
- Metallic stents have longer patency, lower complication rates than plastic stents.
  - Require fewer repeat interventions to maintain patency.

Transjugular Intrahepatic Portosystemic Shunt (TIPS)
Decompression of portal hypertension via creation of a shunt between the portal and hepatic veins. This reduces portal pressures and blood flow, effectively "bypasses" the liver.

Indications
- Variceal hemorrhage refractory to endoscopic treatment.
- Refractory ascites due to end stage liver disease, requiring frequent paracentesis.
- Hepatic hydrothorax requiring recurrent thoracentesis.

Pre-procedure care
- Review cross sectional imaging studies.
  - Establish patency of portal vein.
  - Assess for focal mass lesions (should avoid these).
- Check labs and correct coagulopathy/thrombocytopenia.

Technique
- Internal jugular access using Seldinger technique.
- Hepatic venography and wedged portal pressure measurements obtained to confirm portal hypertension.
- Wedge portogram (catheter wedged into a small tributary to the hepatic vein. CO_2 or contrast is injected, which will traverse the capillaries and fill the portal system) performed to provide roadmap of portal vein.
- Through a long sheath, a needle is passed from the hepatic vein into the portal vein, and a wire passed through this into the splenic vein.
- Angiography performed to assess anatomy and measure length of stent needed (see Figure 10.9).
- Stent placement and angioplasty performed over the wire.

Risks
- Hemorrhage, infection, damage to arteries, liver, death.
- Stent stenosis or occlusion, which may require re-intervention.

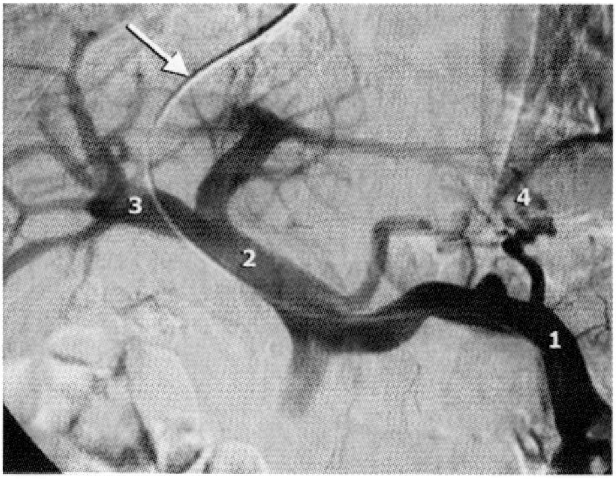

Figure 10.9 Portogram from TIPS procedure. The catheter (arrow) extends from the right hepatic vein through the liver, into the portal vein, with tip in the splenic vein. Contrast opacifies the splenic vein (1), portal vein (2), right portal vein (3), and varices (4).

Aspiration, biopsy, and drainage

Most common modalities used for imaging guidance are CT and ultrasound, although MRI is being used with increasing frequency, particularly in breast interventions. Bone lesions require fluoroscopic or CT guidance.
- The lesion of interest must be visible on the modality selected for imaging guidance.
- In obese patients or for deep lesions, CT is preferable to US.

Biopsies

Patient preparation
It is often deep structures that are being biopsied with imaging guidance, and manual compression is not effective if bleeding occurs. Consequently, coagulopathy should be corrected prior to procedure.

General techniques
Choosing approach
- Shortest path to the target, avoiding other organs, major vessels, and other important structures.
- If heterogeneous lesion, avoid areas of necrosis or cavitation.
  - PET/CT images may aid in selecting most metabolically active portion of lesion to target.

Technique
- Using imaging guidance, a needle is placed into the lesion.
- Co-axially, core biopsies are obtained with specialized needles (spring loaded). Gauge varies:
  - Chest/abdomen/pelvis biopsies 18–20g most common.
  - Bone biopsies up to 11g- special needle used to traverse cortex.
  - Breast biopsies up to 9g (with vacuum).

Complications
Bleeding, infection, puncture of non-target structures.

Lung biopsy
Historically performed with fluoroscopic guidance, now supplanted by CT guidance. Enables successful biopsy of even small lesions.

Technique
- Avoid traversing a fissure and bulla if possible (increased risk of PTX).
- Puncture the pleura perpendicularly (decreases risk of PTX).
- If cavitary lesion, biopsy the thickest wall.

Post procedure
- CXRs must be performed to evaluate for PTX prior to discharge.

Solid organ biopsy
- Liver, renal, and other lesions may be accessible via US or CT.
  - In young patients, consider US to avoid radiation.
  - In large patients, lesion may not be conspicuous enough for US.
- Adrenal masses usually poorly seen with US; CT is required. Often, the gantry must be angled such that needle can be advanced from caudal to cranial to access the adrenal gland, to avoid traversing the lung base.
- If there is ascites, there is higher risk of hemorrhage from liver biopsy. Consider paracentesis prior to biopsy.

Drains, aspirations, and tube placement
CT and US guidance most commonly used; decision based on the age of the patient, operator preference, and conspicuity of the abnormality.

See "General Techniques of Interventions," p. 459, for procedural technique.

Abscess drainage
The walls of an abscess are often thick and fibrous.
  - Must progressively dilate the tract.
  - Procedure can be quite painful in this setting
- Drain placement may result in transient bacteremia.
- Catheter is left in place until abscess is no longer draining.

Paracentesis
- Largest pocket of fluid selected for access.
- Use Doppler to ensure no abdominal wall vessels will be traversed.
- Large volume paracentesis (> 5 L): administer albumin intravenously (6–8g/L removed) to prevent impairment in circulating blood volume and associated renal impairment +/− hyponatremia.

Thoracentesis
- US used to confirm fluid in the pleural space and identify loculations; these may preclude complete drainage.
- Largest pocket selected for access; typically in costophrenic recess with patient upright during procedure.
- US guidance is especially helpful with small pleural fluid collections that would be difficult to sample blindly.

Chest tube
- Placed for the management of effusions or PTX.
  - Effusions typically drained with US guidance. Because these are usually located dependently, chest tube is usually placed in inferior thorax.
  - PTX may be treated with fluoroscopic or CT guidance. Usually, tube is placed in anterior and superior thorax.
- After placement, the tube is connected to a Pleur-Evac™ device and initially connected to low wall suction.

Image guided tumor ablations

These are regional therapies for malignant disease. The goal is cell death, including the entirety of the tumor and a small surrounding zone of normal tissue.

Indications
Historically reserved for non-operative candidates or non-resectable tumors. As more data on long term efficacy is collected, indications have expanded:
- Renal cell carcinoma: curative intent, as an alternative to partial nephrectomy.
- Hepatocellular carcinoma and hepatic metastatic disease
  - When non-resectable.
  - Curative intent when poor operative risk.

General techniques
Performed under imaging guidance; most commonly US and CT, although MRI also used. May be performed with conscious sedation or general anesthesia.

Patient preparation
- Antibiotics: use varies from institution to institution.
  - If patient has a biliary catheter or stent, antibiotics are typically given for hepatic radiofrequency ablation (RFA).
- General anesthesia widely utilized in USA; less so in Europe.

Follow-up
All ablation techniques require regular follow-up imaging (CT or MRI) to assess for residual tumor, local recurrence, and/or new lesions.

Radiofrequency ablation (RFA)
High frequency alternating current is delivered to the target via a needleprobe.
- Many different probe sizes, types, and designs exist.
- Induces thermal coagulation necrosis.

Cryoablation
Tissue is frozen by using high pressure argon gas delivered to the tip of the delivery probe. The gas expands and cools to extremely low temperature.
- CT or MRI guidance are preferred, as they demonstrate the ice-ball that is produced during the procedure.

Vascular access

Temporary central venous lines
- Commonly used in inpatients and for short term use.
- Internal jugular vein preferred, femoral acceptable, but higher infection rate.
- PIC (peripherally inserted central) lines are also considered temporary. They can be placed with US and/or fluoroscopic guidance via the cephalic or basilic veins.
- Desired tip location: superior vena cava.

Tunneled central venous lines
- Used for long term access. Catheters have a cuff on the shaft that is placed near the exit site.
  - The cuff incites fibrosis and scarring to the SQ tissues, to aid in catheter retention and limit the spread of infections arising at the insertion site.
- Hemodialysis and hemopharesis catheters are large bore dual lumen tunneled catheters, which can tolerate high flow rates; used for both aspiration and injections.

Technique
- Antibiotics given pre-procedure
- Catheter is tunneled subcutaneously from infraclavicular chest wall to the internal jugular puncture site and delivered intravascularly via a peel-away sheath.

Subcutaneous port catheters
Used for intermittent vascular access on a long term basis (e.g., administration of chemotherapy). These are convenient for the patient, and likely have lower infection rates than tunneled catheters.
- Device is entirely SQ with no external portion.
- The port reservoir has a silicone diaphragm that can be punctured repeatedly with specialized needles designed for this purpose.

Technique
- Skin incision made (can be placed in the arm or chest) and pocket dissected in the SQ tissues large enough to hold the port reservoir.
- Port is attached to the catheter, placed in the pocket, and the catheter is then tunneled and delivered as for tunneled lines.

References

Baum S, Pentecost MJ, *Abrams' Angiography* Vols. I-III, 4th ed., Boston, Little, Brown and Company, 1997.

Dartmouth Human Anatomy website (for vascular anatomy) www.dartmouth.edu/~anatomy.

Hirsch AT, Haskal ZJ, Hertzer NR, et al., ACC/AHA 2005 practice guidelines for the management of patients with peripheral arterial disease (lower extremity, renal, mesenteric, and abdominal aortic). A collaborative report from the American Association for Vascular Surgery/Society for Vascular Surgery, Society for Cardiovascular Angiography and Interventions, Society for Vascular Medicine and Biology, Society of Interventional Radiology, and the ACC/AHA task force on Practice Guidelines. *Circulation*. 2006; 113(11): e463.

Seddon M, Saw J, Review. Atherosclerotic renal artery stenosis: Review of pathophysiology, clinical trial evidence, and management strategies *Canadian Journal of Cardiology*, 27(4): S1–S60, available online May 6, 2011).

Survival handbook for interventional radiology (Dartmouth-Hitchcock Medical Center). https://docs.google.com/View?id=dhmdczz8_4c2z5smj2

Waybill PN, Brown DB, *Patient Care in Vascular and Interventional Radiology.*, 2nd ed. Fairfax, VA: SIR, 2010.

Chapter 11

Breast Imaging

Petra Lewis, MBBS and Elizabeth W. Dann, MD

Mammography *470*
  How are images acquired? *470*
  Mammographic screening *472*
  Diagnostic mammography *474*
  Normal anatomy *474*
  How do I read a mammogram? *475*
  Patterns of disease on mammography *476*
  Breast imaging reports *482*
Ultrasound *483*
  When do you do breast ultrasound? *483*
  How do you do a breast ultrasound? *484*
  Normal breast ultrasound *484*
  Patterns of disease on breast ultrasound *485*
MRI *487*
  How do you do breast MRI *487*
  When do you do breast MRI? *487*
  Patterns of disease on breast MRI *489*
Other modalities *490*
Common conditions *491*
  Cysts *491*
  Ductal carcinoma in situ (DCIS) *492*
  Invasive carcinomas *493*
  Fibroadenomas *495*
Procedures *496*
  Cyst aspiration *496*
  Needle/wire localizations (NLOC) *496*
  Percutaneous core biopsy *497*
  Sentinel node injection *498*
  Galactography (ductography) *499*
Management problems *499*
  Palpable masses *499*
  Man with a breast lump/tenderness *499*
  Breast pain *500*
  Cellulitis/mastitis *500*
  Nipple discharge *500*
References *500*

Mammography

Mammography images the breast using x-rays. It is used for detecting asymptomatic breast cancer *(screening mammography)*, and for the workup of clinical and mammographic-detected abnormalities *(diagnostic mammography)*.

How common is breast cancer?

Age 25 1:19,608
Age 35 1:622
Age 45 1:93
Age 55 1:33

Age 65 1:17
Age 75 1:11
Age 85 1:9
Age 95 1:8

(NCI data from 1990s)

How are images acquired?

Technology

Film-screen mammography

Uses low energy x-rays to expose radiographic film.

Digital mammography

The x-rays "expose" a digital receptor plate, which allows for later image adjustment and analysis, e.g., magnification, computer detection software.
- Increased sensitivity for breast cancer shown in denser breasts and younger women compared to film screen, however, benefits are still controversial.
- Most modern mammographic units are digital.

Tomosynthesis

Also called 3D mammography, tomosynthesis involves taking a series of low dose exposures across an arc, with post-processing reconstruction that resembles a CT scan, producing "slices" through the breast.
- This reduces the problem of tissue overlap called superimposition and may improve lesion detection.
- Recent FDA approved and clinical usage is growing.

Radiation to the breast

Women get very concerned about the risks of radiation exposure to the breast. The radiation exposure from a mammogram is approximately 0.1 mSv/view.
- The theoretical potential risk of 10 years of mammography inducing a fatal breast cancer is approximately 1:10,000 (compared to a 1:33 baseline risk).
- After the age of 40 the breast is actually quite insensitive to the effects of radiation.
- Mammography should be avoided in teens and 20s when breasts are more sensitive to radiation.

Views

The breast is firmly compressed between plastic plates during the x-ray exposure. Some women find this uncomfortable and it is important that they are reassured about the importance of this compression to:
- Minimize motion.
- Spread tissues to improve visualization of abnormalities.
- Decrease breast thickness to reduce radiation exposure.

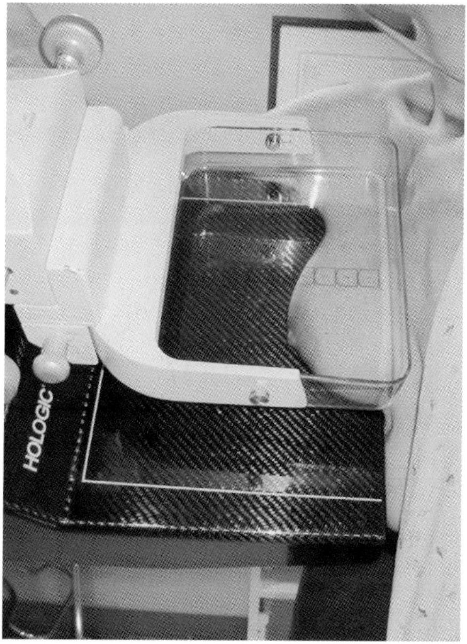

Figure 11.1 Patient positioned in a mammography unit for an MLO view.

Standard Views

Used for screening and diagnostic mammography.

Two orthogonal views are obtained of each breast to maximize inclusion of as much breast tissue as possible (see Figure 11.2).
- Medial-lateral oblique (MLO)—imaging the breast along the long axis of the pectoralis major. The x-ray beam passes from the medial breast to the image receptor laterally.
- Cranial-caudal (CC)—imaging the breast from top to bottom. The x-ray beam passes from above the breast to the image receptor below.

What is a "call back" or "recall"
Screening mammograms are usually read after patients have left the mammographic facility. Patients whose studies are felt to be abnormal (BI-RADS 0 [see p. 489]) are "called back" for diagnostic mammography (additional views and/or ultrasound).
- Call-back rates vary widely, but generally accepted rates are 5–10% in the United States but lower in Europe.
- Call-back rates are monitored by federal mandate both by imaging center and individual radiologist.

Supplementary views
Used for diagnostic mammography
Other views are used to evaluate a possible abnormality seen on screening mammograms or to address an area of clinical concern. These include:

Other angles of rotation:
- From 0 degrees (CC) to 90 degrees (ML or LM).

Magnification views (Mag):
- Small area or whole breast. Increases fine detail but is more susceptible to motion and provides a higher radiation dose to the breast.
- Obtained by increasing distance from breast to receptor plate.
- Used for visualizing calcifications and margins of small masses.

Focal compression:
- Small paddle used to compress overlying tissue away from area of interest.

Rolled views:
- The top of the breast is rolled relative to the bottom to spread out the tissues and provide localization for images only seen in one plane.

Extended CC view (XCC):
- To see axillary or far-lateral tissue.

Computer Assisted Detection (CAD)
Many centers use post-processing software as an adjunct or "second reader." Computerized algorithms identify suspicious regions of interest for the radiologist to re-review.

Can we image patients with breast implants?
Yes, implants can be imaged safely; the risk of rupture is very small. Specialized views will be obtained ("implant displaced" or "Ekland" views) to maximize visualization. Mammograms have reduced sensitivity in implant patients.

Mammographic screening
Mammography has been the primary means of screening for breast cancer since the mid 1980s. It meets the World Health Organization (WHO) criteria for a screening test.

Evidence for benefits from screening mammography

Despite >30 years of trials, screening mammography remains controversial, particularly in the 40–49 age group.

- Based on the USPSTF (U.S. Preventive Services Task Force) 2009 meta-analysis, there is a known reduction in breast cancer mortality due to screening mammography:

Table 11.1

Ages	Mortality Reduction	Number of women screened to save one life
40–49	14%	1904
50–59	17%	1334
60–69	32%	377
70–79	10%	Not defined from data

- Randomized clinical trials (RCTs) have overall demonstrated a 25–30% reduction in breast cancer mortality in women 40–69 years who are screened annually or biennially with mammograms.
- More recent data has brought into question how much of this effect is due to mammography and how much to improvements in treatment.

Limitations of screening mammography

Breast density
Increased breast density is associated with both a lower sensitivity for screening mammography and a higher risk of breast cancer.

Screening interval
Longer screening intervals decrease the chance of catching faster growing cancers earlier.

Outcome
May provide earlier diagnosis without change in outcome.

"Overtreatment"
Potential identification of low grade cancers (and in-situ cancers) that may not be clinically significant but leads to overtreatment ("pseudo-disease").

Reader/expertise dependent
- Sensitivity: 60% to >90%.
- Specificity from 90% to 95%.

Impact of false positives
False positives lead to increased anxiety and benign biopsies (cost and complications).

> Mammography can never "rule out" breast cancer, and concerning clinical abnormalities should be further evaluated by alternative imaging and biopsy, even if imaging is normal.

CHAPTER 11 Breast imaging

Current screening protocols
The age that screening starts and stops and the frequency of screening is not clearly defined, and recommendations vary between medical society and change with time.
- The American College of Radiology and American Cancer Society currently recommends, for women at an average risk, annual mammography from age 40.
- USPSTF recommends biennial from 50–74 years.
- In women with a first degree relative with pre-menopausal breast cancer, screening usually starts 10 years before the age of diagnosis of the relative, but not before age 30.

> **When should screening stop?**
> There is no upper age limit defined by ACR/ACS/AMA, but screening is unlikely to be of benefit if life expectancy is <5–7 years on basis of age or co-morbidities.

Diagnostic mammography

This is an exam consisting of additional mammographic views, which is performed in certain situations:

> **DIAGNOSTIC mammography should be performed when:**
> Abnormality found on screening mammogram.
> Short interval follow-up of a probably benign but abnormal mammogram.
> Patient/physician identified breast lump.
> <u>Focal</u> breast pain/tenderness.
> Suspected abscess.
> Spontaneous nipple discharge.
> New nipple changes (e.g., inversion).

Normal anatomy

Breasts consist of glandular tissue and mammary ducts arranged into 15–20 lobules radiating out from the nipple. These are interspersed by fat and fibrocollagenous septa ("Cooper's ligaments"). Posterior to the breast are the pectoral muscles.
- The ratio of glandular/fibrous tissue to fat varies widely from one woman to another, and changes with age (generally but not always becoming fattier with age).

Normal mammogram
Fatty tissue will appear dark (lucent), and glandular tissue/fibrotic tissue as radiopaque (white). The fibrocollagenous septa appear as fine white lines.
- By convention, labeling of the projection used is placed on the lateral or cephalad aspect of the patient on the film.

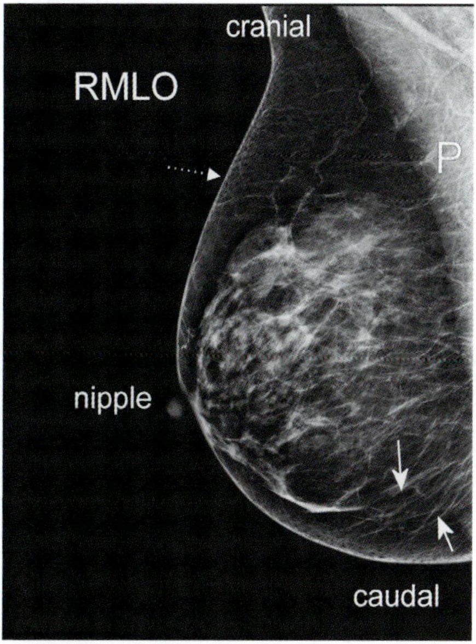

Figure 11.2 Normal MLO mammogram P = pectoralis muscle. Solid arrows = fibrocollagenous septa (Cooper's ligaments), dashed arrow = skin.

How do I read a mammogram?

Mammographic interpretation is almost all pattern recognition due to the limited anatomy present.

Assess technical adequacy

There are strict federal quality control standards regulating all aspects of screening mammography.
- Adequate tissue within field of view on both views.
- The nipple should be in profile on either/both the MLO or CC view.
- No motion.
- Adequate penetration of tissue.

Search pattern

The entire mammogram needs to be searched in a systematic manner:
- Each breast from cranial to caudal on MLO view and lateral to medial on the CC view.
- Each breast from nipple to chest wall left to right.
- Compare one breast to other zone by zone.
- *Compare each view with multiple older mammograms.*

Don't forget!:
- The axilla for normal and abnormal nodes.
- The inframammary fold.
- The retroareolar region.

Comparison films

Comparison films are key in mammography due to the lack of normal anatomy and inter-patient variability. Comparison with films 2+ years ago decreases call back rates and *may* help detect smaller cancers.
- Breast cancers grow slowly and may only be recognized when compared to studies several years ago.
- If patients obtain mammograms at the same center each year this markedly aids this process.
- Centers are federally mandated to send older comparison mammograms either digitally or on film to other centers at no cost to patient.

Breast density

Assessed in all patients according to set criteria from the American College of Radiology.
1. Fatty: <25% glandular tissue.
2. Scattered: 25–50% glandular tissue.
3. Heterogeneously dense: 51–75% glandular tissue.
4. Extremely dense: >75% glandular tissue.

What are we looking for?
- Breast density (see preceding).
- Symmetry—most breasts have a relatively symmetrical distribution of glandular and fatty tissue.
- Signs of cancer that may include:
  - Asymmetrical tissue or density.
  - Masses.
  - Architectural distortion.
  - Calcifications.

Patterns of disease on mammography

When an abnormality is detected, individual characteristics are evaluated to assess the level of concern for malignancy.

The most worrisome feature determines management with any abnormality.

If the abnormality has some features that appear "benign" but some that are more suggestive of a malignant process, we are likely to biopsy the lesion.

Masses

Defined as a space occupying lesion seen in two projections.
- Benign masses include cysts, fibroadenomas, papilloma, and intramammary lymph nodes.

Table 11.2			
Features	Shape	Margins	Density
Benign	Round	Circumscribed	Fat containing
↓	Oval	Obscured	Low
	Lobular	Microlobulated	Equal
	Irregular	Indistinct	High
Malignant		Spiculated	

Skin lesions can look like masses on a mammogram so a technologist may put a radiopaque marker around them to identify them on the study.

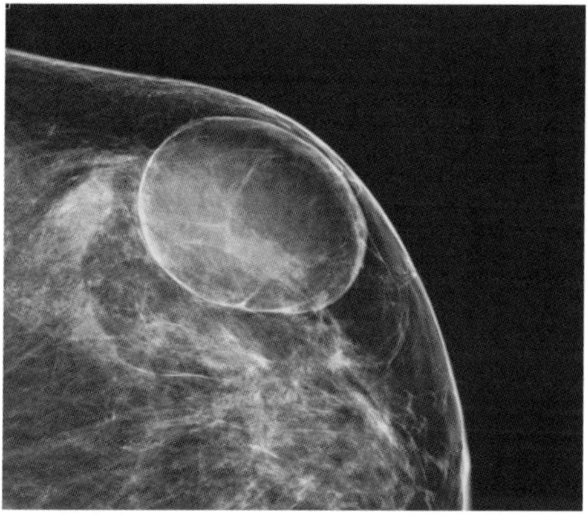

Figure 11.3 This patient's mass is round, circumscribed, and contains lucent material (fat) consistent with a benign oil cyst.

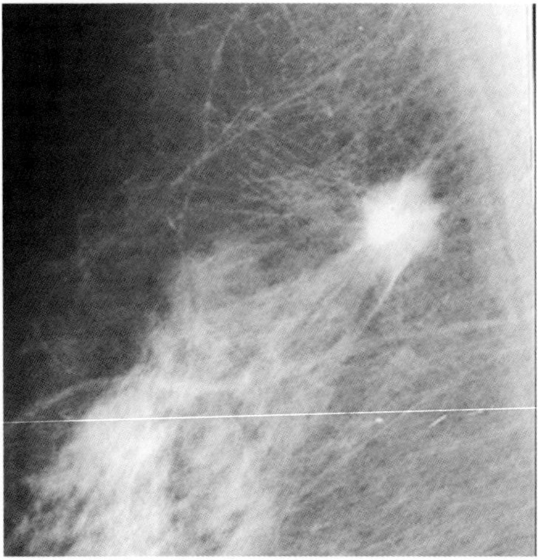

Figure 11.4 In this patient, the mass is lobular, spiculated, and of high density and was an invasive ductal carcinoma.

Calcifications
Some calcification patterns are classic of benign disease. Others need to be evaluated for the likelihood of cancer based on the presence or absence of "benign" or "worrisome" features. The decision to biopsy is usually made on the presence of the most concerning feature and change from prior studies.

Definitely benign calcifications
Some calcifications are definitely benign, including:
- All those with lucent centers (e.g., skin, fat necrosis, oil cysts—latter look like egg shells).
- Vascular (tram track).
- Secretory (coarse, rod like, directed toward nipple, may be centrally lucent).
- Dystrophic (large, coarse, irregular at sites surgery/trauma).
- Milk of Ca++ (form in microcysts and layer on true lateral views).
- Popcorn (coarse, irregular, form typically in fibroadenomas).

"Benign" features
- Round shape.
- Few particles.
- Coarse (larger).
- Scattered distribution.
- Symmetrical distribution.

"Worrisome" features
- Small size (> 0.1 mm).
- More particles.
- Fine linear or branching shapes.
- Pleomorphic (varying in size and shape).
- Clustered distribution (> 5 in a cm^3).
- Segmental, ductal branching or linear distribution.

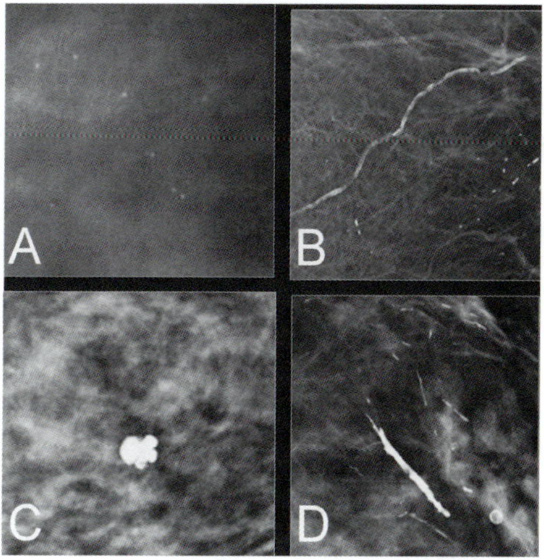

Figure 11.5 Four benign types of calcifications. A = adenosis (round, scattered). B = vascular (tram track). C = calcified fibroadenoma (popcorn). D = secretory (coarse, rod like).

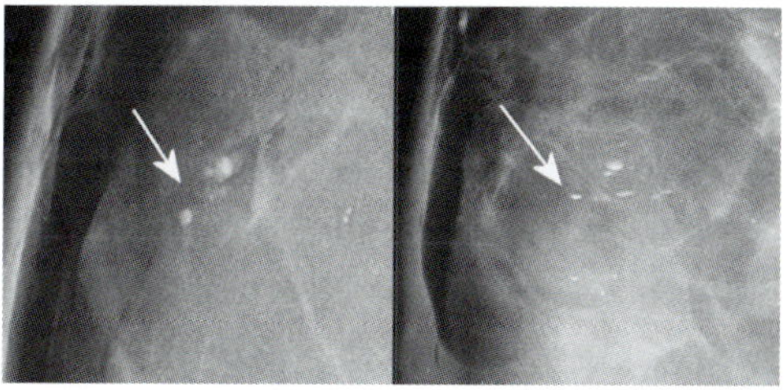

Figure 11.6 Milk of calcium has a characteristic appearance: round and somewhat amorphous on the CC projection (left), and layering dependently in the bottom of cysts in the lateral projection (right).

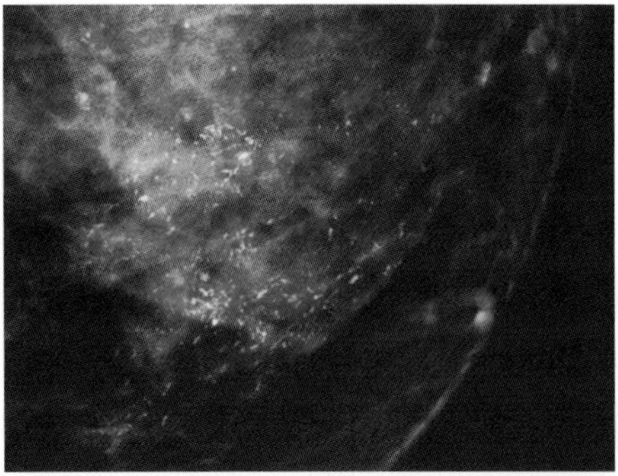

Figure 11.7 Branching, pleomorphic malignant calcifications in a patient with DCIS.

Architectural distortion
Breast architecture is distorted with **no** definite mass visible. Highly suspicious for malignancy if no prior surgery. Specific features include:
- Spiculations radiating from a point.
- Focal retraction of the glandular tissue, i.e., pulling in of the tissue making acute angles rather than smooth curves.
- Distortion of the edge of the glandular tissue.

Benign etiologies include surgery, radial scar (complex sclerosing lesion) and rarely trauma.

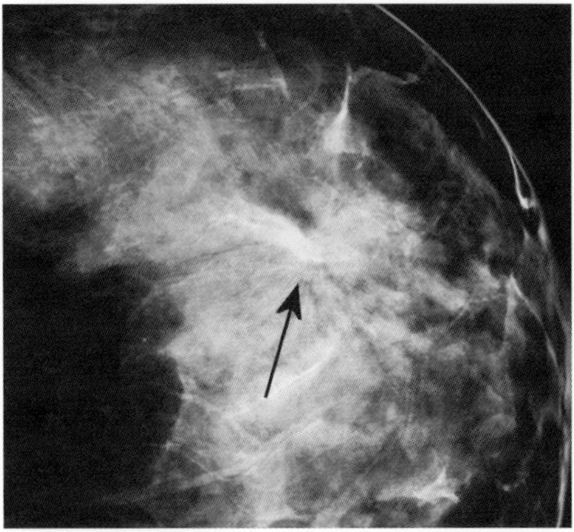

Figure 11.8 Architectural distortion (arrow) can be subtle. See how the glandular tissue is "pulled in" making a sharp angle.

Asymmetries
Most patients' right and left breast tissue is reasonably symmetrical. An asymmetric tissue density can sometimes be a sign of malignancy, especially a new or developing asymmetry.
- Invasive lobular cancer may present this way (although it has many presentations).

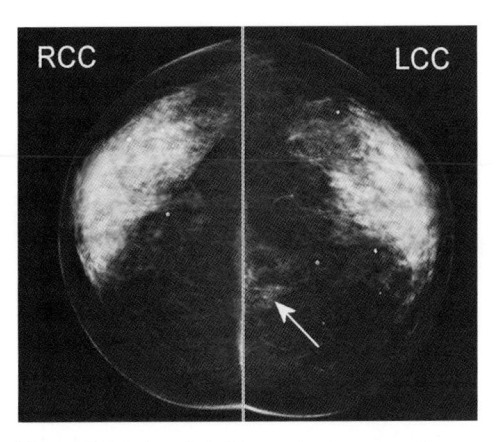

Figure 11.9 Right and left CC views showing an area of asymmetry in the medial left breast (arrow). In this case this was a normal variant.

Associated findings that can be signs of malignancy
- Nipple retraction.
- Skin retraction.
- Skin thickening.
- Trabecular thickening – the fibrocollagenous septa become coarser and widened.
- Abnormal axillary adenopathy.

Communicating the location of a finding
Accurate communication between the referring physician and the radiologist of the location of a clinical finding, and from radiologists (to surgeons, PCPs, and other radiologists, etc.) of radiographic findings is extremely important.

A history of surgery or other breast procedures, and personal/family history of breast cancer may affect the interpretation of a mammogram.

Common descriptors used include:
- Clock face and distance from nipple (see Figure 11.10).
- Quadrant
  - Upper inner, upper outer, lower inner, lower outer
- Additional descriptors:
  - Peri or subareolar, deep central, axillary tail

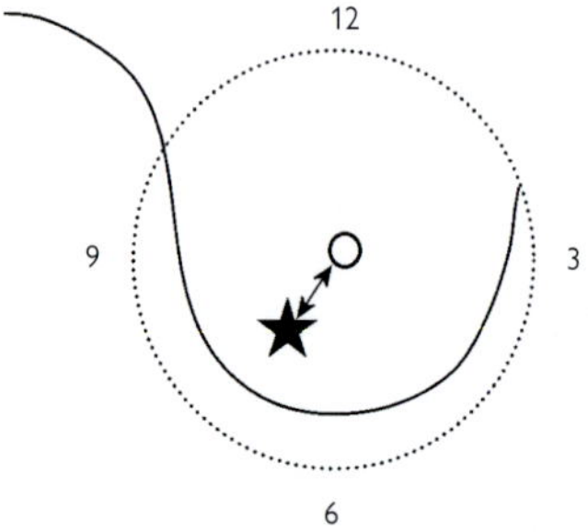

Figure 11.10 Abnormalities in the breast are given a "clockface" localization, as if you were looking at a clock. The right breast is shown with the star at 7:00 in the lower outer quadrant, the double arrow shows the distance from nipple.

Breast imaging reports

Mammographic Quality Standards Act (MQSA) 1992
There are federal mandates controlling image quality and outcome/auditing data at all mammography centers. There also is a requirement that all reports must include a final Breast Imaging-Reporting and Data System (BI-RADS) category after interpretation (see following section).

> **Components of a breast imaging report**
> - Indication for exam.
> - Breast composition (radiographic density).
> - Significant findings (e.g., calcifications, architectural distortion, asymmetric densities).
> - Summary/assessment (BI-RADS category).
> - Management recommendation.

American College of Radiology: Breast Imaging-Reporting and Data System (ACR BI-RADS)
The ACR has developed a lexicon and reporting system that is designed to standardize terminology and classification of mammography, breast ultrasound, and MRI reports (see Table 11.3).
- Allows communication with the referring physician in a clear fashion with a final assessment that indicates a specific course of action.

Table 11.3 BI-RADS Reporting System

Category	Assessment	Recommendation
0	Incomplete	Needs additional imaging and/or prior mammograms for comparison
1	Negative	Routine screening mammography
2	Benign	Routine screening mammography
3	Probably Benign *	Short-interval follow-up recommended
4	Suspicious	Biopsy should be considered
5	Highly Suggestive of Malignancy	Appropriate action should be taken (usually biopsy)
6	Known Biopsy-Proven Malignancy	Appropriate action should be taken (usually surgery)

* A finding placed in this category should have less than a 2% risk of malignancy and cannot be a new finding compared to prior exams

BI-RADS Category 3 Probably Benign
BI-RADS Category 3 should be used as little as possible and not as an alternative to deciding if a lesion is benign or needs biopsy.

BI-RADS Category 4 can be subdivided into:
4a: low concern, 4b: intermediate concern, or 4c: moderate concern

Screening mammograms
Should be ONLY categorized as BI-RADS 0, 1, or 2.

Diagnostic mammograms
May be any category, but the use of BI-RADS 0 should be avoided unless waiting for prior mammograms.

Ultrasound

Ultrasound evaluates different tissue properties than mammography.

When do you do breast ultrasound?
- Focal clinical abnormalities.
  - Lump, <u>focal</u> pain.
- Primary study in evaluating a palpable mass in young (<35), lactating, or pregnant patient.
- Evaluation of a mammographic abnormality.
  - Mass—solid versus cystic, characteristics of a solid mass.
- Focal or regional asymmetric tissue.
- Evaluation of an MRI abnormality.
- Evaluation for abscess or seroma.
- Guidance for interventional procedures.

CHAPTER 11 **Breast imaging**

Screening breast ultrasound
Whole breast screening ultrasound is still controversial and under assessment. There may be an adjunct role in screening higher risk patients with dense breasts (in addition to mammography). ACRIN 6666 trial evaluated screening US <u>only</u> in patients at higher than average risk and with dense breasts.

In this study:
- Supplemental cancer detection over mammography consistently produced 3–4 cases per 1000.
- PPV of biopsy prompted by US approximately 9% (PPV based on mammography = 25–30%).

How do you do a breast ultrasound?
A high frequency linear transducer must be used. Position the patient supine with her arm above her head, with a wedge under her back to rotate her away from the side you are imaging.
- You are aiming to flatten her breast as much as possible.
- Use moderate pressure to reduce artifacts.

Images are obtained in radial and antiradial planes relative to the nipple, scanning systematically through the area of interest. Unless screening is being performed, generally a <u>focused</u> ultrasound is performed of the specific site of concern, usually including that entire quadrant.
- Make sure you image as deep as the pectoralis muscle, but you do not usually need to image deeper.
- On gray scale set the gain so that fat appears a medium gray.
- Do not take random images—very easy to make mass-like artifacts from fat lobules that will become part of the patient's record.

Use of color and pulsed Doppler
See chapter 5, Ultrasound, "Doppler," p. 243 for technical details. Both color and power Doppler are used in the breast.
- The presence of flow within a mass confirms that it is solid.
- Both benign and malignant masses can be hypovascular, or hypervascular.
- Used as an aid to direct biopsy away from large vessels to decrease risk of bleeding.

Normal breast ultrasound
Fat is relatively hypoechoic (mid-gray).
- Fibrous tissue is echogenic (white).
- Glandular tissue is intermediate-echogenic (whiter than fat).
- Lesion echogenicity is described relative to fat echogenicity.

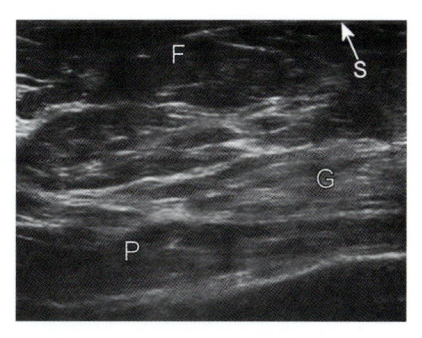

Figure 11.11 Normal breast ultrasound F = fat, G = glandular tissue, P = pectoralis muscle, S = skin.

As with mammography, findings are classified based on their imaging characteristics and a BI-RADS assessment made.

Limitations of ultrasound and pitfalls
- High false positive rate for screening.
- High inter-user variability due to experience and equipment which affects both the sensitivity and specificity of technique.
- Ultrasound parameters incorrectly set can obscure abnormalities or produce artifacts that are misinterpreted as lesions.
- Limited penetration; deep lesions hard to image, especially in large breasts with fatty composition.
- Pseudo-lesions can be seen:
  - Fat lobules.
  - Cooper's ligaments may shadow.
  - Chest wall "pseudo-lesions"—e.g., ribs misinterpreted as lesions.
- Nipple shadowing—difficult to assess behind the nipple (special techniques required).

Patterns of disease on breast ultrasound

The reference for echogenicity in the breast is the echogenicity of the breast fat (i.e., all other substances are described as either hyperechoic or hypoechoic to fat).

Masses

Table 11.4	
Benign Features	**Malignant Features**
Anechoic (= simple cyst)	Hypoechoic
Homogeneously hyperechoic (fat, vascular lesions)	Spiculation
Parallel to chest wall	Not parallel to chest wall
Oval shape	Microlobulation
Gently lobulated	Angular margins
Thin echogenic pseudocapsule (e.g., fibroadenoma)	Shadowing
	Duct extension
	Branching pattern

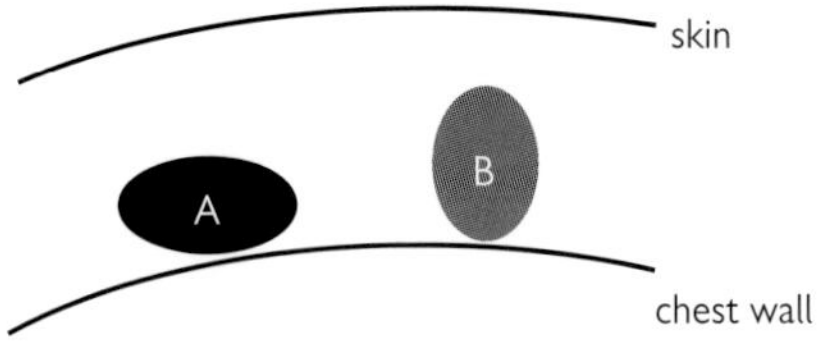

Figure 11.12 The long axis of lesion A is "parallel" to the chest wall—a benign feature of solid masses such as fibroadenomas. Lesion B is perpendicular to the chest wall, a feature that is more suspicious for malignancy.

Simple cyst
- Anechoic.
- Smooth posterior wall.
- Round/oval shape.
- Thin, avascular septations.
- No internal vascularity.
- Increased through transmission (appears "bright" behind cyst as the fluid conducts more sound than the surrounding tissue).

Complex cysts
- Contain internal echoes from blood or proteinaceous fluid.
- Echoes may be mobile under real-time ultrasound.
- No internal vascularity.
- May require aspiration to exclude a solid mass.

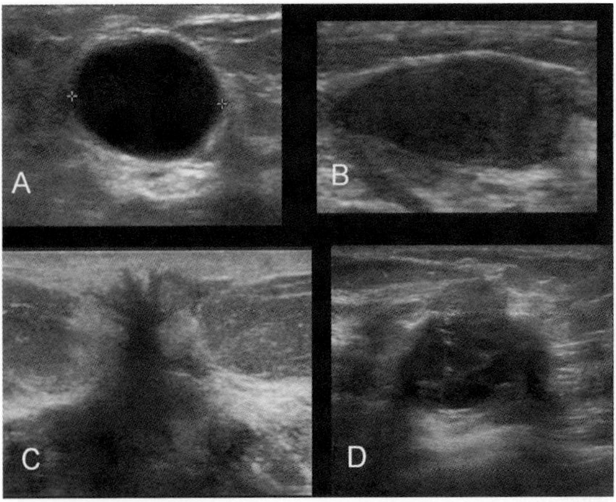

Figure 11.13 Contrasting benign versus malignant features: A: benign simple cyst—imperceptibly thin rim, completely anechoic, enhanced through transmission (brighter behind the cyst/fluid). B: Fibroadenoma—smooth walls, echogenic capsule, oval shape parallel to chest wall. C: Invasive ductal carcinoma—angular, spiculated mass with thick and indistinct margins and decreased sound transmission (dark behind) D: focal fibrocystic changes—indeterminate by US with mixed benign and malignant features.

MRI

How do you do breast MRI?

Breast MRI can be performed with contrast to detect malignancy, or without contrast for implant assessment. Breast MRI should only be performed in centers that are able to perform MRI guided interventional procedures.

Contrast enhanced breast MRI adds physiologic information. The breasts are scanned serially (usually 4–5 times) before and after the injection of IV gadolinium to assess for areas of contrast enhancement (increased signal on T1 following contrast). Malignant tumors tend to enhance early and vigorously with fast washout of the contrast.

Technique
- Patients are scanned face-down with their breasts dependent in specialized breast coils that lie close to the breasts.
- Specialized software for the rapid scanning is needed as well as for kinetic analysis of the contrast enhancement (see "CAD," p. 495).

When do you do breast MRI?

These guidelines are developing and vary among facilities and medical societies. The following are based on the recommendations from the American College of Radiology and the American Cancer Society 2010.

Breast cancer staging

Many centers use it routinely to stage all new breast cancer diagnoses.
- Ipsilateral disease: Additional unsuspected malignancies detected in 10–15% patients.
- Contralateral disease: Additional unsuspected malignancies detected in 3–5. %.
- The effect on recurrence rates and survival rates is controversial and under study, survival benefit has not been shown.
- Some centers use it as part of staging in the setting of isolated DCIS.
  - Can show extent of non-calcified portions.

Unknown primary
- Looking for occult breast cancer as a cause of metastatic axillary adenocarcinoma.
- MRI detects the primary cancer in up to 70% of these patients.

High risk screening

Screening breast MRI remains controversial due to its high cost and low specificity (high rate of false positives). No current trials have assessed effect on mortality and have only assessed high risk individuals.

<u>Americal Cancer Society (ACS) recommendations:</u>
Annual MRI screening recommended (based on scientific evidence):
- *BRCA* mutation.
- First-degree relative of *BRCA* carrier, but patient has not been tested.
- Lifetime risk ~20–25% or greater (from calculated models).

Annual MRI screening recommended (based on expert consensus opinion but not confirmed in trials):
- Radiation to chest between age 10 and 30 years.
- Li-Fraumeni syndrome and first-degree relatives.
- Cowden and Bannayan-Riley-Ruvalcaba syndromes and first-degree relatives.

Breast MRI detects approximately twice as many cancers as mammography in high risk individuals.

Evaluation by a genetics unit should be considered before commitment to routine screening by MRI due to the cost involved and the significant risk of false positives (From 20–40% on a first screening exam, dropping to less than 10% on subsequent exams).

Diagnostic
The role of MRI in diagnostic breast imaging is not yet clearly defined.

Patients who are BI-RADS 0 on the basis of screening mammography exams should undergo standard mammographic/ultrasound evaluation before MRI.

Consider in:
- Worrisome nipple discharge (especially bloody) or nipple retraction in a patient with a negative diagnostic mammogram and ultrasound.
- Evaluation for recurrence at lumpectomy site in a patient with negative mammographic work up but clinical suspicion, or an equivocal mammogram.
- Evaluation of implant integrity.

A negative MRI should never exclude biopsy a lesion which is suspicious on mammography or ultrasound.

Implant evaluation
Implants may be silicone, saline, or both (double layered implants).
- Silicone implant integrity can be evaluated using specific pulse sequences that suppress water and fat signal, leaving only the silicone as bright on the image.
- Contrast is not indicated (so does not also evaluate for cancer).
- Saline implants do not require MRI imaging; collapse if ruptured (unlike silicone implants).

Advantages of breast MR
No ionizing radiation.
- Multiplanar imaging, images entire breast volume and chest wall.
- >90% sensitivity for invasive carcinoma.
- Detects occult, multifocal, or residual malignancy.
- May estimate tumor size better than mammography/ultrasound.
- Ability to image regional lymph nodes.

Disadvantages of breast MR
- High equipment and examination costs (~8–10x mammography).
- Injection of gadolinium required.
- Difficult learning curve for interpretation due to physiological enhancement with high false positive rate (specificity ≈ 30–50%).
- May be false negative in low grade DCIS and other slow growing cancers.

ACR BI-RADs for breast MR
- Uniform terminology for interpretation.
- Similar to mammography.
  - BI-RADS 0–6 categories. See earlier BI-RADS section, p. 488

Patterns of disease: breast MRI
- As with other modalities, when reading a breast MRI one evaluates the characteristics of structural abnormalities (masses, distortion, margins).
- Unique to BMRI is evaluation of enhancement patterns (kinetics).
  - Extent, degree, and type of enhancement.

MRI appearances of normal and abnormal breast tissue

Table 11.4

Normal glandular tissue	T1 dark pre-contrast, progressively ↑ signal with contrast
Normal lymph nodes	T2 bright, hypervascular with wash-out kinetics
Cysts	T2 bright
Carcinoma	T2 iso-intense to dark, usually rapidly enhancing and wash-out.
DCIS	Usually clumped enhancement with widely variable kinetics. Low grade may not enhance

Diffuse hormonal enhancement
The enhancement pattern of the breast on MRI is hormonally sensitive and can obscure small foci of malignancy. This is particularly a problem in younger patients.

To minimize the effects of hormones, patients should be scanned in day 7–14 of the menstrual cycle, and preferably off exogenous hormones (HRT, OCP) for 3 months.

Computer assisted analysis (detection)
Many centers use post-processing software to evaluate the kinetics of contrast in the breast tissue.
- It color-codes each voxel on the image according to how fast the contrast flows into and washes out of the breast tissue. This results in an enhancement curve to be displayed for each voxel.
- One typical display is shown in Color Plate 15.

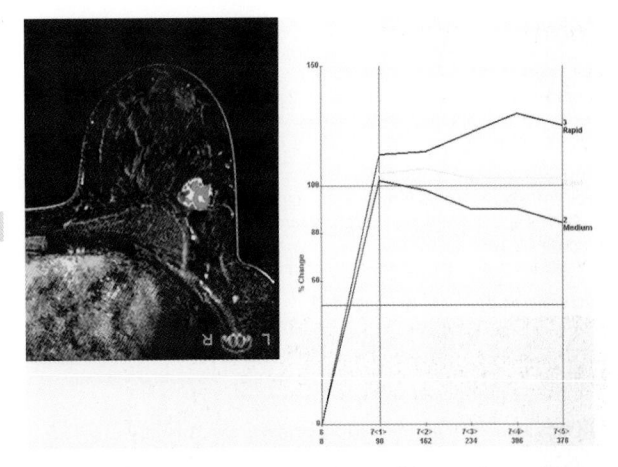

Figure 11.14 Computer-assisted analysis of breast MRI contrast kinetics. Left image is an invasive ductal carcinoma showing "malignant" or rapid wash-out of contrast (red). Right image demonstrates the typical contrast wash-out curves for benign (blue), malignant (red) and indeterminate (yellow) processes. See Color Plate 15.

- *Benign curve*: slowly accumulates contrast (as seen in normal tissue and fibrocystic tissue) with no significant wash-out during imaging period.
- *Malignant curve*: rapid peak enhancement followed by rapid washout.
- *Indeterminate or "Plateau"*: in between the prior two.

Unfortunately, there is considerable overlap between these kinetic curves.
- "Benign" curves may be seen in DCIS, invasive lobular and low-grade invasive ductal cancers.
- "Malignant" curves may be seen in normal lymph nodes and vascular tumors such as papillomas and hemangiomas.

Other modalities

Other functional imaging modalities such as FDG-PET and "scintomammography" with Tc-99m sestamibi using dedicated breast imaging devices are being investigated and may have a role to play in the future in the diagnosis of breast cancer. FDG-PET is commonly used for staging in advanced breast cancers.

Common conditions

Cysts

Breast cysts are very common, especially in the fourth decade (although seen in all ages), may present with a palpable mass, focal tenderness, or be asymptomatic. They are often multiple.

Mammography

Well defined mass or often multiple masses.
- May change in size significantly in short time interval, or one year to another ("waxing and waning").
- Variable density, may be fairly low density.

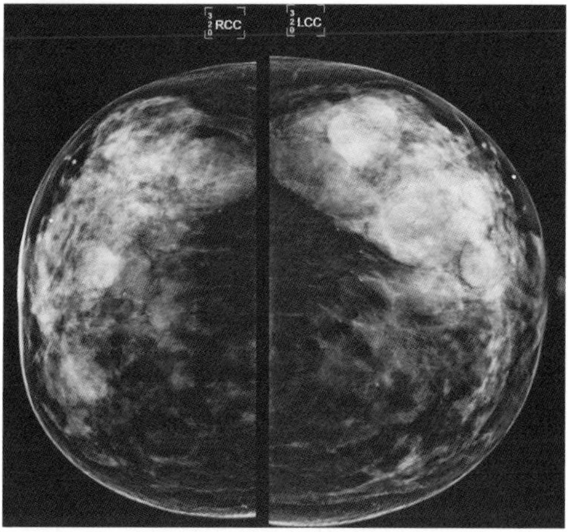

Figure 11.15 Multiple bilateral breast cysts on CC mammograms.

Ultrasound

Well defined anechoic mass (see Figure 11.13 and detail p. 492) with increased through transmission.
- May have internal echoes if complex (e.g., hemorrhage into cyst).

MRI

A simple cyst is well circumscribed, very bright on T2, and shows no internal enhancement.
- A cyst with proteinaceous debris can have variable internal signal, but it will not show internal enhancement.

Ductal carcinoma in situ (DCIS)
Mammography
DCIS has a variable appearance on mammography, partly dependent on its grade and presence of any intra-ductal necrosis. It may be occult or appear as:
- Multiple clustered or segmental micro calcifications that may be: fine linear, branching, pleomorphic (see Figures 11.7 and 11.16).
  - These may be distributed along ducts (lying in a line, often branching) directed toward the nipple.
  - Not all DCIS calcifications "follow the rules," and even quite benign appearing calcifications may end up being DCIS.
- A focal density or mass (rarely).

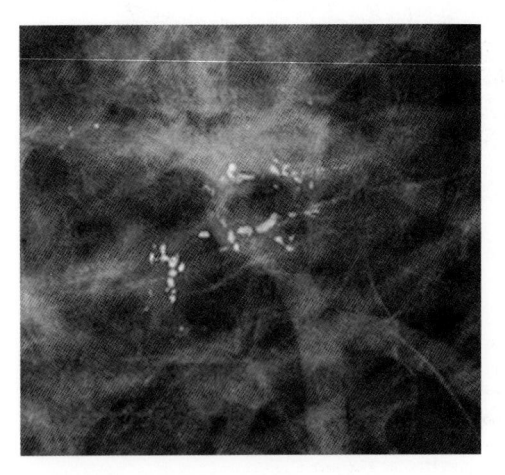

Figure 11.16 DCIS. Pleomorphic calcifications lying along a ductal branching distribution.

Ultrasound
DCIS is often not visible on ultrasound, but may be seen as a hypoechoic mass that may be linear and/or branching, following a ductal distribution.
- Sometimes distended ducts are seen containing hypoechoic, material with vascular flow.
- Clustered microcalcifications may be sometimes be seen as echogenic foci.

MRI
Clumped enhancement in a ductal distribution is a hallmark of DCIS. The enhancement can be low grade and have "benign" kinetics.

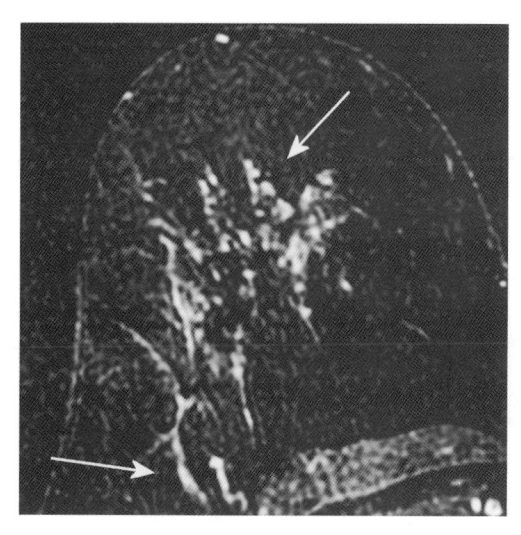

Figure 11.17 Subtraction (contrast minus non-contrast) MRI image showing extensive clumped enhancement in a ductal distribution in a patient with biopsy proven DCIS.

Invasive carcinomas
Invasive cancers have highly variable appearances, depending on the type of cancer and the grade. Although a few malignancies (e.g., mucinous and medullary) may present as well defined masses, most invasive cancers have irregular, spiculated, or poorly defined borders on all imaging modalities.

Mammography (see Figures 11.8 and 11.18).
- Masses that are as dense or denser than surrounding tissue.
- May grow relatively slowly over years.
- May have associated pleomorphic calcifications.
- +/− architectural distortion.
- Developing asymmetric density.

Other cancer subtypes
- Invasive lobular cancers have a greater tendency to appear as subtle architectural distortion or a subtle asymmetric density and may be mammographically occult.
- Inflammatory breast cancer may present with diffuse skin and fibrocollageous septa (trabecular) thickening.

500 CHAPTER 11 **Breast imaging**

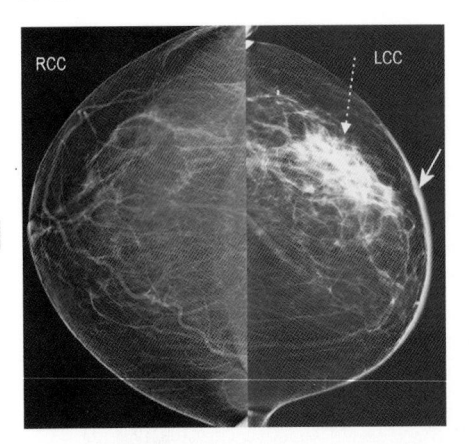

Figure 11.18 Inflammatory breast cancer in the left breast with normal right for comparison. Note the skin (solid arrow) and trabecular (dotted arrow) thickening.

Ultrasound (see Figure 11.13).
- Solid hypoechoic masses, usually with internal vascularity.
  - May have an echogenic "halo" around the mass.
- Occasionally appears as more ill-defined hypoechogenicity.

MRI
- Invasive ductal carcinomas typically have intense enhancement and rapid ("malignant") wash-out.
- Lower grade ductal and lobular carcinomas may have less enhancement and "benign" kinetics.

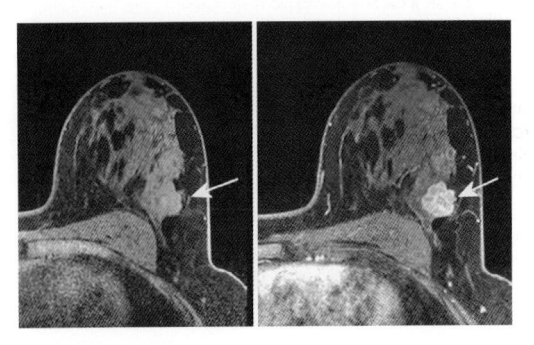

Figure 11.19 (Left) Pre and (right) post contrast T1 weighted images of a 3 cm invasive ductal carcinoma in the left breast showing intense enhancement. See also kinetic analysis Color Plate 15.

Fibroadenomas

Fibroadenomas are the most common mass in young women (teens upward), are commonly palpable and have certain features common on all imaging modalities:
- Typically oval or gently lobulated with smooth sharp margins.
- Grow slowly with time premenopausally (1–2 mm a year) then may shrink.
- Can grow fast in young women especially when pregnant.

Mammography
- As dense or denser than surrounding tissue.
- Coarse internal calcifications common ("popcorn").

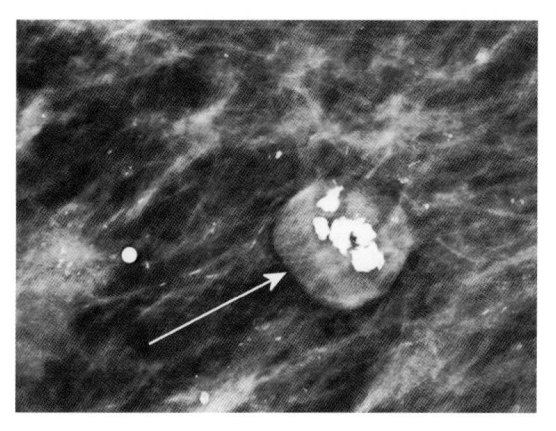

Figure 11.20 Fibroadenoma on mammography. Well defined mass with popcorn calcifications.

Ultrasound (see Figure 11.13)
- Hypo to isoechoic.
- Avascular to occasionally intensely vascular.
- Echogenic "pseudocapsule."

MRI
- Homogenous progressive enhancement.
- +/− dark internal septa.
- May be T2 bright.
- Imaging features often not diagnostic.

Procedures

Cyst aspiration

Indications
- If a patient's cyst is tender and not resolving spontaneously.
- If a hypoechoic mass is suspected to be a complex cyst (internal echoes but no perfusion).
- Cysts with internal masses or vascular septa are best biopsied with a vacuum assisted device.

Technique
- 18G needle under US guidance, aspirating with a syringe.
- Contents usually only sent to cytology if frankly bloody as cytology often confusing if cysts are inflamed.
- If cytology sent, marker must be left at aspiration site so the area can be identified if surgical excision required.
- Failed aspirations need core biopsy as they are likely solid masses.

Needle/wire localizations (NLOC)
"Marks" lesions with a wire so surgeons can find them in the breast.

Indications
- Lesions not amenable to percutaneous biopsy due to:
  - Location in the breast (e.g.. calcifications close to the chest wall).
  - Lesions very close to the nipple.
- Medical conditions that preclude lying prone for the 20 minutes required for a stereotactic biopsy.
- Localizing lesions that need surgical excision (e.g., known cancer or atypia) (see Figure 11.21).

Technique
A needle is placed into the lesion under either ultrasound guidance or using an x-ray grid.
- A wire with a hook on the end is placed through the needle and the needle removed.
- Usually performed an hour or two before surgery.
- At surgery, a piece of tissue around the hook of the wire is removed.

Percutaneous core biopsy
Minimally invasive tissue diagnosis for any BI-RADS 4 or 5 lesion.
- Guidance may be by ultrasound, stereotactic, or MRI (see later sections).
- Modality chosen by ease of visualization and patient factors.
- 2 basic needle types:
  - Spring loaded, cutting.
  - Vacuum assisted ("sucks" tissue into the cutting chamber and provides larger samples).

Techniques common to all biopsies
- Sterile preparation.
- Lidocaine +/− epinephrine for local anesthesia.
- 2–5 mm skin incision with a scalpel.
- A tiny metallic clip is left at the biopsy site to confirm sampling site and allow NLOC if further excision is needed.

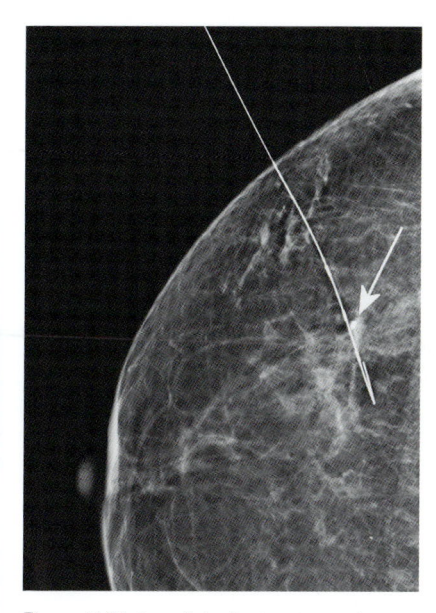

Figure 11.21 A needle localization wire tip adjacent to the needle biopsy marker (arrow).

> **Patients on anticoagulants**
> Patients usually need to discontinue anticoagulant therapy for core needle biopsies. This may involve them transferring to injectable anti-coagulants temporarily, for example, lovenox (enoxaparin) bridge. Some centers stop aspirin and plavix (clopidogrel) for a week before biopsy.

Ultrasound guided biopsy

Ultrasound biopsy is the method of choice if lesions can be seen by ultrasound—cheapest, fastest, and the most comfortable for patients.
- Fine needle aspiration
  - 18–23 g needles.
  - Generally, core biopsy (if available) is preferred over FNA due to its much higher sensitivity (98+% compared to 80%).
- Core cutting needles
  - Well defined solid lesions > 5 mm.
- Vacuum assisted needles
  - Ill-defined or largely cystic lesions (due to large samples).

- Very small lesions.
- Lesions against chest wall (difficult to biopsy safely with cutting needles).

Stereotactic biopsy

Stereotactic biopsy uses x-ray guidance to guide core needle biopsy placement. Generally, this is performed for calcifications, masses, or suspicious densities with no ultrasound correlate.

<u>Technique:</u>
- Patient lies prone on stereo table with breast through hole in table in light compression.
- Two images taken 15 degrees from center with digital mammography.
- Computer calculates x, y, and z coordinates of lesion.
- Local anesthesia applied.
- Vacuum assisted needle takes 9 or 10g samples.
- Sample is x-rayed to confirm sampling of lesion.
- Image pairs repeated after each needle adjustment to check position from x-rays via the control unit.

> **Stereotactic biopsy cannot be performed if:**
> - The patient exceeds table weight limit (>300–350 lb).
> - Lesion is not visible when imaged on the stereo unit.
> - Patient cannot lie prone or climb up to table.
> - Some very posterior lesions close to chest wall.
> - Very thin breasts (under 15–20 mm compressed).

MRI guided biopsy

If lesions are only seen on MRI (usually after mammo/US workup), an MRI guided biopsy can be performed.

<u>Technique:</u>
- Specialized biopsy coil/grid on MRI table.
- Patient in prone position.
- Non-ferromagnetic vacuum assisted needle system.
- Patient is slid in the bore for images, and slid out of the bore for tissue sampling.

Sentinel node injection

The "sentinel node(s)" is the node or nodes that malignant cells first drain to from a tumor. By removing and testing this node(s)—usually by immunohistochemical studies—surgeons may avoid the need for an axillary dissection.

The sentinel nodes (usually 1–3) can be identified by using one or more of these tests:
- Injecting blue dye around the tumor at surgery and following the lymphatics visually.

- Injecting Tc-99m sulfur colloid around the tumor +/– intradermally above the tumor or even subareolar (the breast drains to the areolar then outwards to the axilla +/– the internal mammary nodes).
  - The sentinel nodes are then localized by a gamma probe at the time of surgery.

Galactography (ductography)
This involves injecting contrast into a nipple duct and obtaining mammograms. Usually performed for patients with suspicious nipple discharge (e.g., bloody or spontaneous).
- Performed when conventional imaging is negative.
- Technically challenging procedure because duct orifices cannot normally be seen.
- Aims to see filling defects in ducts usually due to DCIS or papillomas.

Management problems

Palpable masses
- Refer for DIAGNOSTIC mammography and ultrasound.
- Although rare, imaging can be negative in palpable malignant masses.
- In patients <35, ultrasound is usually the initial investigation.
- Diffusely "lumpy bumpy breasts" should have routine screening mammography because diagnostic imaging is rarely helpful unless this is a new finding.

> **Palpable masses**
> Discrete lumps if new/growing should be referred to a clinical provider such as a breast surgeon for consideration of biopsy even if imaging negative.

Man with a breast lump/tenderness
Male patients are managed similarly to women when they have breast symptoms. Tender retroareolar breast lumps are most commonly due to gynecomastia (uni or bilateral), but men do develop breast cancer (0.05% of all breast cancers), the vast majority of which are infiltrating ductal cancers.
- Mammography is performed bilaterally (for comparison).
  - Breast cancers are similar in appearance to female tumors.
  - Gynecomastia appears as a flame shaped subareolar opacity, often bilateral but asymmetrical.
- Ultrasound may or may not be performed—not usually needed if classic mammographic features of gynecomastia are present.
  - Breast cancers are similar in appearance to female tumors.
  - Gynecomastia appears as subareolar flame shaped hypoechoic tissue.

Breast pain
- Rarely, a tumor can be painful; much more commonly pain is due to fibrocystic changes, cysts, or hormonal changes.
- Diffuse, bilateral, or regional breast pain should have routine screening mammography only.
- Focal pain ("can you point to it with a finger?") should have mammography plus ultrasound.

> It is vital that physicians accurately convey the site of concern (mass, pain) to the radiologist, recording breast side, size, position (clock face), and distance from nipple.

Cellulitis/mastitis
Most times, this is managed clinically. However, imaging should be considered when symptoms do not resolve or an abscess is considered possible (e.g., post surgical, palpable mass).
- Usually this involves ultrasound as mammography is usually unhelpful and painful.
- Always consider inflammatory breast cancer in "mastitis" that does not resolve (in this case mammography may be performed).

Nipple discharge
- Bloody nipple discharge is the most concerning, but cancer-associated nipple discharge can also be clear or serous.
- Unilateral spontaneous is more concerning than bilateral or expressible only.
- Mammography +/− magnified views and/or peri-areolar ultrasound.
- Ductography may be helpful.
- Consider MRI for bloody nipple discharge.
- Many patients require surgical duct exploration/excision.

References

American Cancer Society guidelines for breast screening with MRI as an adjunct to mammography. *CA Cancer J Clin.* 2007; 57:75–89.

Nelson HD, Tyne K, Naik A et al. Screening for Breast Cancer: An Update for the U.S. Preventive Services Task Force. Ann Int Med 2009; 151:727–737

Index

A

Abdominal aortic aneurysm (AAA)
 defined, 164
 follow-up, 164
 post endovascular repair of, 164–5
 pre-operative evaluation of, 164
 ruptured, 181
 ultrasound imaging of, 258–9
Abdominal aortic dissection, 165–6
 computed tomography for, 165–6
 magnetic resonance angiography for, 166
Abdominal calcification, 126–8
 patterns of, 127
Abdominal compartments, normal CT anatomy on, 140
Abdominal pain, 34–5
Abdominal radiographs, in neonates, 300–3
 bowel obstruction, 303
 calcifications, 301
 necrotizing enterocolitis, 302–3
 normal film, 300–1
 pneumoperitoneum, 301–2
Abdominal series, acute, 116
Abdominoperineal resection (APR), 354
Abnormal intraluminal air, 143
 portal venous gas, 143
Abortion
 diagnosing, 272
 spontaneous, 271–2
Abscess, 146, 154, 399
 acute diverticulitis with peri-diverticular, 147
Achalasia, 346–7
 primary, 346
 secondary, 347
Acoustic window, 240
Acromioclavicular joint, dislocations/subluxations in, 229
Adenomas, 169
 adrenal, 177

computed tomography for, 169
 magnetic resonance imaging for, 169
Adenomyosis, 179
Adnexal tubal ring sign, 272–3
Adrenal adenomas, 177
Adrenal masses, 176–8
 computed tomography for, 176, 177
 incidentally discovered, workup of, 178
 magnetic resonance imaging for, 176
Adrenal metastases, 178
Adrenocortical carcinoma, primary, 178
Air, 19, 247
 abnormal intraluminal, 143
 bronchograms, 56
 enema, for intussusception, 313–14
 extra-luminal, 142–3, 181
 free intraperitoneal, 143
 in large intestine, 117
 mesenteric, 143
 retroperitoneal, 121, 143
  in lower abdomen, 121
  in upper abdomen, 121
 in soft tissues, 210
 in stomach, 117
Airspace opacification, 55–7
 air bronchograms, 56
 differential diagnosis of, 55
 silhouettes, 56–7
 spine sign, 57
 subtypes of, 55
Airway, 53
 children, 308–9
 infants, 308–9
ALARA (As Low As Reasonably Achievable) principle, 22, 191
Albuterol, for bronchospasm, 21
Allergies
 contrast, 2, 20–1
 GBCA, 17
Alveolar opacities, 82
 chest CT for, 82

Alveolar pulmonary edema, 91–4
American Association for the Surgery of Trauma (AAST), 158
American College of Radiology: Breast Imaging-Reporting and Data System (ACR BI-RADS), 488–9
American College of Radiology Appropriateness Criteria® (ACR AC), 31–40
Amniocentesis, 275
Amnionicity, 273–4
Amniotic fluid abnormalities, 280–1
Amniotic fluid index (AFI), 280–1
Anaphylactoid reaction, 20–1
Anaphylaxis, treatment for, 21
Anechoic masses, 248
Anembryonic pregnancy, 272
Aneuploidy screening, 275
Aneurysms
 chest CT for, 88–9
 pseudoaneurysms, 454
Angiography, 456–7
 conventional, 374
 CT. See CT angiography
 of dialysis fistulas, 462–3
 magnetic resonance. See Magnetic resonance angiography
 renal/mesenteric, 463–5
Angiomyolipoma (AML), 176
Angulation fracture, 202
Anisotropy, 199
Ankle injuries, 225–7
 computed tomography for, 227
 fractures, 226
 magnetic resonance imaging for, 227
 missing areas in, 227
 radiographic findings of, 225
Ankle mortise, disruption of, 226
Anomaly screening, 275

INDEX

Anterior cruciate ligament (ACL), 224
Anterior mediastinal masses, 66–7
  differential diagnosis of, 67
  radiographic findings for, 66
Anterior-posterior (AP) chest radiographs, 42
  technical considerations for, 42
Anticoagulation reversal, 452
Antrum, 340–1
Aorta, anatomy of, 252
Aortic aneurysm, 112
  abdominal, 164–259
  indications for, 112
  magnetic resonance angiography for, 112
Aortic dissection, 104–5, 112
  abdominal, 165–6
  for chest pain, 32
  CT angiography for, 163–6
  diagnosis of, 181
  indications for, 112
  magnetic resonance angiography for, 112
  on non-contrast MRI, 167
Apophyses, 317
Apparent diffusion coefficient maps (ADC maps), 372–3
Appendicitis, 28, 160–1
  acute, 161
  computed tomography for, 29
  magnetic resonance imaging for, 28
  perforated, 161
  ultrasound imaging of, 28, 258
Arterial ultrasound, 288–9
Arterio-venous malformations (AVM), 385, 386
Arthritis, 207–9, 234
  inflammatory, 208–9
  musculoskeletal MRI for, 196
  musculoskeletal ultrasound for, 198
  osteoarthritis, 207–8, 219, 234
  radiographic evaluation for, 207
  rheumatoid, 215, 234
Arthrography, 238
Arthroplasty, 234–6

hemiarthroplasty, 235
infection and, 236
open reduction internal fixation, 235
osteolysis, 236
total, 234–6
Artifacts, computed tomography, 6
Artifactual cardiomegaly, 54
Ascites, 255–6
Asthma, 306
Atelectasis
  chest CT for, 84
  distinguished from pleural effusions, 73
Atlanto-axial dislocation, 410
Atropine, for hypotension, 21
Automated implantable cardioverter-defibrillators (AICDs), 25, 53
Avascular necrosis (AVN), 219–21
  magnetic resonance imaging for, 221
  predisposing factors, 219–21
  radiographic findings of, 219

B

Babies, imaging in, 292–3
  cooperation, 293
  embarrassment, 293
  fear, 293
  radiation exposure in, 292–3
  size and age, 292
Back pain, 36
Bacterial pneumonia, atypical, 96
  on computed tomography, 96
  findings of, 96
Bacterial pneumonia, typical, 95
  chest x-ray for, 96
  on computed tomography, 95–6
  findings of, 95
Bariatric surgery, 343
Barium, 331
  contraindications, 331
  indications, 331
  swallow, 338, 339
    double contrast, 339
    single contrast, 339
Barium sulfate, 19

risks and contraindications of, 20
Benign hepatic tumors, 168–9
  adenoma, 169
  focal nodular hyperplasia, 169
  hemangioma, 168
β-Blockers, for anaphylaxis, 21
Bicarbonate infusion, for contrast induced nephropathy, 16–17
Bile duct strictures, 172
Biliary interventions, 468–9
  biliary stent, 469
  cholecystostomy, 468
  percutaneous cholangiogram and drainage, 468–9
  techniques and patient preparation, 468
  transjugular intrahepatic portosystemic shunt, 469
Biliary obstruction, 257
  extrahepatic biliary ductal dilatation, 257
  intrahepatic biliary ductal dilatation, 257
Biliary stent, 469
Biophysical profile (BPP), 281
Biopsies, 470–1
  general techniques, 470–1
  lung biopsy, 471
  patient preparation, 470
  solid organ biopsy, 471
Bladder injuries, 158–9
  CT cystography, indications for, 159
  findings of, 159
  techniques, 159
Bladder masses, 364–6
Bladder rupture, 366
Bleeding
  vaginal, 276
  postpartum, 279
Blood, 146
  extraperitoneal, 146
  intraperitoneal, 146
  retroperitoneal, 146
Blunt traumatic aortic injury (BTAI), 105–6
  CT angiography for, 105–6
  radiographic findings of, 105–6
Bones, 54
  abdominal radiography of, 118

extremity/joint radiograph of, 185
heterotopic, 210
imaging, 426–30
  metastatic cancer, 427–9
  radiotracers and protocols, 427
  time for, 426–7
marrow
  abnormalities, 214
  marrow conversion, 214
  marrow infiltration, by malignancy/infection, 214
pathology for, 194
trauma, 214
within masses, 210
radiodensity, decreased, 206
scintigraphy, 447
tumors, computed tomography for, 193
Bosniak classification, of renal cysts, 176
Bowel gas pattern, 301
Bowel obstruction, 130–2
  small, 130–2
  colon obstruction, 132
  neonates, 303
Bowel wall
  assessment of, 142
  inflammation in, 143
  normal CT anatomy on, 142
  walls, trauma in, 159–60
  wall thickening, 122–3
    causes of, 144
    colon, 123
    defined, 144–5
    differential diagnosis of, 144–5
    small bowel, 123
Brain MRI, pulse sequences used in, 13
Breast imaging, 475–506
  common conditions, 497–501
  cysts, 497–501
    aspiration, 502–5
  ductal carcinoma in situ (DCIS), 498
  fibroadenomas, 501
  galactography (ductography), 505
  invasive carcinomas, 499–500
  magnetic resonance imaging, 493–6
  mammography, 476–89
  management problems, 505–6
  modalities, 496

MRI-guided biopsy, 504
needle/wire localizations (NLOC), 502
percutaneous core biopsy, 502–4
procedures, 502–5
sentinel node injection, 504–5
stereotactic biopsy, 504
ultrasound, 489–92
ultrasound-guided biopsy, 503–4
Breasts, normal anatomy of, 480
Breath holding, 151–2
Bronchiectasis, 101
Bronchiolitis, 306
Bronchoalveolar carcinoma (BAC), 103
Bronchospasm, treatment for, 21
Bronchovascular markings, 59–60
Buckle fractures, 317
  of distal radius, 321
  handle, 327
Bursal effusion, 221
Bursitis, 221

C

Calcification, 76–7
  abdominal, 126–8
  extrapulmonary, 77
  lung, 76
  mediastinum, 76
  neonatal abdomen, 301
  pleural, 76–7
Calcific tendonopathy, 211
Calcium, 210, 247
  within masses, 210
  within tendons, 210
Call back, 478
Capillary telangiectasia, 385
Carcinoid tumors, 148
Cardia, 340–1
Cardiac CT
  applications of, 107–10
  strengths and limitations of, 111
Cardiac imaging, 41–41
  cardiac CT, 107–10, 111
  cardiac MRI, 110–11
  common conditions, 439–41
  coronary calcium scoring, 107, 108, 110
  coronary CTA, 107–10
  radiotracers and protocols, 436–9
  time for, 436
  vascular MRA, 112–13

Cardiac MRI, 110
  indications for, 110
  strengths and limitations of, 111
  technique, 110–11
Cardiomyopathy, 441
Cardiothoracic ratio, 295
Carotid angiograms, 415
Carotid artery
  ultrasound, 289
Cartilage, 221
Cavernous angioma, 385
Cavitary masses, in lungs, 98
Cecal volvulus, 133, 136, 357
Central nervous system, 447
Central vascular access, 459
Central venous catheters, 53
Cerebral angiograms, 415
Cerebral metastases, 397
Cerebral perfusion tracers, 27, 447
Cerebritis, 399
Cerebrovascular disease, 38
Chagas disease, 347
Chest CT, 77–107
  accessory series, 78
  algorithms, 78
  contrast-enhanced, 77
  disease patterns
    abnormal air on, 81
    lung abnormalities, 82–6
    mediastinal abnormalities, 87–8
  non-enhanced, 77–8
  normal anatomy, 79
  pericardial abnormalities, 90–1
  pitfalls and problems of, 81
  pleural abnormalities, 89–90
  search strategies, 79, 80–1
  vascular abnormalities, 88–9
  windows, 78
Chest pain, 32–3
  acute cardiac-type, 33
  aortic dissection for, 32
  chronic cardiac-type, 33
  pulmonary embolus, 32–3
Chest radiographs, in neonates, 295–9
  congenital thoracic abnormalities, 299
  normal film, 295–6
  pneumothorax, 296–7
  pulmonary interstitial emphysema, 297

Chest radiographs, in neonates (Cont'd)
surfactant deficiency, 298
transient tachypnea of the newborn, 298
Chest tubes, 53
Chest x-ray (CXR), 52–5
abnormal air on, 68–72
initial quality check, 52
older children, 306
older infants, 306
pulmonary emboli, 29
search patterns, 52–5
 airway, 53
 bones, 54
 diaphragm, 53
 heart, 53–4
 hila, 53
 lines and tubes, 52, 53
 lungs, 53
 mediastinum, 53
 pleura, 53
 soft tissues, 55
solitary pulmonary nodule on, 33
traumatic aortic injury, 113
typical bacterial pneumonia, 96
upright, for, pneumoperitoneum, 120
Child abuse, 39, 324
diagnosis of, 152
imaging of, 325–6
 fractures, dating, 325
 head CT, 326
 head MRI, 326
 radiographic skeletal survey, 325
 radionuclide bone scan, 325
pathognomonic findings of, 326–7
 musculoskeletal, 327
 neurological, 326
reporting, 324
timing of, 324
Children, imaging in, 292–3
cooperation, 293
embarrassment, 293
fear, 293
older, 306–24
 airway, 308–9
 asthma, 306
 bronchiolitis, 306
 chest, 306–7
 croup, 308
 developmental dysplasia of the hip, 321
 epiglottitis, 308–9, 328

foreign body aspiration, 307
fractures. See Fractures, in infants/children
gastroesophageal reflux, 310
hypertrophic pyloric stenosis, 310–11
intussusception, 313–14
Legg-Calve-Perthes disease, 323
malrotation, 311–12, 328
normal CXR, 306
round pneumonia, 307
slipped capital femoral epiphysis, 317–19
tracheoesophageal fistula, 309
transient synovitis of the hip, 323
vesicoureteral reflux, 314–15
radiation exposure in, 292–3
size and age, 292
Cholecystitis
acute, 442–3
chronic, 443
Cholecystostomy, 468
Choledocholithiasis, 172, 173
Cholelisthiasis, 128, 253, 254
acute, 254
chronic, 254
Chondrosarcoma, 213
Chorionicity, 273–4
Cimetidine
for anaphylaxis, 21
for urticaria, 21
Cirrhosis, 166
Cisterns, 371
Claustrophobia patients, MRI scanning for, 26
Clavicular fractures, 228
Closed fracture, 202
Cobblestoning, 135
Coils, magnetic resonance imaging of, 11
Colitis, 145, 356
Collateral ligaments, 223
Colon
cancer, 345, 355
micro-colon, 304
normal sized, 304
obstruction, 132
small left. See Meconium plug syndrome
unused, 304
wall thickening in, 123
Colonic aganglionosis, 304

Colonic anatomy on lower GI fluoroscopic studies, 353–4
Colonic inertia. See Meconium plug syndrome
Colonic strictures, 355
Colonic volvulus, diagnosis of, 181
Color Doppler ultrasound, 243, 288, 490
Combined swallow, 338, 340
Comminuted fracture, 202
Common bile duct (CBD), size of, 257
Compound fracture, 202
Computed tomography (CT), 6
of abdomen/pelvic, 136–51
 acquisition and reconstruction of, 136–7
 bowel, 142
 conditions evaluated with, 154–78
 disease patterns, 142–51
 lymph nodes, 142
 mesentery, 142
 normal anatomy on, 140
 peritoneal compartment, 142
 phases of, 137–8
 pitfalls of, 142
 protocols of, 137–8
 retroperitoneal compartment, 142
 search strategies, 141
 solid organs, 141
 timings of, 137–8
abdominal aortic dissection, 165–6
acquisition of images in, 6
adenoma, 169
adrenal masses, 176, 177
ankle injuries, 227
appendicitis, 29
atypical bacterial pneumonia, 96
diverticulitis, 162
dose, reduction of, 24
elbow, 233
femoral neck fracture, 219
guiding interventional procedures, 451
hand, 234
head, 326, 370–2
 brain perfusion, 370
 CT angiography, 370
 head CT, 370, 371–2

image acquisition, 370
neck CT, 370
normal anatomy, 371
orbits, face, temporal bones, sinuses, 370
spine CT, 370
hepatocellular carcinoma, 170–1
Hounsfield Units, 7
hydronephrosis, 174
image display, 7
interpretation in oncology patients, 151
intraluminal agents indications, 18
of knee, 225
of labral injuries, 230
motion, 14–15
multidetector, 8
musculoskeletal, 191–5
  image acquisition, 191–2
  pitfalls and problems of, 193–4
  reading, 194–5
  timing of, 192, 193
pancreatic masses, 171
physical properties, 6
pregnant patients, 27
protocols, 9–10
pulmonary edema, 94
pulmonary emboli, 29, 107
reformatting techniques, 8
renal calculi, 29
renal cell carcinoma, 176
renal cysts, 175–6
renal masses, 175
risks of, 22
role in musculoskeletal masses, 213–14
signal-to-noise ratio, 14
trauma, 30
traumatic aortic injury, 113
typical bacterial pneumonia, 95–6
urolithiasis, 173
wrist, 234
Computer assisted detection (CAD), 478
Congenital abnormalities, 172
  major, 275
  minor, 275
Congenital diaphragmatic hernia (CDH), 299
Congenital thoracic abnormalities, 299
Consolidation, 55
  distinguished from pleural effusions, 73
Contrast, 16–19

administration, risks associated with, 22
allergies, 2, 20–1
  reactions of, 21
  risk factors for, 20
  pretreatment protocols for, 21
  prevention of, 21
  treatment for, 21
computed tomography, 6
enhancement, 8
enema, 351–2
  contraindications to, 352
-enhanced chest CT, intravenous, 77
enhancement, 12, 153
extravasation/ infiltration, 21, 22
gadolinium-based contrast agents, 17
intraluminal agents, 18
intravenous iodinated, 16–17
magnetic resonance angiography with, 14
magnetic resonance angiography without, 13–14
uses of, 20
Contrast induced nephropathy (CIN), 16
  alternative exam for, 16
  prevention of, 16–17
Contusion, 154
Conventional angiography, 374
COPD, 99–100
Corner fractures, 327
Coronary calcium scoring, 108
Coronary CTA
  applications of, 107–10
  findings of, 110
  indications for, 108
  performance of, 110
  radiation dose for, 110
  technique, 108
Costs for imaging, 30–1
Cranial-caudal (CC), 477–8
Crohn disease, 162, 163, 350–1
  CT enterography for, 162
  MR enterography for, 162
Crohns enteritis, 145
Cross sectional imaging, 191–9
Croup, 308
Cruciate ligaments, 224
Cryoablation, 473
CT angiography (CTA), 10

for aortic dissection, 104–66
for blunt traumatic aortic injury, 105–6
coronary, 107–10
CT Arthrography, 193
CT colonography, 139–40
  image interpretation, 140
  indications for, 139
  patient preparation, 140
CT cystography, for bladder injuries, 159
CT enterography (CTE), 137, 138
  for Crohn disease, 162
CT urography, 139
Curved maximum intensity projection reformats, CTA, 10
Curved planar reformats, CT, 8
Cystic renal cell carcinoma, 176
Cystogram, 360–1, 363
Cysts, 247
  breast, 497–501
    ductal carcinoma in situ (DCIS), 498
    magnetic resonance imaging, 497
    mammography, 497
    ultrasound, 497
  musculoskeletal ultrasound for, 198
  ovarian, 264
  renal, 259
Cytotoxic edema, 377

D

Decubitus abdomen
  pneumoperitoneum in, 120
  radiograph findings of, 116
Degenerative disc disease, 406
Degenerative joint disease (DJD). *See* Osteoarthritis
Dementia, imaging of, 38
Dens fracture, 411
Detectors, in x-rays, 3
Developmental dysplasia of the hip (DDH), 321
  clinical presentation of, 321
  diagnosis of, 321
  risk factors of, 321
Device screening, 26
Dialysis fistulas, angiography of, 462–3

INDEX

Diaphragm, 53
Diazepam, for seizures, 21
Diet, interventional procedures and, 451–2
Digital Imaging and Communications in Medicine (DICOM), 15
Digits, musculoskeletal radiograph of, 187
Dilated bowel, air in, 124
Diphenhydramine
  for anaphylaxis, 21
  for contrast allergies, 21
  for urticaria, 21
Disc bulge, 407
Disc extrusion, 407
Disc herniation, 406–7
Dislocation
  internal derangements in, 206
  shoulder, 228–9
Disofenin (DISIDA), 441–2
Displacement fracture, 202
Dissection, 455
Distal femoral fractures, 223
Distal humeral fractures, 231
  supracondylar, 320
Distal radial fractures, 233–4
  buckle/torus, 321
Distal tibial fracture, 193
Distraction fracture, 202
Diverticulitis, 161–2, 356
  acute, with peri-diverticular abscess, 147
  computed tomography for, 162
Diverticulosis, 356
Dobhoff tube-DHT. See Feeding tubes
Doppler ultrasound, 243–4
  color, 243, 288, 490
  power, 243
  pulsed wave, 244, 490
  umbilical artery, 279
Double contrast barium enema, 353
Drainage catheters, 120
Drain/pigtail catheter placement, 459
Drains, aspirations, and tube placement, 471–2
  abscess drainage, 471
  chest tube, 472
  paracentesis, 471
  thoracentesis, 471
Ductal carcinoma in situ (DCIS), 498
  magnetic resonance imaging for, 498–9
  mammography, 498
  ultrasound, 498
Duodenal cancer, 350
Duodenal ulcers, 348–9
Duodenum, 341

E

Echogenicity, 244–5
Ectopic pregnancy, 272–3
Edema, 376–7
  cytotoxic edema, 377
  vasogenic edema, 376–7
Elbow, 230–3
  computed tomography for, 233
  epicondylitis, 232–3
  fractures, 231
  joint effusions in, 231
  magnetic resonance imaging for, 233
  radiographic findings of, 231
Embolization, 458
Emission versus transmission scanning, 420
Emphysema, 99–100
  warning, 100
Emphysematous cholecystitis, diagnosis of, 181
Emphysematous pyelonephritis, diagnosis of, 182
Empyema, 75
Enchondroma, 200
Endocrine imaging, 432–6
  common conditions, 434–5
  therapeutic uses of, 435–6
  time for, 432
  radiotracers and protocols, 432–4
Endoleak classification, 165
Endometrial thickening, 267–8
  benign causes of, 268
  malignant causes of, 268
  postmenopausal endometrium, normal, 267–8
  premenopausal endometrium, normal, 267
Endometriosis, 265–6
Endoscopy, 352
Endotracheal tubes (ETT), 53, 294
Entire lung atelectasis, 62–4
Epicondylitis, 232–3
Epididymis, 282
Epididymitis, 283
Epidural hematoma (EDH), 392
Epiglottitis, 308–9
  diagnosis of, 328
Epinephrine
  for anaphylaxis, 21
  for bronchospasm, 21
Erosions, radiographic evaluation of, 207
Esophageal strictures
  benign causes of, 345
  malignant causes of, 346
Esophagectomy with gastric pull up, 343
Esophagitis, 346
Esophagram, 340
Esophagus, 340
  motility disorders of, 336–7
Essentials of radiology, 1–40
  imaging modalities, 2–15
  requisition, 1–2
Expiratory studies, of chest radiographs, 44
Extracellular contrast agents, 17
Extrahepatic biliary ductal dilatation, 257
Extra-luminal air, 142–3
  diagnosis of, 181
Extraperitoneal space, normal CT anatomy on, 140
Extrapulmonary, calcification in, 77
Extravasation, active, 155, 156
Extremity
  arteriography, 459–62
  anatomy and terminology, 460
  common conditions, 460–2
  technique, 459–60

F

F-18 FDG PET, 423–6, 439, 447
  for advanced breast cancers, 496
  glucose metabolism PET scan, 436
Facial trauma, 402–3
  medial orbital wall fractures, 402
  orbital floor fractures, 402–3
  zygomaticomaxillary complex fracture (ZMC), 403

Falciform ligament, 120–1
FAST (Focused Assessment with Sonography in Trauma) scan, 30, 256
Fat, 209–10
  saturation, 12, 152
  suppression techniques, 152
Fatigue fracture, 203
Fatty liver, 255
Feeding tubes, 53, 120, 367
Femoral neck fractures, 217–18
Femoral vascular catheters, 120
Fetal anomalies, 281
Fibroadenomas, 501
  magnetic resonance imaging, 501
  mammography, 501
  ultrasound, 501
Filling defects on fluoroscopy, 335
Films, 4–6
  comparison of, 482
  intradepartmental films, radiography of, 4–6
  plain. See Radiography
  portable, 4–6, 14
  supine-supine, 44
First trimester pregnancy, 269–71
  aneuploidy screening, 271
  dating, 270
  early OB ultrasound, anatomy on, 270–1
  intrauterine pregnancy, diagnosing, 270
  ultrasound imaging, timing of, 269–70
Fluid, 146, 246
  collections, 154
  extraperitoneal, 146
  intraperitoneal, 146
  retroperitoneal, 146
Fluoroscopic-guided lumbar puncture, 414
Fluoroscopy
  barium, 331
  contrast choices, 331–2
  disease patterns, 333–7
  display, 330
  double contrast technique, 332
  versus endoscopy of GI tract, 332–3
  extrinsic masses, 333–5
  filling defects on, 335
  fold thickening, 337
    characterizing, 337
    differential diagnosis, 337

for guiding interventional procedures, 450
GU tract. See GU tract fluoroscopy
intraluminal agents indications, 18
leaks, 336
lesion localization, 333–5
lower GI tract. See Lower GI tract fluoroscopy
motility disorders, 336–7
  esophagus, 336–7
  small bowel, 337
  stomach, 337
mucosal abnormalities, 333
obstruction, 335–6
pregnant patients, 27
radiation risk, 330–1
single contrast technique, 332
strictures, 335–6
submucosal masses, 333
technology, 330–3
tube studies, 367–8
T-tube cholangiogram, 367–8
upper GI tract. See Upper GI tract fluoroscopy
water soluble contrast, 331–2
Focal ileus, 133
Focal nodular hyperplasia (FNH), 169
Fold thickening, 337
  characterizing, 337
  differential diagnosis, 337
Foot, musculoskeletal radiograph of, 187
Football sign, 120–1
Forearm, musculoskeletal radiograph of, 187
Foreign bodies, 210
  aspiration diagnosis of, 113
  infants, 307
  neonates, 307
  finding, 286
Fractures, 155, 200, 201–3
  angulation, 202
  ankle, 226
  apophyses, 317
  bone scanning for, 429
  bucket handle, 327
  buckle, 317
  closed, 202
  comminuted, 202
  compound, 202
  corner, 327
  dating, 325
  displacement, 202

distal humeral supracondylar, 320
distal radius, buckle/torus fracture of, 321
distraction, 202
elbow, 231
fatigue, 203
femoral neck, 217–18
greenstick, 202, 316
hip, 217
impacted, 202
incomplete, 316
in infants/children, 315–17
insufficiency, 37, 203
intra-articular, 202
involving physis, 202
knee, 223
maisonneuve, 226
multiple, 327
open, 202
override, 202
pathologic, 203
pelvic ring, 216–17
radial head dislocation, 321
reduction of, 204
rib, 327
rotation, 202
Salter-Harris classification of, 315
secondary ossification centers, avulsion of, 317
shoulder, 227–8
simple, 202
skull fracture, unexplained, 326
stress, 203
toddlers, 319–20
torus, 317
Free intraperitoneal air, 143
Functional MRI, 11
Fundoplication, 343
Fundus, 340–1

G

Gadolinium-based contrast agents (GBCA), 17
  extracellular agents, 17
  hepatobiliary specific MRI agents, 17
  risks, 17–18
Galactography (ductography), 505
Gallbladder, anatomy of, 251
Gallium-67, 447
Gamma cameras, 421
Gas, 19
  abdominal radiography for, 119

INDEX

Gasless abdomen, 129
Gastric adenocarcinoma, 349
Gastric banding, 343
Gastric bypass, 343
Gastric emptying studies, 442
Gastric lymphoma, 350
Gastric metastatic disease, 350
Gastric motility, 337
Gastric tubes (G tube), 367
Gastric ulcers, 348–9
 benign ulcers, 348
 ulcerating malignancy, 348
Gastric volvulus, 135, 348
Gastroesophageal reflux (GER), 310
Gastroesophageal reflux (GERD), 348
Gastrograffin, 133, 331
Gastrointestinal bleeding, 444
Gastrointestinal imaging, 441–4
 common conditions, 442–4
 radiotracers and protocols, 441–2
 time for, 441
Gastrointestinal interventions, 466
Gastrointestinal perforations, patterns of, 336
Gastrointestinal stromal tumors (GIST), 350
Gastrointestinal tract, contrast examinations of, 332
 double contrast technique, 332
 single contrast technique, 332
Gastro-jejunostomy tube (GJ tube), 367
Gastrostomy and gastrojejunostomy tubes, 466
Gated blood pool scans, 436
Glenohumeral (GH) joint, dislocations/subluxations in, 228–9
Glioblastoma multiforme, 396
Glucagon, for anaphylaxis, 21
Gradient recalled echo (GRE), 372–3
Grave disease, 434
Gray-scale imaging, 287

Greenstick fracture, 202, 316
Ground glass opacity, 55
Growth disorders, 278
 LGA fetus, 278
 SGA fetus, 278
GU interventions, 467–8
 percutaneous nephrostomy (PCN), 467
 ureteral stents, 467–8
GU perforations, patterns of, 336
GU tract fluoroscopy
 bladder masses, 364–6
 bladder rupture, 366
 cystogram, 360–1, 363
 hydronephrosis, 364
 hysterosalpingogram, 362–3
 intravenous pyelogram, 361–2, 363
 retrograde urethrogram, 361, 363
 VCUG, 363
 voiding cystourethrogram, 360
 renal masses, 364
 vesicoureteral reflux (VUR), 364

H

Hand, 233–4
 computed tomography for, 234
 fractures, 233–4
 magnetic resonance imaging for, 234
 musculoskeletal radiograph of, 187
 radiographic findings of, 233
Hangman's fracture, 410
Headache, imaging of, 37
Head-and-neck lymph-node-classification system, 403
Head and neck radiology, 401
Head CT, 370, 371–2
Head trauma, 391–5
Heart, 53–4
Hemangioma, 168
Hemarthroplasty, 235
Hemoperitoneum, 146, 154, 155
Hemorrhage, 154
Hepatobiliary scans, 441–2
Hepatobiliary specific MRI agents, 17

Hepatocellular carcinoma, 170–1
 computed tomography for, 170–1
 magnetic resonance imaging for, 170–1
Hepatomegaly, abdominal radiography for, 128
Hepatosplenomegaly, 129
Hernias, inguinal, 284
Herniation
 tonsillar, 380
 transtentorial, 379
 uncal, 379–80
Heterotopic bone, 210
Heterotopic ossification, 211
Hibernating myocardium, 439
Hila, 53
Hip
 developmental dysplasia of, 321
 fractures, 215, 217
 computed tomography for, 219
 magnetic resonance imaging for, 219
 transient synovitis of, 323
Hirschprung disease, 304
HOCM agents, 331
Hollow viscera, anatomy of, 116–17
Hounsfield Units (HU), 7
Humeral fractures, 227–8
Hyaline membrane disease (HMD). See Surfactant deficiency
Hyaluronidase injection, for contrast extravasation/ infiltration, 22
Hybrid scanners, 422
Hydramnios, 280–1
Hydroceles, 283
Hydronephrosis, 173–4, 364
 causes of, 174
 computed tomography for, 174
 pitfalls of, 174
 right, 175
 ultrasound imaging of, 261
Hydropneumothorax, 74
Hydrosalpinx, 268
Hypertrophic pyloric stenosis (HPS), 310–11
Hypervascular masses, 167
 enhancement pattern of, 167
Hypoechoic masses, 248
 noncalcified, 248
Hypoperfusion shock bowel complex, 160

INDEX

Hypotension, treatment for, 21
Hypovascular masses, 166
  enhancement pattern of, 167
  liver, 147–8
Hysterosalpingogram (HSG), 362–3
Hysterosonography, 262

I

I-123, 420
  endocrine imaging, 433
I-131
  endocrine imaging, 433
  therapeutic uses of, 435–6
Ileum, 341
Ileus, 132–3
  focal, 133
Image display, computed tomography, 7
  standard windows, 7
  window level, 7
  window width, 7
Image guidance
  methods of, 450–1
  computed tomography, 451
  fluoroscopy, 450
  magnetic resonance imaging, 451
  ultrasound, 450
  use of, 450
Image-guided tumor ablations, 472–3
Imaging
  algorithms, 31–40
  factors affecting quality of, 14–15
  risks of, 22–6
Impacted fracture, 202
Implanted metallic structures, safety of, 25
In-111 labeled white blood cells, 447
Incomplete fractures, 316
Indicatins for imaging, 30
Indium-111 labeled pentetreotide, 426
Infants
  imaging in, 306–24
  airway, 308–9
  asthma, 306
  bronchiolitis, 306
  chest, 306–7
  croup, 308
  developmental dysplasia of the hip, 321
  epiglottitis, 308–9
  foreign body aspiration, 307
  fractures. See Fractures, in infants/children
  gastroesophageal reflux, 310
  hypertrophic pyloric stenosis, 310–11
  intussusception, 313–14
  Legg-Calve-Perthes disease, 323
  lines and tubes, 294
  malrotation, 311–12
  normal CXR, 306
  round pneumonia, 307
  slipped capital femoral epiphysis, 317–19
  tracheoesophageal fistula, 309
  transient synovitis of the hip, 323
  vesicoureteral reflux, 293, 314–15
  vomiting, 39–40
Infection, 94–399
  imaging, 447
  musculoskeletal MRI for, 196
  musculoskeletal ultrasound for, 198
Infertility, 269
Inflammation, 143–4, 153, 206, 398–9
  bowel wall, 143
  mesenteric, 143
  peribronchial, 59–60
  retroperitoneal, 143
  radiological findings of, 206
  solid organ, 144
Inflammatory
  arthritis, 208–9
  radiographic findings of, 209
  types of, 208–9
Inguinal hernias, 284
Inspiratory studies, of chest radiographs, 44
Insufficiency fractures, 37, 203
Internal
  derangements, 204–6
  dislocation, 206
  magnetic resonance imaging, 205–6
  musculoskeletal MRI for, 196, 221
  radiography, 204
  subluxation, 206
  ultrasound, 206
Interstitial abnormalities, chest CT for, 84
Interstitial patterns, 58–60
  bronchovascular markings, 59–60
  differential diagnosis of, 58–60
  Kerley lines, 60
Interventional radiology, 449–74
  aneurysms, 454
  angiography, 456–7
  aspiration, biopsy and drainage, 470–2
  biliary interventions, 468–9
  central vascular access, 459
  dialysis fistulas, angiography of, 462–3
  diet, 451–2
  dissection, 455
  drain/pigtail catheter placement, 459
  embolization, 458
  extremity arteriography, 459–62
  general techniques of, 456–9
  GI interventions, 466
  GU interventions, 467–8
  image guidance, use of, 450
  image-guided tumor ablations, 472–3
  imaging guidance methods, 450–1
  leak/extravasation, 455
  occlusion, 453
  patient preparation for, 451–2
  percutaneous stent placement, 457–8
  percutaneous transluminal angioplasty, 457
  pre-procedure considerations, 452
  pre-procedure labs, 452
  pre-procedure medications, 452
  pseudoaneurysms, 454
  renal/mesenteric angiography, 463–5
  Seldinger technique, 456
  stenoses, 454
  thrombolysis, 458–9
  vascular access, 473
  vascular disease, patterns of, 452–5
  venography, 462
Intestinal
  malrotation, 311–12
Intra-aortic balloon pump, 53
Intra-articular fracture, 202

I

Intracranial hemorrhage (ICH), in neonates, 305
Intradepartmental films, radiography of, 4–6
Intrahepatic biliary ductal dilatation, 257
Intraluminal agents, 18
  contraindications of, 20
  indications of, 18
  risks of, 20
  types of, 18–19
Intraperitoneal compartment, anatomy of, 117
Intravenous iodinated contrast, 16–17
  administration contraindications to, 17
  screening for CRI before, 16
  risk, 16
Intravenous pyelogram (IVP), 361–2, 363
  for renal calculi, 29
Intussusception, 313–14
  diagnosis of, 313–14
  etiology of, 313
Iodine-131 scanning, 423, 426
Islet cell tumors, 172

J

Jaundice, management of, 35–6
Jefferson's fracture, 410
Jejunostomy tubes (J tube), 367
Jejunum, 341
Joints, 236–7
  arthrography, 238
  aspiration, 237
  biopsies, 238
  effusions, 206, 209
    in elbow, 231, 232
    hip, 323
    radiological findings of, 209
  injection-pain study, 237
  injections, 238
  risks of, 236
  soft tissue aspirations, 238
  spaces
    extremity/joint radiograph of, 186
    radiographic evaluation of, 207
Jumped facets, 410

K

Kerley lines, 60
  etiology of, 60

Kidney
  anatomy of, 251
  injuries, 158
    fracture, 158
    grading of, 158
Knee, 221–5
  computed tomography for, 225
  fractures, 223
  internal derangement, 223–5
  joint effusion, 222
    radiographic findings of, 222
  magnetic resonance imaging for, 225
  osteoarthritis, 223
  radiographic findings of, 221–2

L

Labral injuries, 230
  computed tomography for, 230
  magnetic resonance imaging for, 230
Labral tears, 221
Laceration, liver, 154, 156
Ladd bands, 312
Large intestine, air in, 117
Laryngeal edema, treatment for, 21
Lateral chest radiographs, 42
Lateral collateral ligament complex (LCLC), 223
Lateral decubitus chest radiographs, 42
Leak/extravasation, 455
Left lower lobe, lung atelectasis in, 62
Left upper lobe, lung atelectasis in, 62
Legg-Calve-Perthes disease, 323
Leiomyomas, 179
  magnetic resonance imaging for, 179
  ultrasonography for, 179
Leptomeninges, 389
Lesions
  internal characteristics of, 200–1
  margins of, 200
LGA fetus, growth disorders in, 278
Ligaments, 223–4
  collateral, 223
  cruciate, 224
Linear/subsegmental atelectasis, 64

Lines and tubes, 52, 53
  for abdominal radiographs, 120
  malpositioned, diagnosis of, 114
  in neonates/infants, 294
Linitis plastica, 350
Lipohemarthrosis, 222
Liver
  anatomy of, 251
  hemangioma, 256
  injuries, grading of, 157
  laceration, 154, 156
  lesions, imaging characteristics of, 171
  masses, 166–71
    computed tomography for, 168
    enhancement pattern of, 167
    hypervascular masses, 167
    hypovascular masses, 166
    magnetic resonance angiography for, 168
    ultrasound imaging of, 256
  trauma in, 155–7
Lobar atelectasis/collapse, patterns of, 61–4
  entire lung atelectasis, 62–4
  left lower lobe, 62
  left upper lobe, 62
  linear/subsegmental atelectasis, 64
  right lower lobe, 61–2
  right middle lobe, 61
  right upper lobe, 61
Loculated effusions, 74
Lordotic chest radiographs, 44
Low anterior resection of the rectum (LAR), 354
Lower GI tract fluoroscopy, 351–60
  abdominoperineal resection, 354
  cecal volvulus, 357
  colitis, 356
  colon cancer, 345
    screening, 355
  colonic anatomy on, 353–4
  colonic strictures, 355
  contrast enema, 351–2
    contraindications to, 352
  diverticular disease, 356
  diverticulitis, 356
  diverticulosis, 356

INDEX

double contrast barium enema, 353
double contrast enemas, 352–3
endoscopy, 352
low anterior resection of the rectum (LAR), 354
partial colectomy, 353–4
polypoid lesions, 359
sigmoid volvulus, 357
single contrast, 353
single contrast barium enema, 353
volvulus, 356–7
water soluble enema, 353
Low lung volumes
causes of, 44
production of, 44
Luminal dilatation, 249
Lungs, 52
abnormalities, chest CT for, 82–6
abscess, 98
biopsy, 471
calcification in, 76
cancer, 102–4
imaging findings of, 102
primary, 65
screening of, 104
staging of, 103–4
subtypes of, 102
cavitatory masses in, 98
chest radiograph of, 296
imaging of, 444–6
adiotracers and protocols, 445
common conditions, 445–6
time for, 444
masses/nodules, 64–6, 85
characteristics of, 85
on CT, management of, 86
defined, 85
differential diagnosis of, 65
management of, 66
metastases, 65
primary lung cancer, 65
worrisome features, 65
Lymphadenitis, 148
Lymphadenopathy, 148, 403
sites of, 88
Lymph nodes, 87–8
computed tomography of, 149–50
locations of, 150
enlarged, 149–50
neoplastic, 150
normal, 149, 151
appearance of, 87

normal CT anatomy on, 142
pathologic, features of, 150
Lymphoma, 148

M

Magnetic resonance angiography (MRA), 13, 153
for abdominal aortic dissection, 166
with contrast, 14
without contrast, 13–14
vascular, 112–13
Magnetic resonance imaging (MRI), 10, 372–496
of abdomen/pelvic, 151–4
breathing, dealing with, 151–2
conditions evaluated with, 154–78
disease patterns on, 153–4
motion artifact, 151–3
normal structures, look of, 153
protocols of, 152–3
pulse sequences in, 152
technical considerations for, 152–3
of acute abdomen
in pregnant women, 178–9
in young patient, 178–9
acquisition of images in, 10–11
adenoma, 169
adenomyosis, 179
adrenal masses, 176
ankle injuries, 227
appendicitis, 28
avascular necrosis, 221
breast, 493–6
computer assisted analysis, 495–6
cysts, 497
ductal carcinoma in situ (DCIS), 498–9
fibroadenomas, 501
invasive carcinomas, 500
need for, 493–5
patterns of disease, 495–6
procedure, 493
cardiac, 110–11
claustrophobia patients, 26
coils, 11
contrast enhancement, 12
elbow, 233

epicondylitis, 233
fat saturation, 12
femoral neck fracture, 219
functional MRI, 11
-guided biopsy, 504
for guiding interventional procedures, 451
hand, 234
head, 326
hepatocellular carcinoma, 170–1
image acquisition, 372–4
implanted metallic structures, safety of, 25
internal derangements in, 205–6
intraluminal agents indications, 18
of knee, 225
of labral injuries, 230
leiomyomas, 179
menisci, 224
motion, 14–15
musculoskeletal, 195–7
image acquisition, 195
pitfalls and problems of, 196–7
timing of, 195–6
obesity patients, 26
pancreatic masses, 171
patient inside, 25
pregnant patients, 26, 28
protocols, 12–14
pulse sequences, 12, 13
renal calculi, 29
renal cell carcinoma, 176
renal cysts, 175–6
renal masses, 175
risks of, 25
risk reduction of, 26
device screening, 26
patient screening, 26
surroundings, checking, 26
role in musculoskeletal masses, 214
rotator cuff injuries, 229
safety, 14
signal generation, 11
signal-to-noise ratio, 14
spectroscopy, 11
T1 and T2 relaxation, 10
3D acquisition & reformatting, 11
3T imaging, 11
tissue composition, 11
trauma, 30
wrist, 234
Magnification, in x-rays, 3
Maisonneuve fracture, 226

INDEX

Malpositioned tubes and lines, diagnosis of, 114
Mammographic Quality Standards Act (MQSA) 1992, 488–9
Mammography, breast, 476–89
 architectural distortion, 486
 associated findings that can be signs of malignancy, 487
 asymmetries, 487
 calcification patterns, 484–5
 comparison films, 482
 cysts, 497
 diagnostic, 480
 ductal carcinoma in situ, 498
 fibroadenomas, 501
 finding location, communicating, 487–8
 image acquisition, 476–8
 invasive carcinomas, 499
 masses, 483
 patterns of disease on, 482–5
 radiation to breast, 476
 reports, 488–9
 screening, 478–80
Marrow abnormalities, musculoskeletal MRI for, 196
Marrow conversion, 214
Marrow infiltration, by malignancy/ infection, 214
Masses, 248
 abdominal radiography for, 119, 128
 adrenal, 176–8
 anechoic, 248
 bone within, 210
 calcium within, 210
 hypoechoic, 248
 noncalcified, 248
 liver, 166–71
  computed tomography for, 168
  enhancement pattern of, 167
  hypervascular masses, 167
  hypovascular masses, 166
  magnetic resonance imaging for, 168
  ultrasound imaging of, 256
 in lung, 64–6
 cavitatory, 98
 characteristics of, 85
 on CT, management of, 86
 defined, 85
 differential diagnosis of, 65
 management of, 66
 metastases, 65
 primary lung cancer, 65
 worrisome features, 65
 mediastinal, 66–8, 87
  anterior mediastinal masses, 66–7
  middle mediastinum, 67
  posterior mediastinum, 68
 mesenteric, 148
 musculoskeletal, 212–14
  aggressive features of, 212
  benign features of, 212
  computed tomography, role of, 213–14
  interpretation of, 212
  magnetic resonance imaging, role of, 214
  ultrasound for, 198
 pancreatic, 171
  computed tomography for, 171
  enhancement pattern of, 171
  islet cell tumors, 172
  magnetic resonance imaging for, 171
  pancreatic adenocarcinoma, 171–2
  protocols and techniques for, 171
 renal, 175–6, 260
 solid organ, 147–8
 solid ovarian, 264
 testicular, 284
Maximum intensity projection (MIP), computed tomography, 8
Mebrofenin, 441–2
Meconium plug syndrome, 304
Medial collateral ligament (MCL), 223
Medial-lateral oblique (MLO), 477–8
Mediastinal abnormalities, chest CT for, 87–8
 lymph nodes, 87–8
 masses, 87
Mediastinal masses, 66–8, 87
 anterior mediastinal masses, 66–7
 middle mediastinum, 67
 posterior mediastinum, 68
Mediastinum, 53
 calcification in, 76
 chest radiograph of, 295
 middle, 67
Meningeal disease, 389
Meningioma, 397
Meningitis, 398–9
Menisci
 internal derangement in, 224
 magnetic resonance imaging for, 224
Mesenteric air, 143
Mesenteric bowel infarction, diagnosis of, 181
Mesenteric inflammaion, 143
Mesenteric ischemia, diagnosis of, 181
Mesenteric masses, computed tomography of, 148
Mesenteroaxial volvulus, 348
Mesentery
 normal CT anatomy on, 142
 trauma in, 159–60
Metastases, 65
 adrenal, 178
 cerebral, 397
 characteristics of, 65
 imaging characteristics of, 171
Methylcellulose, 19
Methylprednisolone, for contrast allergies, 21
Meullerian duct anomalies, 179
MIBG, 423
Micro-colon, 304
Middle mediastinum, 67
Midgut volvulus, 311–12
Mineralization, radiographic evaluation of, 207
Minimum intensity projection (MinIP), computed tomography, 8
M mode ultrasound, 242
Modalities, imaging, 2–15
Modified swallow, 340
Motility, 336–7
 disorders, 336–7
 esophagus, 336–7
 small bowel, 337
 stomach, 337
Motion, 14–15
MR arthrogram, for rotator cuff injuries, 230

INDEX

MR cholangiopancreatography (MRCP), 153
  indications for, 153
  protocols for, 153
  techniques, 153
MR enterography (MRE), 153
  for Crohn disease, 162
Mucosal defects, 333
Multidetector computed tomography (MDCT), 8, 9–10
Multiplanar reformats (MPR), computed tomography, 8, 9
Multiple pregnancies, 273–4
  ultrasound imaging for, 281
Multiple sclerosis, 399
Musculoskeletal imaging, 183–238
  computed tomography, 191–5
    image acquisition, 191–2
    pitfalls and problems of, 193–4
    reading, 194–5
    timing of, 192, 193
  disease patterns, 199–214
  magnetic resonance imaging, 195–7
    image acquisition, 195
    pitfalls and problems of, 196–7
    timing of, 195–6
  normal anatomy, 184
  radiography. See Radiography, musculoskeletal
  ultrasound, 197–9
    image acquisition, 197
    pitfalls and problems of, 198–9
    timing of, 197–8
Mycobacterium tuberculosis, 97
  military, 97
  post-primary, 97
  primary, 97
Myelination, assessing, 374–5
Myelogram, 414
Myocardial infarction, 439–41
Myocardial ischemia, 439

N

N-acetyl cysteine, for contrast induced nephropathy, 16–17
Nasogastric tube (NGT), 120
National Lung Cancer Screening Trial (2011), 104
Neck CT, 370
Necrotizing enterocolitis (NFC), 302–3
Needle/wire localizations (NLOC), 502
Negative agents, 19
Negative intraluminal agents, 19
Neonatal contrast enemas, 304
Neonatal UGI, 304
Neonates, imaging in, 293–305
  abdominal radiographs. See Abdominal radiographs, in neonates
  chest radiographs. See Chest radiographs, in neonates
  GI tract fluoroscopy, 303–4
  lines and tubes, 294
  neuroimaging, 305
  radiographic views, 293
Nephrogenic systemic fibrosis (NSF)
  GBCA, 18
  prevention strategies, 18
Nephroprotective agents, for contrast induced nephropathy, 16–17
Nervous system, 37–8
Neuroimaging, 369–417
  blood, 383–5
  carotid angiograms, 415
  cerebral angiograms, 415
  cerebral metastases, 397
  computed tomography, 370–2
    brain perfusion, 370
    computed tomography angiography, 370
    head CT, 370, 371–2
    image acquisition, 370
    neck CT, 370
    normal anatomy, 371
    orbits, face, temporal bones, sinuses, 370
    spine CT, 370
  conventional angiography, 374
  degenerative disc disease, 406
  diagnoses, 416
  disc herniation, 406–7
  edema, 376–7
  facial trauma, 402–3
  fluoroscopic guided lumbar puncture, 414
  head and neck radiology, 401
  head CT, pitfalls of, 400–1
  head trauma, 391–5
  herniation patterns, 377–80
  hydrocephalus and CSF dynamics, 382–3
  infection, 398–405, 412
  inflammation, 398–9
  lymphadenopathy, 403
  magnetic resonance imaging, 372–4
    image acquisition, 372–4
    pitfalls of, 400–1
  masses, 348, 377–408
  meningeal disease, 389
  midline shift, 377–80
  multiple sclerosis, 399
  myelogram, 414
  myelography, 408
  neonatal, 305
  normal aging, 374–5
  peripheral nerve-sheath tumors, 398
  primary brain tumors, 396–7
  seizure disorders, 399–400
  sinus disease, 401–2
  spine, 405–6
    anatomy on CT, 405
    anatomy on MRI, 405
    computed tomography, 405–6
    imaging test, 405–6
    magnetic resonance imaging, 406
    radiography, 405–6
  stroke/cerebral infarction, 389–91
  therapeutic intracranial procedures, 415–16
  trauma, 409–12
  vertebroplasty, 414–15
Neuropathies, musculoskeletal ultrasound for, 198
Nodules in lung, 64–6
  characteristics of, 85
  on CT, management of, 86
  defined, 85
  differential diagnosis of, 65
  management of, 66
  metastases, 65
  primary lung cancer, 65
  worrisome features, 65

INDEX

Non-accidental injury (NAI). See Child abuse
Non-enhanced chest CT (NECT), 77–8
 high resolution, 77–8
 low dose, 77–8
Non-small cell carcinoma, 102
Normal pressure hydrocephalus (NPH), 383
Normal sized colon, 304
Nuchal translucency screening, 271
Nuclear medicine, 419–48
 bone imaging, 426–30
  radiotracers and protocols, 427
  time for, 426–7
 cardiac imaging, 436–41
  common conditions, 439–41
  radiotracers and protocols, 436–9
  time for, 436
 central nervous system, 447
 endocrine imaging, 432–6
  common conditions, 434–5
  radiotracers and protocols, 432–4
  therapeutic uses of, 435–6
  time for, 432
 GI imaging, 441–4
  common conditions, 442–4
  radiotracers and protocols, 441–2
  time for, 441
 infection imaging, 447
 lung imaging, 444–6
  common conditions, 445–6
  time for, 444
 physiologic imaging, principles of, 420–2
  diagnosis versus therapy, 420
  radioisotopes and radiopharmaceuticals, 420
  reading nuclear medicine images, 422
 renal imaging, 430–1
 specific radiation precautions related to, 422–3
  nursing mothers, 423
 tumor imaging/PET scans, 423–6
Nuclear studies, pregnant patients, 28
Nursing mothers, radiation precautions, 423

O

Obesity patients, 15
 magnetic resonance imaging for, 26
Obstruction, 335–6
Occlusion, 453
 acute versus chronic, 453
 angiographic findings, 453
Octreotide, 423
Olecranon fracture, 231, 232
Oligohydramnios, 280
Omenatal metastasis, 150, 151
Oncology patients, CT scan interpretation in, 151
Open fracture, 202
Open reduction internal fixation (ORIF), 235
Opposed-phase imaging, 152
Oral/naso-gastric tubes, 53
Oral agents, for magnetic resonance imaging, 19–22
Orchitis, 283
Organ enlargement, 249
Organoaxial volvulus, 348
Organomegaly, abdominal radiography for, 128
Orthopedic hardware and fixation devices, radiography of, 235–6
 follow-up imaging, 236
 immediate post-operative imaging, 235
Osseous metastatic disease, 215
Osteoarthritis, 207–8, 219
 in hand, 234
 in hip, 219
 in knee, 223
 radiographic findings of, 208
 risk factors of, 207–8
 in wrist, 234
Osteoarthritis, 234
Osteolysis, 236
Osteomyelitis
 bone scanning for, 429–30
 computed tomography for, 192
 in diabetic patient foot, 36–7
Osteosarcoma, 213
Ovarian cysts, 264
 complex, 264
 simple, 264
Ovarian lesions, magnetic resonance imaging for, 179–80
 protocol and techniques for, 179–80
 findings of, 180
Ovarian torsion, 265
Ovaries, anatomy of, 262
Override fracture, 202
Overuse tendinosis. See Epicondylitis

P

Pacemakers, 25
 wire, 53
PA chest x-ray, risks of, 23
Pachymeninges, 389
Pancreas
 anatomy of, 252
 trauma in, 157
Pancreatic abnormalities, ultrasound imaging for, 258
Pancreatic adenocarcinoma, 171–2
Pancreatic contusion, 157
Pancreatic masses, 171
 computed tomography for, 171
 enhancement pattern of, 171
 islet cell tumors, 172
 magnetic resonance imaging for, 171
 pancreatic adenocarcinoma, 171–2
 protocols and techniques for, 171
Pancreaticoduo-denectomy, 343
Pancreatic pseudocyst, 164
Pancreatitis, 163
 complications of, 163
 computed tomography for, 163
Paraesophageal hernia, 347
Partial colectomy, 353–4
Pathologic fracture, 203
Patient's device safety, 26
Patient screening, 26
Pediatric patients, radiation risks in, 24
Pediatrics, 38–28
Pelvic fracture, 215
 computed tomography for, 219
 magnetic resonance imaging for, 219
 ring, 216–17

Pelvic pain, 34–5
Pelvis, ultrasound imaging of, 261–9
  common conditions, 264–8
  normal anatomy, 262
  prostate, 269
  protocols, 262
Percutaneous cholangiogram (PTC) and drainage, 468–9
Percutaneous core biopsy, 502–4
Percutaneous nephrostomy (PCN), 467
Percutaneous stent placement, 457–8
Percutaneous transluminal angioplasty (PTA), 457
Perforated appendicitis, 161
Perforation, diagnosis of, 181
Perfusion imaging, 437
Peribronchial cuffing due to edema, 91–4
Peribronchial inflammation, 59–60
Peribronchial thickening, 59–60
Pericardial abnormalities chest CT for, 90–1
  differential diagnosis of, 91
Pericardial calcification, chest CT for, 90–1
Pericardial effusions, 75
Pericardial fluid, 90
Pericardial thickening, chest CT for, 90
Periosteal reaction, 199–200, 202
Peripheral nerve-sheath tumors, 398
Peripheral vascular occlusive disease (PVOD), 460–1
Peripheral venous thrombosis, ultrasound imaging for, 286–8
Peritoneal cavity, normal CT anatomy on, 140
Peritoneal compartment, normal CT anatomy on, 142
Peritonsillar abscess, 404
PET (positron emission tomography) scanners, 422
Physiologic imaging, principles of, 420–2
  diagnosis versus therapy, 420
  images, acquiring, 420–1

radioisotopes and radiopharmaceuticals, 420
  reading nuclear medicine images, 422
Physis, fractures involving fracture, 202
Picture Archiving and Communication System (PACS), 15–16
Placenta, accessory lobes of, 279
Placental abruption, 279
Placental cord insertion, of umbilical cord, 279
Placental disorders, 278
  location, 278–9
  pitfalls, determining, 279
Plain films. See Radiography
Pleura, 53
Pleural abnormalities, chest CT for, 89–90
Pleural calcification, 76–7
  chest CT for, 90
Pleural effusions, chest CT for, 89
  distinguished from pleural consolidation/atelectasis, 73
  and pulmonary edema, 94
  supine radiographs, 73–4
  types of, 74–5
  upright radiographs, 72–3
Pleural masses, chest CT for, 90
Pleural thickening, chest CT for, 89
  differential diagnosis of, 89
Pneumatosis intestinalis, 121–2, 129
  portal venous gas, c
Pneumobilia, 122, 143
Pneumomediastinum, 71
  etiologies of, 71
  radiographic findings for, 71
Pneumonia, round, 307
Pneumopericardium, 72
  etiologies of, 72
Pneumoperitoneum, 120–302
  diagnosis of, 152–3
  decubitus abdomen, 120
  supine abdomen, 120–1
  upright CXR, 120
Pneumothorax, 68–297
  chest CT for, 89
  small, 68
  on supine images, 70
  tension, 70–1

  on upright images, 68
Polypoid lesions, 359
Popliteal vein thrombosis, 287
Portable films, radiography of, 4–6, 14
Positive intraluminal agents, 18–19
Posterior-anterior (PA) chest radiographs, 42
  technical considerations for, 42
Posterior cruciate ligament (PCL), 224
Posterior mediastinum, 68
Postmenopausal endometrium, normal, 267–8
Power Doppler ultrasound, 243
Prednisone, for contrast allergies, 21
Pregnancy(ies), 269
  anembryonic, 272
  ectopic, 272–3
  first trimester, 269–71
    aneuploidy screening, 271
    dating, 270
    early OB ultrasound, anatomy on, 270–1
    intrauterine pregnancy, diagnosing, 270
    ultrasound imaging, timing of, 269–70
  multiple, 273–4
  second trimester, 274–8
    aneuploidy screening, 275
    anomaly screening, 275
    biometric measurements, 275
    bleeding, 276
    normal anatomy, 276–8
    size/date discordance, 275
    ultrasound imaging, timing of, 274
  third trimester, 274–8
    aneuploidy screening, 275
    anomaly screening, 275
    biometric measurements, 275
    bleeding, 276
    normal anatomy, 276–8
    size/date discordance, 275
    ultrasound imaging, timing of, 274
  twin, 274

INDEX

Pregnant women, imaging in, 27–30
- acute abdomen in, MRI scanning of, 178–9
- safety of, 179
- computed tomography, 27
- fluoroscopy, 27
- general considerations, 27
- magnetic resonance imaging, 26, 28
- nuclear studies, 28
- radiography, 27
- risk to mother, 28
- ultrasound, 28

Premenopausal endometrium, normal, 267
Primary brain tumors, 396–7
Prospective Investigation of Pulmonary Embolism Diagnosis (PIOPED) criteria, 446
Prostate, ultrasound imaging of, 269
Prosthesis imaging, 193
Proximal fibular fractures, 223
Pseudopolyps, 135
Pseudotumor, 75
Pulmonary edema, 91–4
- cardiogenic pulmonary edema with cardiomegaly, causes of, 91
- computed tomography findings in, 94
- noncardiogenic, 91
- with normal heart size, causes of, 91
- signs of, 91–4

Pulmonary emboli (PE), 29, 106–446
- chest x-ray for, 29
- computed tomography for, 29, 107
- magnetic resonance angiography for, 113
- radiographic findings of, 106
- VQ scan for, 29

Pulmonary embolus, 32–3
Pulmonary hypertension, 59–60
Pulmonary interstitial emphysema (PIE), 297
Pulmonary venous flow, cephalization of, 91–4
Pulmonary venous hypertension, 59–60

Pulsed wave Doppler ultrasound, 244, 490
Pus, 146
Pylorus, 340–1

R

Radial head
- dislocation, 321
- fractures in, 231

Radiation
- dose, reduction of, 24–5
- during procedures, 25
- exposure, 330–1
- risks of, 22, 330–1

Radiofrequency ablation (RFA), 472
Radiographic skeletal survey, 325
Radiographs,
- abdominal, 116–35
- computed tomography. See Computed tomography, of abdomen/pelvic
- disease patterns, 120–9
- indications for, 116
- lines and tubes for, 120
- normal anatomy, 116–17
  - hollow viscera, 116–17
  - intraperitoneal compartment, 117
  - retroperitoneal compartment, 117
  - solid viscera, 117
- pitfalls of, 129
- search strategies for, 118–19
- views of, 116

Radiography, 3, 42–77
- acquisition of images in, 3–4
- airspace opacification, 55–7
- for ankle injuries, 225
- anterior-posterior chest radiographs, 42
- calcifications, 76–7
- chest CT. See Chest CT
- chest x-ray. See Chest x-ray
- common views, 4
- developmental dysplasia of the hip, 321
- disease patterns, 55–77
- epicondylitis, 233
- expiratory studies, 44
- for femoral neck fractures, 218
- foreign body aspiration, 113, 210

- infection, 94–8
- inspiratory studies, 44
- internal derangements in, 204
- interstitial patterns, 58–60
- intussusception, 313
- lateral, 55
  - chest radiographs, 42
  - decubitus chest radiographs, 42
- lobar atelectasis/collapse, patterns of, 61–4
- lordotic chest radiographs, 44
- lung masses/nodules, 64–6
- malpositioned tubes and lines, 114
- mediastinal masses, 66–8
- motion, 14–15
- normal anatomy, 47–52
- patient position, 44
- patient rotation, 45
- pelvic ring fractures, 216–17
- pericardial effusions, 75
- physical properties, 4
- pleural effusions, 72–5
- posterior-anterior chest radiographs, 42
- potable vs. intradepartmental films, 4–6
- pulmonary edema, 91–4
- shape/form, 4, 5
- signal-to-noise ratio, 14
- slipped capital femoral epiphysis, 318–19
- study penetration, 46
- tension pneumothorax, 114
- thickness, 4
- toddler fractures, 320
- trauma, 30
- traumatic aortic injury, 113
- volume loss, 61

Radiography,
- musculoskeletal, 184–91
- acute findings of, 189
- chronic findings of, 189
- extremity/joint radiograph, 185–6
- image acquisition, 184–5
- negative films with high clinical suspicion, in trauma, 189
- pitfalls and problems of, 191
- requesting radiographs, 184
- semantics, 187

terminology, 188
views of, 184, 185
Radioisotopes, 420
Radionuclide bone
  scan, 325
Radiopharmaceuticals/
  radiotracer, 420
  and protocols, 427
Raynaud's
  phenomenon, 462
Reactive airways disease
  (RAD). See Asthma
Reactive bone formation,
  radiographic evaluation
  of, 207
Recall, 478
RECIST criteria, 151
Reformatting
  computed tomography, 8
  magnetic resonance
    imaging, 11
Reimbursement for
  imaging, 31
Renal angiography, 463–5
  anatomy, 463
  GI bleed, 464
  mesenteric ischemia, 464
  renal artery
    stenosis, 464–5
  technique, 463
Renal artery stenosis, 465
Renal calculi, 29, 258–9, 364
  computed tomography
    for, 29
  intravenous pyelogram
    for, 29
  magnetic resonance
    imaging for, 29
  ultrasound for, 29
Renal cell carcinoma
  (RCC), 176
  computed tomography
    for, 176
  magnetic resonance
    imaging for, 176
Renal cysts, 175–6, 259
  Bosniak classification
    of, 176
  complex, 176
    computed tomography
      for, 175–6
    magnetic resonance
      imaging for, 175–6
  simple
    computed tomography
      for, 175
    magnetic resonance
      imaging for, 175
Renal imaging, 430–1
  radiotracers and
    protocols, 430–1

time for, 430
Renal masses, 175–6, 260
  computed tomography
    for, 175
  magnetic resonance
    imaging for, 175
Reproduction, 269–82
  common
    conditions, 278–82
  first trimester, 269–71
    aneuploidy
      screening, 271
    dating, 270
    early OB ultrasound,
      anatomy on, 270–1
    intrauterine pregnancy,
      diagnosing, 270
    ultrasound imaging,
      timing of, 269–70
  second/third trimester
    pregnancy, 274–8
    aneuploidy
      screening, 275
    anomaly screening, 275
    biometric
      measurements, 275
    bleeding, 276
    normal anatomy, 276–8
    size/date
      discordance, 275
    ultrasound imaging,
      timing of, 274
Requisition, 1–2
  elements of, 2
Respiratory gating, 151–2
Respiratory
  triggering, 151–2
Reticular patterns. See
  Interstitial patterns
Retrograde urethrogram
  (RUG), 361, 363
Retroperitoneal air, 121,
  143
  in lower abdomen, 121
  in upper abdomen, 121
Retroperitoneal
  compartment
  anatomy of, 117
  inflammation in, 143
  normal CT anatomy
    on, 142
Retroperitoneal space,
  normal CT anatomy
  on, 140
Retropharyngeal
  abscess, 404
Rheumatoid arthritis
  (RA), 215, 234
  radiographic findings
    of, 215
Rib fractures, 54, 327

Right lower lobe, lung
  atelectasis in, 61–2
Right middle lobe, lung
  atelectasis in, 61
Right upper lobe, lung
  atelectasis in, 61
Rigler's sign, 120–1
Rotation fracture, 202
Rotator cuff (RC) injuries,
  shoulder, 229–30
  magnetic resonance
    imaging for, 229
  mechanism of, 229
  MR arthrogram for, 230
  radiographic findings
    of, 229
  ultrasound for, 230
Round pneumonia, 307
Ruptured abdominal aortic
  aneurysm, diagnosis
  of, 181
Ruptured aneurysms, 387

S

Sail sign, 231
Salter-Harris classification,
  of fractures, 315
Sarcoidosis, 101
SBFT, 340, 345–9
Scaphoid fractures, 234
Scapula fractures, 228
Scatter, in x-rays, 3
Scrotal ultrasound, 282–4
  anatomy on, 282
  common
    conditions, 283–4
Secondary ossification
  centers, avulsion of, 317
Second trimester
  pregnancy, 274–8
  aneuploidy screening, 275
  anomaly screening, 275
  biometric
    measurements, 275
  bleeding, 276
  normal anatomy, 276–8
  size/date discordance, 275
  ultrasound imaging, timing
    of, 274
Seizure disorders,
  399–400
  treatment for, 21
Seldinger technique, 456
Semi-supine films, effect
  of, 44
Sentinel clot sign, 155
Sentinel node
  injection, 504–5
SGA fetus, growth disorders
  in, 278

INDEX

Short T1 inversion recovery (STIR), 372–3
Shoulder, 227–30
 dislocations/subluxations, 228–9
 fractures of, 227–8
 radiographic findings of, 227
 rotator cuff injuries, 229–30
Sigmoid volvulus, 133, 357
Signal-to-noise ratio, 14
Silhouettes, 56–7
 loss of, 57
 normal, 56
Simple cyst, imaging characteristics of, 171
Simple fracture, 202
Single contrast barium enema, 353
Sinus disease, 401–2
Skull fracture, unexplained, 326
Sliding/axial hiatal hernia, 347
Slipped capital femoral epiphysis (SCFE), 317–19
Small bowel
 motility disorders of, 337
 obstruction, 130–2
 thickening, 123
Small-bowel follow-through (SBFT), 340
Small cell carcinoma, 102
Small intestine, air in, 117
Soft tissues, 55
 abnormalities, radiological findings for, 206
 air in, 210
 extremity/joint radiograph of, 186
 radiographic evaluation of, 207
Solid organs
 biopsy, 471
 inflammation in, 144
 masses, 147–8
 normal CT anatomy on, 141
Solid ovarian masses, 264
Solid viscera, anatomy of, 117
Solitary pulmonary nodule (SPN), 33
Solumedrol, for anaphylaxis, 21
Sonohysterography, 262, 268

Spinal epidural hematoma, 411–12
Spine, 405–6
 anatomy on CT, 405
 anatomy on MRI, 405
 computed tomography, 405–6
 imaging test, 405–6
 magnetic resonance imaging, 406
 radiography, 405–6
Spine CT, 370
Spine sign, 57
Spleen
 anatomy of, 253
 injuries, 155–7
 grading of, 157
Splenomegaly, abdominal radiography for, 128
Spontaneous abortion, 271–2
Stenoses, 454
 chest CT for, 89
Stents, ureteral, 467–8
Stereotactic biopsy, 504
Stomach, 300
 air in, 117
 motility disorders of, 337
Stones, abdominal radiography for, 118
Stool, air within, 129
Stress, 37
 fracture, 203
 injuries, 194
 methods of, 438
 myocardial perfusion imaging, 436
Strictures, 335–6
Subarachnoid hemorrhage (SAH), 393, 394
Subcapsular hematoma, 154
Subdural hematoma, 393
Subdural hemorrhage, 326
Subfalcine herniation, 379
Subluxation
 internal derangements in, 206
 radiological findings of, 206
 shoulder, 228–9
Subpulmonic effusions, 74–5
Supine
 abdominal radiographs, 116
 pneumoperitoneum in, 120–1
Supine-supine films, 44

Supraglottitis. See Epiglottitis
Surfactant deficiency, 298
Surgery, for contrast extravasation/infiltration, 22
Surroundings, checking, 26
Synovitis, 221

T

T1 relaxation, magnetic resonance imaging, 10
T2 relaxation, magnetic resonance imaging, 10
Tc-99m DMSA, 431
Tc-99m DPTA, 430–1
Tc-99m DTPA aerosol, 445
Tc-99m hepatobiliary scan, 441–2
Tc-99m labeled RBC GI bleeding scan, 442
Tc-99m labeled RBC MUGA, 436
Tc-99m labeled white blood cells, 447
Tc-99m MAA, 445
Tc-99m MAG3, 430–1
Tc-99m methylene diphosphonate (Tc-99m MDP)
 bone imaging, 427
Tc-99m pertechnetate endocrine imaging, 433
Tc-99m sestamibi, 434, 437
Tc-99m sulfur colloid (DPTA), 431
Teardrop fracture, 410
Temporal bone fractures, 395
Tendons
 calcium within, 210
 injury, 221
 internal derangement in, 225
Tension pneumothorax, 70
 diagnosis of, 114
 radiographic findings for, 70–1
Testicles, anatomy of, 282
Testicular masses, 284
Testicular torsion, 283
Testicular trauma, 284
Tetrofosmin perfusion imaging, 437
Thallium-201, 437–8, 447
Therapeutic intracranial procedures, 415–16

Third trimester
  pregnancy, 274–8
  aneuploidy screening, 275
  anomaly screening, 275
  biometric measurements, 275
  bleeding, 276
  normal anatomy, 276–8
  size/date discordance, 275
  ultrasound imaging, timing of, 274
Thoracic and lumbar spine fractures, 411
  burst fracture, 411
  compression fracture, 411
3D mammography. See Tomosynthesis
3D ultrasound, 242
Thrombolysis, 458–9
Thumbprinting, 123, 135
Thymus, chest radiograph of, 295
Thyroid cancer, 436
  endocrine imaging, 436
Thyroid nodule evaluation, 435
Thyroid ultrasound, 284–5
Thyrotoxicosis, 436
  endocrine imaging, 436
Tibial plateau fractures, 223
Toddlers
  fractures, 319–20
  wheezing in, 306
Tomosynthesis, 476
Tonsillar abscess, 404
Tonsillar herniation, 380, 381
Torus fractures, 317
  of distal radius, 321
Total arthroplasty, 234–6
Toxic megacolon, 135, 181
Toxic multinodular goiters (TMNG), 435
Toxic nodular goiter, 434–5
Tracheoesophageal fistula (TEF), 309
Tracheostomy tube, 53
Transabdominal ultrasound, 262
Transient synovitis of the hip, 323
Transient tachypnea of the newborn (TTNB), 298
Transjugular Intrahepatic Portosystemic Shunt (TIPS), 469, 470
Transrectal ultrasound, 262
Transtentorial herniation, 379

Transvaginal ultrasound, 262
  early pregnancy findings on, 270
Trauma, 30, 154–60, 214
  bladder, 158–9
  bowel, 159–60
  computed tomography for, 30, 192
  contusion, 154
  extravasation, active, 155
  fracture, 155
  hemoperitoneum, 154
  kidneys, 158
  laceration, 154
  liver, 154, 155–7
  magnetic resonance imaging for, 30
  mesentery, 159–60
  musculoskeletal MRI for, 195–6
  musculoskeletal ultrasound for, 197–8
  pancreas, 157
  radiographs for, 30
  sentinel clot sign, 155
  spleen, 157
  subcapsular hematoma, 154
  testicular, 284
  ultrasound for, 30
Traumatic aortic injury, diagnosis of, 113
T-tube cholangiogram, 367–8
Tube studies, 367–8
  Dobhoff tube, 367
  gastric tubes, 367
  gastro-jejunostomy tube, 367
  jejunostomy tubes, 367
Tumors
  musculoskeletal MRI for, 196
  musculoskeletal ultrasound for, 198
Twin pregnancies, 274
2D ultrasound, 242

U

UGI, 340, 345–9
  neonatal UGI, 304
Ultrasonography
  foreign bodies, 210
  leiomyomas, 179
Ultrasound, 489–92
  acoustic window, 240
  advantages and disadvantages of, 240
  appendicitis, 28
  applications of, 290
  arterial, 288–9
  breast, 489–92
    benign versus malignant features, 491–2
    cysts, 497
    ductal carcinoma in situ (DCIS), 498
    fibroadenomas, 501
    invasive carcinomas, 500
    normal breast ultrasound, 490–1
    patterns of disease on, 491–2
    procedure, 490
    screening breast ultrasound, 490
    time for, 489–90
  disease patterns, 246–9
  Doppler, 243–4
  -guided biopsy, 503–4
  guided procedures, 289
  for guiding interventional procedures, 450
  image acquisition, 240–6
  image display, 244–6
    real time, 245
    static, 245
  internal derangements in, 206
  intussusception, 313
  measurements in, 245–6
  M mode, 242
  musculoskeletal imaging using, 197–9
    image acquisition, 197
    pitfalls and problems of, 198–9
    timing of, 197–8
  pregnant patients, 28
  probes, 241
  renal calculi, 29
  rotator cuff injuries, 230
  soundwave, 240
  3D, 242
  thyroid, 284–5
  tissue characteristics, 246–9
  transducers, 241
  trauma, 30
  2D, 242
  vascular, 286–9
  venous, 286–8
Umbilical artery catheters (UACs), 294
Umbilical artery Doppler, 279

U

Umbilical cord, placental cord insertion of, 279
Umbilical venous catheters (UVCs), 294
Uncal herniation, 379–80
Unused colon, 304
Upper GI series, 339
 double contrast, 339
 single contrast, 339
Upper GI tract fluoroscopy, 338–51
 achalasia, 346–7
  hiatal hernias and reflux, 347
  primary, 346
  secondary, 347
 anatomy on studies of
  duodenum, 341
  esophagus, 340
  jejunum and ileum, 341
  stomach, 340–1
 barium swallow/esophagram, 339
  double contrast, 339
  single contrast, 339
 combined swallow, 338, 340
 Crohn disease, 350–1
 duodenal cancer, 350
 duodenal ulcers, 349
 esophageal strictures
  benign causes of, 345
  malignant causes of, 346
 esophagitis, 346
 esophagram, 340
 gastric adenocarcinoma, 349
 gastric banding, 343
 gastric bypass, 343
 gastric lymphoma, 350
 gastric metastatic disease, 350
 gastric ulcers, 348–9
  benign ulcers, 348
  ulcerating malignancy, 348
 gastric volvulus, 348
 gastroesophageal reflux, 348
 gastrointestinal stromal tumors, 350
 linitis plastica, 350
 mesenteroaxial volvulus, 348
 modified barium swallow, 338
 modified swallow, 340
 neoplasms of, 349–50
 organoaxial volvulus, 348
 pancreatico-duodenectomy, 343
 paraesophageal hernia, 347
 patient preparation, 338
 post surgical anatomy, 343
  bariatric surgery, 343
  esophagectomy with gastric pull up, 343
  fundoplication, 343
 SBFT, 340, 345–9
 sliding/axial hiatal hernia, 347
 small-bowel follow-through (SBFT), 340
 UGI, 340, 345–9
 upper GI series, 339
  double contrast, 339
  single contrast, 339
Upper limb, vasospastic disorders of, 462
Ureteral stents, 467–8
Urinary tract infections (UTIs), 38–9
Urolithiasis, 173
 computed tomography for, 173
 pitfalls of, 173
Urticaria, treatment for, 21
Uterine fibroids, 266
Uterus, anatomy of, 262
Uterus tumors, magnetic resonance imaging for, 179

V

Vaginal bleeding, 276
Vascular abnormalities, chest CT for, 88–9
 aneurysms, 88–9
 stenoses, 89
Vascular access, 473
 subcutaneous port catheters, 473
 temporary central venous lines, 473
 tunneled central venous lines, 473
Vascular conditions, 104–7
Vascular disease patterns, 452–5
 aneurysms, 454
 dissection, 455
 leak/extravasation, 455
 occlusion, 453
 pseudoaneurysms, 454
 stenoses, 454
Vascular MRA, 112–13
Vascular ultrasound, 286–9
Vasogenic edema, 376–7
Venography, 462
Venous angioma, 385
Venous ultrasound, 286–8
 color Doppler, 288
 Doppler spectral imaging, 288
 gray-scale imaging, 287
 peripheral venous thrombosis, 286–8
ventilation–perfusion (VQ) scanning, 444
Vertebroplasty, 414–15
Vesicoureteral reflux (VUR), 314–15, 364
Virtual colonoscopy. See CT colonography
Visipaque, for contrast induced nephropathy, 16–17
Voiding cystourethrogram (VCUG), for vesicoureteral reflux, 314–15, 360, 363
Volume averaging, 9
Volume loss, 61
 signs of, 61
VoLumen™, 19, 137
Volvulus, 133–57
 cecal, 133, 136
 gastric, 135, 348
 midgut, 311–12
 sigmoid, 133, 135
VQ scan, for pulmonary emboli, 29

W

Wall thickening, 248–9
Water, 19
 soluble agents, 19
  risks and contraindications of, 20
 soluble contrast, 331–2
 soluble enema, 353
Wavelength, of x-rays, 3

Weber type ankle injuries, 226
Wrist, 233–4
  computed tomography for, 234
  fractures, 233–4
  magnetic resonance imaging for, 234
  musculoskeletal radiograph of, 187
  radiographic findings of, 233

X

Xe-133, 445
X-rays
  features of, 3
  radiation doses from, 22–3
    background radiation, 23–4
    effective doses of, 23–4
    modes of measurement, 22–3

Y

Young child with hip/leg pain, 323–4
  pain, localization of, 323–4
Young patient
  acute abdomen in, MRI scanning of, 178–9